TECHNOLOGY, COMMUNICATION, DISPARITIES AND GOVERNMENT OPTIONS IN HEALTH AND HEALTH CARE SERVICES

RESEARCH IN THE SOCIOLOGY OF HEALTH CARE

Series Editor: Jennie Jacobs Kronenfeld

Recent Volumes:

Volume 21:   Reorganizing Health Care Delivery Systems: Problems of Managed Care and Other Models of Health Care Delivery, 2003

Volume 22:   Chronic Care, Health Care Systems and Services Integration, 2004

Volume 23:   Health Care Services, Racial and Ethnic Minorities and Underserved Populations, 2005

Volume 24:   Access, Quality and Satisfaction with Care: Concerns of Patients, Providers and Insurers, 2007

Volume 25:   Inequalities and Disparities in Health Care and Health: Concerns of Patients, Providers and Insurers, 2007

Volume 26:   Care for Major Health Problems and Population Health Concerns: Impacts on Patients, Providers, and Policy, 2008

Volume 27:   Social Sources of Disparities in Health and Health Care and Linkages to Policy, Population Concerns and Providers of Care, 2009

Volume 28:   The Impact of Demographics on Health and Healthcare: Race, Ethnicity, and Other Social Factors, 2010

Volume 29:   Access to Care and Factors that Impact Access, Patients as Partners in Care and Changing Roles of Health Providers, 2011

Volume 30:   Issues in Health and Health Care Related to Race/ Ethnicity, Immigration, SES and Gender, 2012

Volume 31:   Social Determinants, Health Disparities and Linkages to Health and Health Care, 2013

RESEARCH IN THE SOCIOLOGY OF HEALTH CARE
VOLUME 32

TECHNOLOGY, COMMUNICATION, DISPARITIES AND GOVERNMENT OPTIONS IN HEALTH AND HEALTH CARE SERVICES

EDITED BY

JENNIE JACOBS KRONENFELD

*Department of Sociology, Arizona State University,
Tempe, AZ, USA*

United Kingdom – North America – Japan
India – Malaysia – China

Emerald Group Publishing Limited
Howard House, Wagon Lane, Bingley BD16 1WA, UK

First edition 2014

Copyright © 2014 Emerald Group Publishing Limited

Reprints and permission service
Contact: permissions@emeraldinsight.com

British Library Cataloguing in Publication Data
A catalogue record for this book is available from the British Library

ISBN: 978-1-78350-645-3
ISSN: 0275-4959 (Series)

ISOQAR certified
Management System,
awarded to Emerald
for adherence to
Environmental
standard
ISO 14001:2004.

ISOQAR
REGISTERED
Certificate Number 1985
ISO 14001

INVESTOR IN PEOPLE

CONTENTS

LIST OF CONTRIBUTORS *ix*

PART I: INTRODUCTION TO VOLUME

TECHNOLOGY, COMMUNICATIONS,
GOVERNMENT ROLES AND HEALTH
DISPARITIES
Jennie Jacobs Kronenfeld *3*

PART II: TECHNOLOGY

CAN INFORMATION TECHNOLOGY IMPROVE
HEALTH CARE EQUITY IN THE UNITED STATES?
LESSONS FROM TAIWAN
Claudia Chaufan and Yi-Chang Li *19*

PATTERNS OF ONLINE HEALTH SEARCHING
2002–2010: IMPLICATIONS FOR SOCIAL
CAPITAL, HEALTH DISPARITIES AND THE
DE-PROFESSIONALIZATION OF MEDICAL
KNOWLEDGE
Timothy M. Hale, Melinda Goldner, *35*
Mike Stern, Patricia Drentea and
Shelia R. Cotten

PART III: COMMUNICATION

THE IMPLEMENTATION OF PUBLIC HEALTH
COMMUNICATION MESSAGES TO PROMOTE
TEENAGE MOTHERS' SENSE OF SELF AND
AVERT STIGMA
Neale R. Chumbler, Helen Sanetmatsu and   63
John Parrish-Sprowl

VIRTUAL HEALTH: THE IMPACT OF
HEALTH-RELATED WEBSITES ON
PATIENT-DOCTOR INTERACTIONS
Scott V. Savage, Samantha Kwan and   93
Kelly Bergstrand

REJECT, DELAY, OR CONSENT? PARENTS'
INTERNET DISCUSSIONS OF THE HPV VACCINE
FOR CHILDREN AND IMPLICATIONS FOR HPV
VACCINE UPTAKE
Kathy Livingston, Kathleen M. Sutherland and   117
Lauren M. Sardi

PART IV: GOVERNMENT ROLES AND LESSONS FROM OTHER COUNTRIES

DETERMINANTS IN NORWEGIAN LOCAL
GOVERNMENT HEALTH PROMOTION –
INSTITUTIONAL PERSPECTIVES
Marit K. Helgesen and Hege Hofstad   143

SOCIAL IMPLICATIONS OF LONG TERM CARE
INSURANCE IN JAPAN: A REVIEW
Atsuko Kawakami   181

HARM TO THE HEALTH OF THE PUBLIC ARISING
FROM AGGRESSIVE MARKETING AND SALES OF
HEALTH-RELATED PRODUCTS AND SERVICES:
ANOTHER ASPECT OF MEDICALIZATION WHICH IS
A CAUSE FOR CONCERN?
Kai-Lit Phua   199

IMPROVING RESIDENT OUTCOMES IN STATE
MEDICAID NURSING FACILITY LONG-TERM CARE
PROGRAMS: AUGMENTING CMS SURVEYS WITH
MODEST CHANGES TO A FEW STATE PROGRAM
FEATURES
Charles Lockhart, Kristin Klopfenstein,   213
Jean Giles-Sims and Cathan Coghlan

PART V: HEALTH DISPARITIES

FUNDAMENTAL CAUSES OF HEALTH DISPARITIES:
ASSOCIATIONS BETWEEN ADVERSE
SOCIOECONOMIC RESOURCES AND MULTIPLE
MEASURES OF HEALTH
Katie Kerstetter and John J. Green   237

PREDICTORS OF RURAL HEALTH CLINIC
MANAGERS' WILLINGNESS TO JOIN
ACCOUNTABLE CARE ORGANIZATIONS
Thomas T. H. Wan, Maysoun Dimachkie Masri and   259
Judith Ortiz

AGING PUERTO RICANS' EXPERIENCES OF
DEPRESSION TREATMENT: A NEW ETHNOGRAPHIC
EXPLORATION
Marta B. Rodríguez-Galán and Luis M. Falcón   275

LIST OF CONTRIBUTORS

Kelly Bergstrand	School of Sociology, University of Arizona, Tucson, AZ, USA
Claudia Chaufan	Institute for Health & Aging, University of California, San Francisco, San Francisco, CA, USA
Neale R. Chumbler	Department of Health Policy and Management, University of Georgia, Athens, GA, USA
Cathan Coghlan	Institutional Research, TCU, Fort Worth, TX, USA
Shelia R. Cotten	Department of Media and Information, Michigan State University, East Lansing, MI, USA
Patricia Drentea	Department of Sociology, University of Alabama, Birmingham, Birmingham, AL, USA
Luis M. Falcón	College of Fine Arts, Humanities and Social Sciences, University of Massachusetts at Lowell, Lowell, MA, USA
Jean Giles-Sims	Department of Sociology, TCU, Fort Worth, TX, USA
Melinda Goldner	Department of Sociology, Union College, Schenectady, NY, USA
John J. Green	Sociology Department and Center for Population Studies, University of Mississippi, University, MS, USA

Timothy M. Hale	Center for Connected Health, Partners HealthCare and Harvard Medical School, Boston, MA, USA
Marit K. Helgesen	Norwegian Institute of Urban and Regional Research (NIBR), Oslo, Norway
Hege Hofstad	Norwegian Institute of Urban and Regional Research (NIBR), Oslo, Norway
Atsuko Kawakami	Department of Sociology, University of Wisconsin, Oshkosh, WI, USA
Katie Kerstetter	Department of Sociology and Anthropology, George Mason University, Fairfax, VA, USA
Kristin Klopfenstein	Education Innovation Institute, University of Northern Colorado, Greeley, CO, USA
Jennie Jacobs Kronenfeld	Sociology Program, Sanford School of Social and Family Dynamics, Arizona State University, Tempe, AZ, USA
Samantha Kwan	Department of Sociology, University of Houston, Houston, TX, USA
Yi-Chang Li	Department of Healthcare Administration, Chung Shan Medical University, Taichung City, Taiwan
Kathy Livingston	Department of Sociology, Quinnipiac University, Hamden, CT, USA
Charles Lockhart	Department of Political Science, TCU, Fort Worth, TX, USA
Maysoun Dimachkie Masri	Department of Health Management and Informatics, College of Health and Public Affairs, University of Central Florida, Orlando, FL, USA
Judith Ortiz	Rural Health Research Group, College of Health and Public Affairs, University of Central Florida, Orlando, FL, USA

John Parrish-Sprowl	Department of Communication Studies, Global Health Communication Center, Indianapolis, IN, USA
Kai-Lit Phua	School of Medicine and Health Sciences, Monash University (Malaysia), Bandar Sunway, Selangor, Malaysia
Marta B. Rodríguez-Galán	Sociology Department, St. John Fisher College, Rochester, NY, USA
Helen Sanetmatsu	Herron School of Art and Design, Indiana University, Indianapolis, IN, USA
Lauren M. Sardi	Department of Sociology, Quinnipiac University, Hamden, CT, USA
Scott V. Savage	Department of Sociology, University of California, Riverside, Riverside, CA, USA
Mike Stern	NORC at the University of Chicago and the College of Charleston, Chicago, IL, USA
Kathleen M. Sutherland	Department of Sociology, Quinnipiac University, Hamden, CT, USA
Thomas T. H. Wan	Public Affairs Doctoral Program, College of Health and Public Affairs, University of Central Florida, Orlando, FL, USA

PART I
INTRODUCTION TO VOLUME

TECHNOLOGY, COMMUNICATIONS, GOVERNMENT ROLES AND HEALTH DISPARITIES

Jennie Jacobs Kronenfeld

ABSTRACT

Purpose — *This chapter provides both an introduction to the volume and a brief review of literature on technology, communications, and health disparities.*

Methodology/approach — *Literature review.*

Findings — *The chapter argues for the importance of greater examination of technology, communications, and their linkages to health disparities and other related factors.*

Originality/value of chapter — *Reviews the topic of technology, communication, and health disparities and previews this book.*

Keywords: Health disparities; health care disparities; technology; communications; government

Technology, Communication, Disparities and Government Options in Health and
Health Care Services
Research in the Sociology of Health Care, Volume 32, 3–15
Copyright © 2014 by Emerald Group Publishing Limited
All rights of reproduction in any form reserved
ISSN: 0275-4959/doi:10.1108/S0275-495920140000032001

This chapter provides an introduction to Volume 32 in the Research in the Sociology of Health Care series, *Technology, Communication, Disparities and Government Options in Health and Health Care Services*. The beginning of this chapter will review some of the more important material about technology and communications as related to health and health care, and some of the relevant literature on health disparities. The last part of this chapter will review the overall contents of the volume and the structure of the volume.

TECHNOLOGY

Technology can refer to many different things, especially as related to health care in which medical technology is so important. In this chapter, the technology being discussed is mostly information-related technology, not medical technology more broadly. In fact, this section on technology and the next section on communications related to health care are closely related, as so many of the new issues in communication in health care also relate to some aspects of information technology and the Internet, which is also discussed some in this section. One of the definitions for information technology is technology used to collect, store, retrieve, and transfer clinical, administrative, and financial information electronically.

Health technology has become a subject of greater study both because of the growth in new technologies and also because of a hope that new technologies can become one way to improve the delivery of health care and result in more and better health care at lower costs (Schoen et al., 2012). One of the important debates in the literature is whether there is a positive impact of health information technology (HIT) on productivity. Within health, productivity is often understood as a ratio between quality and amount of care and costs. A number of studies support the argument that many types of HIT implementation, such as Electronic Health Records (EHR), will prevent medical errors, increase administrative efficiency, reduce costs, and expand access to quality and affordable care (Hillestad et al., 2005; Palvia et al., 2012; Taylor et al., 2005). The literature on the impact of technology and increases in productivity are older and better established in other sectors of the economy, although the results are not always clear with some experts arguing there are positive results (Buntin et al., 2011) while others dispute those outcomes (Dranove et al., 2012).

The Internet is another example of technology impacting health and health care. In this book, the Internet can be seen both as a technological innovation that increases knowledge about health and health care and one that impacts communication about health and health care. The communication aspects of the Internet are discussed in the next section. The Internet and use of the Internet has been increasing greatly over the past few decades. From its earliest beginnings around 1970 until the late 1980s, the Internet was mostly a means for sending of text-based emails. The first major browser was Mosaic, coming in 1993 and the later appearance of Google as an Internet search engine in 1998 (Conrad & Stults, 2010). Trend data from the Pew Internet and American Life (2014) trend data provide some evidence that Internet usage has increased in the past decade from 46 to 79 percent of all adults in the United States. People use the Internet for all kinds of activities now such as shopping, reading magazines and newspapers, and making airline tickets and travel-based purchases. Use of the Internet for health-related purposes has also grown, and people now routinely turn to the Internet to learn about health problems, potential treatments, and drugs and drug interactions as well as communication purposes of finding others who may be sharing a similar medical problem (Fox & Jones, 2009; Hale, Cotten, Drentea, & Goldner, 2010; Rice, 2006).

Clearly, the shift in technology from the creation and expansion of the Internet means that more traditional sources of health information such as physicians and the mass media are increasingly being supplemented and even replaced by the Internet (Brodie, Kjellson, Hoff, & Parker, 1999; Cotten & Gupta, 2004; Goldsmith, 2000). While people clearly still turn to their physicians for advice, most people also seek out health information online (Ayers & Kronenfeld, 2007; Cotten, 2001; Goldsmith, 2000). In several studies by Fox and colleagues (Fox, 2011; Fox & Fallows, 2003), they found that in 2000, 55 percent of Internet users reported having searched the Internet for health information with an increase to 80 percent of Internet users by 2010.

Demographic characteristics do relate to Internet usage. Women are more likely than men to use the Internet to search for health information (Baker, Wagner, Singer, & Bundorf, 2003; Brodie et al., 2000; Fox, 2005; Fox & Fallows, 2003; Fox et al., 2000; Hale et al., 2010) and at least one study (Stern, Cotton, & Drentea, 2012) reported that while female and male parents were similar in online health searches, women were more likely to actually put the information to use. Aspects of socioeconomic status (SES) also impact usage. People with higher incomes and educational levels are more likely to search for health information online (Ayers & Kronenfeld, 2007; Cotten & Gupta, 2004; Hale et al., 2010) and some studies (Baker et al., 2003) find that education is more important as a predictor of use of the Internet for health reasons. Not surprisingly, age also relates to Internet usage, with younger people being more likely to search for health information online (Ayers & Kronenfeld, 2007; Cotten & Gupta, 2004). Some studies (Baker et al., 2003) find the least usage among the oldest, so that people 75 and older were less likely to use the Internet. Age trends will be likely to decline in future years as new older groups will have more experience with the Internet and would be expected to continue to use it as they grow older.

COMMUNICATION

As the previous section has pointed out, the Internet now enables individuals to locate very large amount of information about many health conditions and medications from sites sponsored by government, hospitals, national disease oriented organizations, medical information collections, and even sites created by individuals and by patients and relatives of patients who have certain diseases. Part of the challenge today is to learn to separate more reliable sources of information from less reliable sources of information. While everyone acknowledges that there is a great deal of inaccurate information available on websites, this is not a well-researched area, but it is one that concerns health care professionals as they interact with patients. Health care professionals are concerned that patients now arrive at sources of care armed with inaccurate information and questioning the information and recommendations provided by the health professionals. Some evidence that this may not be as large a problem as some health care professionals fear is provided in a study in 2008 on websites with information about breast cancer. The authors found that only about 5 percent of the sites contained inaccurate information (Bernstam et al., 2008).

The issue of use of the Internet for information and how this impacts doctor–patient communication is an important one. Hardey (1999) has argued that people use the Internet partially to free themselves of dependence on physicians for health knowledge, and thus this limits the medical profession's control over knowledge. There have been a number of studies examining whether patient use of web-based information negatively impacts the doctor–patient relationship (Broom, 2005b; Kivits, 2004). Broom (2005a) argues that physicians differ, with some embracing the use of the Internet by patients while others view it as harming doctor–patient communication. Most agree that patients who use multiple websites to increase their health-related knowledge do bring greater information into communication with the health professional.

The other main way in which the Internet is used both for communication and information is for support groups. Self-help groups and the self-help tradition are well known in health, but the Internet has changed the development of such groups and the distribution of information through the groups (Borkman, 1999; Conrad & Stults, 2010). Prior to the Internet, illness was much more of a private affair, with some self-help groups that occasionally allowed people to communicate with others with the problem. Sometimes physicians even helped to develop these groups to provide communication and information to patients. With the growth of the Internet, illness has become a more shared experience and people can not only obtain specific information from various sources, but can also usually locate online electronic support groups, blogs written by people with a specific health problem about their experience with the problem, and all types of interactive sources where people can leave questions and have them answered by others with the problem. One study from 2005 estimates that around 9 percent of Internet users have visited online support groups (Berger, Wagner & Baker, 2005). While people use the Internet for all types of health problems, some research emphasizes that it is used the most by people with stigmatized illnesses and disabilities, as well as by people who may be socially awkward, limited in other ways in their abilities to communicate with broader groups, or have multiple chronic illnesses (Ayers & Kronenfeld, 2007; Berger, Wagner, & Baker, 2005; Guo, Bricout, & Huang, 2005). The Internet has clearly become a critical resource for lay people with chronic health problems, other ongoing medical needs, mobility issues, or permanent disabilities (Braithwaite, Waldron, & Finn, 1999). Studies have found positive impacts of the use of the Internet as a support tool in addition to a basic information and communication approach, and that use of online support and sharing of health information is associated with positive changes in health attitudes and behaviors among those managing chronic illness (Ayers & Kronenfeld, 2007; Baker et al., 2003; Cotten, 2001).

HEALTH DISPARITIES

Just as communication and technology and their impact on health and health care services are newer areas of interest that have increased a great deal in the last decade and the last few decades, so has been the increased interest and research in health disparities both in health more broadly and in medical sociology more specifically. The interest in health care disparities has expanded beyond researchers to also become an area of high interest to providers of care and policymakers, especially within the United States. The definition of health disparities or differences in health care is important to review. The Institute of Medicine (IOM) defines health care disparities as differences in treatment or access between population groups that cannot be justified by different preferences for services or differences in health (McGuire, Alegria, Cook, Wells, & Zaslavsky, 2006). Within the United States, much of the focus on health care disparities has turned to differences in access and quality across racial and ethnic groups, although these are not the only social characteristics that are of interest either sociologically or from a policy perspective. Differences based on SES and its components including education and income are of both research and policy interest. Beyond research and thinking about policy implications, health care disparities matter even more if they result in health disparities, defined as differences in health outcomes across population groups (Schnittker & McLeod, 2005).

One interesting study that demonstrates the growth in research about social differences in health and health disparities was summarized well by the Adler and Rehkopf (2008) review of US disparities in health by examining literature for the term "health disparities" and finding that while this was a key word in only one article in 1980, and fewer than 30 in the 1990s, it went up to over 400 articles from 2000 to 2004. If the term "health inequalities" was used instead, the pattern of increase was similar.

There has been a major interest in this topic both in the United States and in Great Britain. In 1980, the Black Report in Great Britain was one of the first in that country to apply the term inequality to an examination of health differences. In the United States in this same time period, studies did link together death and health information with information on SES from sources such as the Current Population Study, the US Census, and Social Security Administration records (Kitagawa & Hauser, 1973; Kliss & Scheuren, 1978). Within the United States, some of these earlier studies and traditions in various fields including sociology of research into variation in health, health care utilization, and health services issues by SES and race/ethnicity led to the now well-known efforts in the United States to examine and try to eliminate health disparities due to race/ethnicity and SES in the *Healthy People* series. From the federal government level, one of the pushes for more research on health care inequalities came from the passage of Public Law 106-129, the Healthcare Research and Quality Act of 1999. A first National Healthcare Disparities Report (2005) built on previous efforts in the federal government, especially Healthy People 2010 (U.S. Department of Health and Human Services, 2000) and the IOM Report, "Unequal Treatment: Confronting Racial and Economic Disparities in Healthcare" (Smedley, Stith, & Nelson, 2003). Elimination of disparities in health was a goal of Healthy People, 2010. Unequal Treatment extensively documented health care disparities in the United States, and focused on those related to race and ethnicity, but not on SES, a weakness of the report. The IOM report on Unequal Treatment also looked at factors related to providers of care and argued that providers' perceptions and, from that, their attitudes toward patients can be influenced by patient race or ethnicity (Smedley et al., 2003).

In 2005, the third National Healthcare Disparities Report (2005) was released. The 2005 report focused on findings from a set of core report measures. The two measures of access covered were facilitators and barriers to care and health care utilization. The overall summary indicated that disparities still exist, but some disparities are diminishing, an encouraging result, but one that clearly leaves opportunities for further improvement. Disparities remain in areas of access, quality, and across many levels and types of care including preventive care, treatment of acute conditions, and management of chronic disease. This applies to a variety of specific clinical conditions including cancer, diabetes, end stage renal disease, heart disease, HIV disease, mental health and substance abuse, and respiratory diseases. Looking at access more specifically, major issues of disparity occur for poor people and Hispanics, with lesser but important issues for Blacks, American Indians, and Asians. Poor people have worse access to care than high-income people for all eight core report measures. Hispanics have worse access for 88 percent of the core report measures, while Blacks and American Indians have worse access on half of the measures. For racial minorities, more disparities in quality of care were becoming smaller rather than larger, while for Hispanics, 59 percent were becoming larger and 41 percent smaller. For poor people, half of disparities were becoming smaller and half were becoming larger (National Healthcare Disparities Report, 2005).

Federal government focus on these efforts has continued, and much of it is discussed in the Healthy People 2020 publication, much of which is now easily obtainable through United States government websites (U.S. Department of Health and Human Services, 2013). For the 2020 effort, the report points out that in Healthy People 2000, the goal was to reduce health disparities among Americans, and in Healthy People 2010 the goal was to eliminate, not just reduce, health disparities. By Healthy People 2020, that goal was expanded even further: to achieve health equity, eliminate disparities, and improve the health of all groups. Healthy People 2020 defines health equity as attaining the highest level of health for all people.

The Centers for Disease Control and Prevention (CDC) is another US federal agency that works on issues linked to health differences and health disparities. In a special report they issued in 2011, the agency consolidated the most recent national data available on disparities in mortality, morbidity, behavioral risk factors, health care access, preventive health services, and social determinants of critical health problems in the United States by using selected indicators (Truman et al., 2011). Persistent gaps between the healthiest persons as well as states as units were reported.

In addition to federal government efforts, some important private foundations such as the Commonwealth Foundation now have programs that focus on health differences and health disparities (Commonwealth Fund, 2013). The goals of the Commonwealth Fund's Program on Health Care Disparities are to improve the overall quality of health care delivered to low-income and minority Americans, and to eliminate racial and ethnic health disparities.

REVIEW OF CONTENTS OF THE VOLUME

Part I of this volume contains only one chapter, this introductory chapter to the volume. Part II of this volume is entitled Technology and contains two chapters. The first chapter by Claudia Chaufan and Yi-Chang Li deals with whether information technology may improve health equity in the United States and uses data from Taiwan to consider that issue. They used the case of implementation of HIT in Taiwan's national health insurance system to help think about issues in the US health care system. They point out that the benefits in a universal and publicly financed system such as in Taiwan may be difficult to achieve in a system such as the United States that has multiple health plans competing for different customers. The second by Timothy M. Hale, Melinda Goldner, Mike Stern, Patricia Drentea, and Shelia R. Cotten uses data from five surveys from 2002 to 2010 to examine changing patterns of online health searching. They find that effects vary by inequality factor and time period examined and that gender, age, and education gaps continue to persist over time and appear to be increasing.

Part III of the volume contains three chapters on the issue of communication, and two of these three also relate to the Internet as a form of communication. The chapter that does not link communication to the Internet is the first chapter in the part by Neale R. Chumbler, Helen Sanetmatsu, and John Parrish-Sprowl. This chapter focuses on the implementation of public health communication messages to promote teenage mothers' sense of self and help to deal with issues of stigma. The chapter uses a qualitative research design with a purposive sample of pregnant adolescents or parenting adolescents. The authors conclude that teen pregnancy overall is still a problem, although these women do appreciate having their own baby. They would like more information and education, but are frustrated with perceived stigma from teachers and their own parents and with the existing service programs. The second chapter in this part by Scott V. Savage, Samantha Kwan, and Kelly Bergstrand examines the impact that health-related websites may have on patient–doctor interactions. They conduct a qualitative study of three health-related websites along with a quantitative analysis of survey data. They find that both the number and type of websites that patients use impact their perception of how well doctors listened or paid attention to them in a patient visit. If patients visited more websites, it decreased the perception of how well doctors listened or answered questions but the use of nonprofit or government health-related websites increased the perception that doctors were listening and answering questions. In the last chapter in this part, Kathy Livingston, Kathleen M. Sutherland, and Lauren M. Sardi examine parents' Internet discussions of the human papilloma virus (HPV) vaccine for their children. They utilize a grounded theory approach to collecting data and formulating research questions. Their findings suggest that familiarity with a disease is central to parents' assessment of risk. In addition, parents seem to focus more on the possible side effects of the vaccine than they do on the seriousness of cervical cancer as a disease.

Part IV covers Government Roles and Lessons from Other Countries and contains four chapters. The first is institutional perspectives on determinants in Norwegian local government and health promotion by Marit K. Helgesen and Hege Hofstad. They use data from different administrative sources connected with Norwegian municipalities. They find that municipalities acknowledge and prioritize health behavior independent of experiences socioeconomic challenges, municipal capacity, and local government political profile. The second chapter is by Atsuko Kawakami on social implications of long-term care insurance in Japan. The chapter reviews the evaluations of the newly developed elderly care system in Japan through a detailed literature review. The new insurance provides more options for different types of services and has a new norm of self-reliance and determination for one's own aging. The chapter concludes that it will be important to also build a community care support system into the Long Term Care Insurance approach to help prevent social isolation and respond to emergency situations for the elderly. The third chapter by Kai-Lit Phua relates to harm that could arise from aggressive marketing and sales of health-related products and services in order to maximize profits. This includes an examination of tobacco products and pharmaceutical drugs. The last chapter in this part is by Charles Lockhart, Kristin Klopfenstein, Jean Giles-Sims, and Cathan Coghlan and examines improving resident outcomes in state Medicaid Nursing Facilities Long Term Care Programs. The authors use a data set containing information from 48 US states. They conclude that regulating not just process but structural features may produce improvement in quality of resident outcomes.

Part V includes three chapters focused on different aspects of health disparities. The first chapter by Katie Kerstetter and John J. Green examines some of the fundamental causes of health disparities and tests two of the parts of fundamental cause theory, that SES influences a variety of risk factors for poor health and also affects multiple health outcomes. They employ 2011 Behavioral Risk Factor Surveillance Survey data from the Centers for Disease Control and Prevention (CDC). The analyses provide support for fundamental cause theory and find that adverse socioeconomic conditions are associated with self-rates health, and two leading causes of death in the United States (cancer and heart disease). Thomas T. H. Wan, Maysoun Dimachkie Masri, and Judith Ortiz look at predictors of rural health clinic managers' willingness to join accountable care organizations using data from a survey conducted in spring 2012 that covered eight southeastern states and California. Rural health clinic managers' personal perceptions of the benefits of the Affordable Care Act and knowledge level about it explained the most variance in the managers' willingness to join an accountable care organization, and these perceptions were more important than organizational and context factors. The last chapter in this part and the volume is by Marta B. Rodríguez-Galán and Luis M. Falcón and looks at aging Puerto Ricans and their experiences of depression treatment using ethnographic research approaches. Respondents were resistant to accepting pharmacological treatment for depression and felt that social stressors such as financial strain, lack of a job, housing problems, and social isolation were important triggering or contributing factors in their depression. These results may help to explain and thus reduce some of the health disparities in depression outcomes among Puerto Ricans living in the mainland of the United States.

REFERENCES

Adler, N. E., & Rehkopf, D. H. (2008). U.S. disparities in health: Descriptions, causes and mechanisms. *Annual Review of Public Health, 29,* 235–252.

Ayers, S., & Kronenfeld, J. J. (2007). Chronic illness and health seeking information on the internet. *Health: An Interdisciplinary Journal for the Social Study of Health, Illness and Medicine, 11*(3), 327–347.

Baker, L., Wagner, T. H., Singer, S., & Bundorf, M. K. (2003). Use of the internet and e-mail for health care information: Results from a national survey. *The Journal of the American Medical Association, 289,* 2400–2406.

Berger, M., Wagner, T. H., & Baker, L. C. (2005). Internet use and stigmatized illness. *Social Science and Medicine, 61,* 1821–1827.

Bernstam, E. V., Walji, M. F., Sagaram, S., Sagaram, D., Johnson, C. W., Meric-Bernstam, F. (2008). Commonly cited website quality criteria are not effective at identifying inaccurate information about breast cancer. *Cancer, 112*(6), 1206–1213.

Borkman, T. (1999). *Understanding self-help/mutual aid: Experiential learning in the commons.* New Brunswick, NJ: Rutgers University Press.

Braithwaite, D., Waldron, V., & Finn, J. (1999). Communication of social support in computer-mediated groups for people with disabilities. *Health Communication, 11*(2), 123–151.

Brodie, M., Flournoy, R. E., Altman, D. E., Blendon, R. J., Benson, J. M., & Rosenbaum, M. D. (2000). Health information, the internet, and the digital divide. *Health Affairs, 19,* 255–265.

Brodie, M., Kjellson, N., Hoff, T., & Parker, M. (1999). Perceptions of Latinos, African Americans, and Whites on media as a health information source. *Howard Journal of Communications, 10*(3), 147–167.

Broom, A. (2005a). Medical specialists' accounts of the impact of the internet on the doctor/ patient relationship. *Health: An Interdisciplinary Journal for the Social Study of Health, Illness, and Medicine, 9,* 319–338.

Broom, A. (2005b). Virtually he@lthy: The impact of internet use on disease experience and doctor–patient relationship. *Qualitative Health Research, 15,* 325–345.

Buntin, M. B, Burke, M. F., Hoaglin, M. C., & Blumenthal, D. (2011). The benefits of health information technology: A review of the recent literature shows predominantly positive results. *Health Affairs, 30*(3), 464–471.

Commonwealth Fund. (2013, March). Retrieved from http://www.commonwealthfund.org/ Program-Areas/Archived-Programs/Health-Care-Disparities.aspx

Conrad, P., & Stults, C. (2010). The internet and the experience of illness. In C. E. Bird, P. Conrad, A. M. Fremont, & S. Timmermans (Eds.), *Handbook of medical sociology* (5th ed., pp. 179–191). Nashville, TN: Vanderbilt University Press.

Cotten, S. R. (2001). Implications of the Internet for medical sociology in the new millennium. *Sociological Spectrum, 21*(3), 319–340.

Cotten, S. R., & Gupta, S. S. (2004). Characteristics of online and offline health information seekers and factors that discriminate between them. *Social Science & Medicine, 59*, 1795–1806.

Dranove, D., Forman, C., Goldfarb, A., & Greenstein, S. (2012). *The trillion dollar conundrum: Complementarities and health information technology*. National Bureau of Economic Research. Retrieved from http://www.nber.org/papers/w18281. Accessed on August 24, 2012.

Fox, S. (2005). *Health information online*. Pew Internet & American Life Project. Retrieved from http://www.pewinternet.org/2005/05/17/health-information-online/

Fox, S. (2011). *The social life of health information, 2011*. Retrieved from http://www.pewinternet.org/2011/05/12/the-social-life-of-health-information-2011/

Fox, S., & Fallows, D. (2003). *Health searches and email have become more commonplace, but there is room for improvement in searches and overall Internet access*. Retrieved from http://www.pewinternet.org/2003/07/16/internet-health-resources/

Fox, S., & Jones, S. (2009). *The social life of health information*. Washington, DC: The Pew Internet & American Life Project. Retrieved from http://www.pewinternet.org/files/old-media//Files/Reports/2009/PIP_Health_2009.pdf

Fox, S., Rainie, L., Horrigan, J., Lenhart, A., Spooner, T., & Burke, M. (2000). *The online health care revolution: How the Web helps Americans take better care of themselves*. Retrieved from http://www.pewinternet.org/2000/11/26/the-online-health-care-revolution/

Goldsmith, J. (2000). How will the internet change our health system? *Health Affairs, 19*(1), 148–156.

Guo, B., Bricout, J. C., & Huang, J. (2005). A common open space or digital divide: A social mobility perspective on the on line disability community in China. *Disability and Society, 20*(1), 49–66.

Hale, T. M., Cotten, S. R., Drentea, P., & Goldner, M. (2010). Rural-urban differences in general and health-related Internet use. *American Behavioral Sciences, 20*, 1–22.

Hardey, M. (1999). Doctor in the house: The internet as a source of lay health knowledge and the challenge to expertise. *Sociology of Health and Illness, 21*, 820–835.

Hillestad, R., Bigelow, J., Bower, A., Girosi, F., Meili, R., Scoville, R., & Taylor, R. (2005). Can electronic medical record systems transform health care? Potential health benefits, savings, and costs. *Health Affairs, 24*(5), 1103–1117.

Kitagawa, E., & Hauser, P. (1973). *Differential mortality in the United States*. Cambridge, MA: Harvard University Press.

Kivits, J. (2004). Researching the "Informed Patient": The case of online health information seekers. *Information, Communication & Society, 7*, 510–530.

Kliss, B., & Scheuren, F. J. (1978). The 1973 CPS-IRS-SSA exact match study. *Social Security Bulletin, 42*, 14–22.

McGuire, T., Alegria, M., Cook, B. L., Wells, K. B., & Zaslavsky, A. M. (2006). Implementing the institute of medicine definition of disparities: An application to mental health care. *Health Services Research, 41*, 1979–2005.

National Healthcare Disparities Report. (2005, December). AHRQ Publication No. 06–0017. Agency for Healthcare Research and Quality, Rockville, MD. Retrieved from www.ahrq.gov/qual/nhdr05/nhdr05.pdf

Palvia, P., Lowe, K., Nematie, H., & Jacks, T. (2012). Information technology issues in healthcare: Hospital CEO and CIO perspectives. *Communications of the Association for Information Systems, 30*(19), 293–312.

Pew Internet and American Life. (2014). *Internet use over time*. Retrieved from http://www.pewinternet.org/data-trend/internet-use/internet-use-over-time/

Rice, R. (2006). Influences, usage, and outcomes of internet health information searching: Multivariate results from the Pew surveys. *International Journal of Medical Informatics, 75*, 8–28.

Schnittker, J., & McLeod, J. D. (2005). The social psychology of health disparities. *Annual Review of Sociology, 31*, 75–103.

Schoen, C., Osborn, R., Squires, D., Doty, M., Rasmussen, P., Pierson, R., & Applebaum, S. (2012). A survey of primary care doctors in ten countries shows progress in use of health information technology, less in other areas. *Health Affairs, 31*(12), 2805–2816.

Smedley, B. D., Stith, A. Y., & Nelson, A. R. (Eds.). (2003). *Unequal treatment: Confronting racial and ethnic disparities in health care*. Institute of Medicine, National Academies Press, Washington, DC.

Stern, M. J., Cotten, S. R., & Drentea, P. (2012). The separate spheres on online health: Gender, parenting, and online health information searching in the information age. *Journal of Family Issues, 33*(10), 1324–1350.

Taylor, R., Bower, A., Girosi, F., Bigelow, J., Fonkych, K., & Hillestad, R. (2005). Promoting health information technology: Is there a case for more-aggressive government action? *Health Affairs, 24*(5), 1234–1245.

Truman, B. I., Smith, C. K. S., Roy, K., Zhuo, C., Moonesinghe, R., ... Zaza, S. (2011, January 14). Rationale for regular reporting on health disparities and inequalities – United States. *Morbidity and Mortality Weekly Report Supplements, 60*(1), 3–10.

U.S. Department of Health and Human Services. (2000, November). *Healthy people 2010* (2nd ed.). With understanding and improving health and objectives for improving health (2 Vols.). Washington, DC: U.S. Government Printing Office.

U.S. Department of Health and Human Services. (2013, March). *Healthy people 2020*. Retrieved from http://www.healthypeople.gov/2020/about/disparitiesAbout.aspx

PART II
TECHNOLOGY

CAN INFORMATION TECHNOLOGY IMPROVE HEALTH CARE EQUITY IN THE UNITED STATES? LESSONS FROM TAIWAN

Claudia Chaufan and Yi-Chang Li

ABSTRACT

Purpose — *Over the last few decades, information technology (IT) has significantly altered the nature of work and organizational structures in many industries, including health care. The purpose of this analysis is to compare how system-level differences affect IT implementation in health care (HIT) and the implications of these differences for health care equity.*

Methodology/approach — *We critically analyzed selected claims concerning the capacity of HIT to provide better care to more individuals at lower costs, thus contributing to health care equity, in the context of current health care reform efforts in the United States. We used the case of*

Technology, Communication, Disparities and Government Options in Health and Health Care Services
Research in the Sociology of Health Care, Volume 32, 19–33
ISSN: 0275-4959/doi:10.1108/S0275-495920140000032000

HIT implementation in Taiwan's National Health Insurance system as a contrasting case.

Findings — *We argue that however much HIT may yield in quality improvements or savings in the context of a universal and publicly financed single payer system, such savings simply cannot be accrued by a system of multiple health plans competing for better customers (i.e., less costly patients) and driven by profit.*

Implications — *It is important to define the level of analysis in debates about the potential of HIT to produce better health care at lower costs and the equity implications of this potential. In these debates, US policy makers should consider the commitment to health care equity that informed the design of Taiwan's health care system and of HIT implementation in that country. HIT merely provides enabling tools that are of little value without major systemic changes*

Originality/value of the chapter — *To our knowledge, the health IT expert literature has overlooked when not ignored the ethical principles informing health care systems, an omission which makes it difficult if not impossible to evaluate the potential of HIT to increase equity in health care.*

Keywords: Health IT; Taiwan; universal health insurance; health care reform; health care equity

INTRODUCTION

Over the last few decades, information technology (IT), that is, technology used to "collect, store, retrieve, and transfer clinical, administrative, and financial ... information electronically," has significantly altered the nature of work and organizational structures in many industries, including health care (Brailer, 2010), where health IT (HIT) is receiving increasing attention (Palvia, Lowe et al., 2012). In an age of increasing health care costs and threatened access and quality, HIT implementation has been proposed as a key strategy to yield more and better health care at lower costs (Schoen, Osborn et al., 2012). While empirical support for the positive effects of HIT on productivity — the ratio between quality and amount of care on the one hand, and costs on the other — is mixed, a phenomenon known as the "IT productivity paradox" (Hu & Quan, 2005), many believe that if types of HIT implementation, such as Electronic Health Records (EHR), are adopted and used effectively, HIT can prevent medical errors, increase administrative efficiency, reduce costs, expand access to quality and afford-able care (Hillestad, Bigelow et al., 2005; Palvia, Lowe et al., 2012; Taylor, Bower et al., 2005) and, importantly for the purpose of our analysis, achieve all these goals in an equitable fashion (California Pan-Ethnic Health Network, 2013).

Debates about the productivity yield of IT, while fairly recent in health care, have a long history in other sectors of the economy, where the virtues of IT are extolled by some, while others remain critical of its purported benefits (Brynjolfsson & Hitt, 2003; Chan, 2007). Thus, while a recent review of studies of HIT show predominantly positive results (Buntin, Burke et al., 2011), others call these claims into question. For instance, one study found that adopting EHR was associated with an *increase* in costs, especially in hospitals in unfavorable conditions (e.g., not in urban area), even after six years, with no compensatory increase in quality (Dranove, Forman et al., 2012). Similarly, a recent study indicated that EHR may be adding billions of dollars to US Medicare, private insurance, and patients' bills, because they make it easier for providers to "game" the system by increasing their billing, whether or not they provide more or better services (Abelson, Creswell et al., 2012). Also, authors have warned that the pre-sumed benefits of HIT, if implemented improperly, could actually have negative implications for equity, by creating technological barriers among underserved communities (California Pan-Ethnic Health Network, 2013).

Given these complexities, some researchers have concluded that IT spending and performance, in health care or elsewhere, are unrelated, or that it is not the amount that is spent on IT, but the way IT is used, that delivers its relative advantage (Strassmann, 1997). Others have suggested that the difficulty to pin down the productivity yield of HIT lies in pro-blems of measurement, and recommend that before reaching any conclu-sions the level of analysis at which productivity is measured – for instance, individual health care workers or establishments – should be made explicit (Ross & Ernstberge, 2006).

How are debates about productivity relevant to health care equity? They are relevant because key goals of health care systems include to improve population health and safeguard fairness in health care by delivering qual-ity health care in an equitable fashion (World Health Organization [WHO], 2000). Because resources to accomplish socially desirable goals such as access to quality health care are always limited, anything that can contri-bute to delivering more and better care and lower costs should be welcome.

So the question becomes, can HIT improve the amount and quality of care delivered and do so at lower costs, as well as contribute to the equitable distribution of this care? More specifically, how can HIT contribute to "the core principle that everybody should have some basic security when it comes to their health care," as enshrined in the Affordable Care Act (ACA) (2010), the new federal legislation ruling health care matters in the United States?

This chapter describes the experience of HIT in the context of Taiwan's health care system, including how HIT has enhanced this system, what challenges remain, and how this experience can inform the implementation of HIT in the United States while contributing to the fulfillment of an ostensive goal of US health reform, that is, health care equity. We believe that there are critical system characteristics that are all too often overlooked when debating the goodness, or lack thereof, of HIT in a US context, and that an analysis of its implementation in the Taiwanese context can shed light on the challenges and realistic possibilities of implementing, not only HIT but other potentially useful tools (e.g., disease management, payment reforms) in the United States, in light of major recent changes in federal health care legislation.

BACKGROUND ON TAIWAN'S
HEALTH CARE SYSTEM

Before launching National Health Insurance (NHI), Taiwan had 10 different public insurance schemes. Each one covered a subset of the population, totaling 59% of a population of 21.4 million at the time, leaving uninsured 8.62 million, or 41% of the population, the majority of who were children under 14 and adults older than 65. On March 1, 1995, the Taiwanese government brought all 10 programs, and the totality of the uninsured population, under the same umbrella. No changes in the delivery system were attempted at the time — just radical cost control through public administration for medically necessary services and fee schedules, and coverage expansion to reach universality. One premium rate was set, a percentage of nominal income, now at 5.17% (per person, up to three individuals per family). Additional funds were secured through tobacco taxes and small copayments and coinsurance. Today, the NHI's total premium revenue comes from three sources: government (25%), employers (37%), and compulsory premiums (i.e., a health tax) from the public (38%) (Cheng, 2003).

Essentially, Taiwan has a publicly financed, single payer health care system, whose primary goal is to achieve health care equity, that is, make the best health care possible available to all Taiwanese residents independently of individuals' ability to pay. The system is organized such that patients carry the cash represented by their government-issued insurance cards to any provider of care, which leads to competition among health care providers based on the quality of their services, not their price. Coverage is comprehensive and includes in-patient care, ambulatory care, laboratory tests, diagnostic imaging, prescription and certain over-the-counter drugs, dental care (except orthodontics and prosthodontics), traditional Chinese medicine, day care for the mentally ill, limited home health care, and certain preventive medicine. Some services, such as prenatal care, well-child checkup, adult health examinations (including pap smears) and Highly Active Antiretroviral Therapy (HAART) for HIV/AIDS, which at the beginning belonged to NHI's budget, since 2005 have been paid for by a special government budget (T.-J. Chen, personal communication, September 23, 2012). Organ transplants, among other expensive treatments, are also covered under NHI. There is no rationing of care based on ability to pay, and little or no wait time (Bureau of National Health Insurance – Department of Health – Executive Yuan, 2011; Lu & Hsiao, 2003). Because the provision of health care is tightly coordinated with the public health system, Taiwan's Center for Disease Control has provided pediatric immunizations since the inception of NHI (T.-J. Chen, personal communication, September 23, 2012).

Unlike US private insurance plans, Taiwan's NHI offers the insured complete freedom of choice of affiliated health professionals (over 90% of Taiwanese health care professionals are affiliated to the program), medical establishments, and therapies, and there is no gatekeeper constraining access to specialists. Thus patients can "shop" for doctors, and they regularly do (Cheng, 2003). Because public insurance is not tied to job, age, location, or income, there is no need for patients to change health care providers when their life circumstances change. For-profit insurance schemes are limited to supplemental, non-medically necessary services, such as cosmetic surgery, private rooms for in-patient care, or special nursing care. Freedom of choice of providers and services, financial risk protection, and quality have made NHI very popular, so it is unsurprising that the system consistently receives over 70% public satisfaction rate (Lu & Hsiao, 2003).

While doctors and hospitals must achieve very high productivity to survive – global budgets capping payments from NHI to different sectors of the health care system have been added to the uniform fee schedule – doctors in Taiwan preserve a relatively high income, around 54,000 US dollars yearly compensation for a first year general practitioner in a public teaching hospital (Tainan Municipal Hospital, *GP recruitment ads*. 2012). This compares favorably to the compensation in other professions, such as academia, where the yearly salary for an assistant professor at a public university is around 30,000 US dollars (Personnel Administrator of National Taiwan University, 2012). Sixty three percent of physicians are employed by hospitals, are paid on a salaried basis, and often receive bonus payments based on productivity. Other physicians are paid fee-for-service, and there is some ongoing experimentation with case payments for in-patient services and bundled fees for hospital services (Cheng, 2009).

Despite sharp increases in health care utilization since the implementation of NHI (Chen, Yip et al., 2007; Cheng & Chiang, 1997), national health spending grew from the pre-NHI three-year average of 4.79% of gross domestic product to only 6.1% today as a result of successful cost containment (Liu, Yang et al., 2006). The fear of runaway costs resulting from a substantial increase in utilization has not been borne by the evidence (Lu & Hsiao, 2003). The single payer, public agency with a streamlined claims submission process, a very low administrative overhead both for the system (1.5% in 2008) and for providers, a fee schedule for medically necessary services, global budgets for selected sectors, and universal access to the same comprehensive benefits package are the main reasons for the system's efficient services and low prices (Liu, Yang et al., 2006), whose benefits are distributed across the population.

RATIONALE AND GROWTH OF IT IN TAIWAN HEALTH CARE

In Taiwan, HIT is viewed as a necessary though not sufficient contributor to the high productivity of NHI. Denmark's HIT ranks number one among OECD countries, yet according to a Danish scholar, Taiwan's HIT surpasses Denmark's (Cheng, 2009). There are two basic components in Taiwan's HIT: the Smart Card, a credit card—size card that acts as a single identification when accessing health care services, and the wider HIT system, which includes the EHR system.

At its inception, the purpose of the Smart Card was solely to facilitate claims processing. Yet because providers submit their claims based on the EHRs they keep, from early on the system was able to identify which patient had visited which provider how many times, thus enabled NHI to do a very detailed profiling of both patients and providers and to keep track of the adequacy of the use of medical resources, thus to prevent potential medical frauds in a timely fashion (Liu, Yang et al., 2006; C. Yang, personal communication, October 7, 2012). For instance, because the initial rationale for HIT was to speed up claims processing, attempts to "game" the system by tailoring submissions to maximize reimbursements were easier to diagnose and address (Y.-H. E. Hsu, personal communication, June 19, 2012). Currently, payment reforms are being tested to prevent the abuses frequent in fee-for-service forms of payment (Cheng, Chen et al., 2012).

More recently, the Smart Card has incorporated information on patients' medical history, including prescribed procedures and exams (C. Yang, personal communication, October 7, 2012). This has allowed NHI to assess quality and providers to provide better quality of care by, for instance, checking drug allergy history to prevent medication errors. In addition, the Department of Health of Taiwan has encouraged hospitals, through financial incentives, to collect and utilize the acute care quality indicators derived from their EHR databases to facilitate improvements in health care quality (Chang, Hsiao et al., 2011).

HIT in Taiwan has also provided very tangible advantages to patients, even when the extent of the savings, either for patients, providers or the system, are yet to be established. For instance, in 2009, 11 major hospitals deployed a template-based EHR system called "Taiwan Prescription Template (TPT)," which has allowed patients to download their prescriptions after their medical visits on to a portable device and to carry around their own medical history, offering opportunities to exchange health records among different providers and helping prevent medical errors (Kuo, Li et al., 2009).

Last, because all health care providers follow the HIT template assigned by NHI, interoperability problems, so common in the US scenario (O'Malley, 2010), are all but non-existent in Taiwan. Indeed, it is the single payer model of financing that has eased HIT implementation and allowed very low administrative costs at the level of the system, as well as at the levels of individual medical establishments and providers (C. Yang, personal communication, October 7, 2012).

LESSONS FROM TAIWAN FOR US HEALTH CARE

The Taiwanese value competition, shared responsibility, and choice, and view their country as a thriving market economy (C.-C. Yeh, personal communication, May 8, 2012). They are also proud of their HIT accomplishments, which have allowed their health care system to flourish (C.-h. Lee, personal communication, May 10, 2012). Yet the successful implementation of HIT in Taiwan, especially its contributions to health equity, *presupposes* a system designed to meet this goal. It was this goal that informed the choice of key attributes of this system – including public administration and financing, compulsory contributions from all users based on ability to pay, no restrictions derived from selective contracting of providers, and universal access to a uniform benefit package based exclusively on medical need – and that has guaranteed that whichever benefits may accrue from HIT will be equitable distributed and enjoyed by patients across the population.

It is unsurprising, then, that since the implementation of NHI Taiwan has made great strides toward health care equity: the country has experienced a reduction in mortality amenable to health care, especially among individuals less likely to have been previously insured (Lee, Huang et al., 2010), and an important increase in life expectancy among those groups that had higher mortality rates prior to the introduction of NHI, thus a narrowing of health disparities, especially in deaths from cardiovascular diseases, ill-defined conditions, infectious diseases, and accidents among groups with worse health status (Wen, Tsai et al., 2008). Access to medically necessary health care is today an inalienable right in Taiwan's constitution, and the Taiwanese find pride in the fact that everyone, "from the president to the poorest person," is entitled to the same amount and quality of medically necessary services (C.-C. Yeh, personal communication, May 8, 2012). The system has a clear goal, health care equity, so it is easy to evaluate whether at any given moment HIT is delivering (or not) better care at lower costs in ways that are universally enjoyed.

The US health care system, even in the age of federal health care reform, presents a dramatically different scenario (Table 1). There has been great hope that HIT will help realize the potential of the ACA (The President's Council of Advisors on Science and Technology, 2010), signed into law by President Obama on March 23 2009. However, by 2016, two years after the implementation of the individual mandate, the cornerstone of ACA, there will still remain at least 30 million Americans, 80% of whom are US citizens, mostly white, and between 100 and 199% of the federal poverty line, and including 4.3 million children and nearly 1 million veterans, with no health insurance (Nardin, Zallman et al., 2013). Six million among these uninsured individuals will be assessed a financial penalty (Congressional Budget Office, 2012). Overall, minorities, poor, working-age, and employed adults will continue to be overrepresented among the uninsured.

Table 1. Key Systemic Differences between the Taiwanese and US Health care Systems.

	US Health care	Taiwan Health care
Payers for medically necessary services	Multiple; public and private (commercial for profit)	Public, single-payer. Commercial insurance for medically necessary services banned. Allowed for services "over and above" basic and comprehensive care package
Benefits	Patchy. Vary according to plan. Ten broad categories indicated by ACA, yet many plans exempt (e.g., grandfathered)	Comprehensive and equal across the board
Financing	• Public funding for low income, over 65, and disabled (Medicare and Medicaid), often organized through commercial insurance plans paid by taxpayers (e.g., Medicare Advantage) • Tax exemptions to purchase commercial insurance • Means-tested subsidies to purchase commercial insurance • Co-pays, co-insurance, and deductibles (vary according to plans' actuarial values and individual use) • Out of pocket for uncovered services or uninsured (substantial)	• Government (25 percent); employers (37 percent); and the public (38 percent, a fixed percentage of income) • Additional funding through tobacco taxes/small copayments and coinsurance • Co-pays and co-insurance (very small) • Out of pocket for uncovered services (very low)
Contributions by users	Compulsory; financial hardship and other exemptions (e.g., religious). Exempted individuals remain uninsured	Compulsory; calculated according to ability to pay
Uninsured	About 30 million by 2019	None
Medical bankruptcies	About 1.2 million families in 2007, at least 62% with insurance	None
Choice of providers	Varies according to plans. Out of network providers usually not covered (or covered at substantially higher costs to users)	Full choice of all eligible providers (>90% of Taiwanese doctors) and medical establishments
Cost control	• No system-wide cost controls. Hope that competition among insurers will drive down prices • Partial cost controls attempts via bundled payments, EMR, control of fraud and abuse of public programs, prevention strategies	• System-wide cost controls. Single payer system minimizes administrative overhead and negotiates prices with providers. Global budgets for different sectors (e.g., hospital care) • Close tracking (via Smart Card) provider and patient profiles to identify and reduce fraudulent claims, overcharges, and duplication of services
Costs in US$ per capita and % of GDP	US$8,006 and 17.7 in 2009 (US$8,507.6 and 17.7 in 2011)	US$2,208 and 6.9 in 2009
HIT	• Multiple HIT norms. Varying degrees of interoperability problems. Little system-wide influence on reporting procedures • HIT implementation encouraged yet effects on system-wide productivity hard to track due to fragmentation of the financial structure of system	• One single norm. No interoperability problems. HIT facilitates one uniform reporting procedure and claim filing system, which has significantly reduced transaction costs • HIT system-wide productivity easy to track via single-paying public agency

This number does not include the underinsured, who are very hard to estimate because being underinsured is not apparent until individuals need specific services, and find out that their coverage is insufficient (Chaufan, 2011). However, a low estimate of the number of underinsured is the high percentage of individuals, around 80%, who have health insurance yet still file for bankruptcy because they are unable to pay their medical bills (Himmelstein, Thorne et al., 2009), a number likely to grow as plans with low actuarial values — an estimate of the overall financial protection provided by a health plan — and high deductibles become the new norm.

According to the Kaiser Family Foundation, HIT offers the promise of potential improvements in quality of care as well as increased efficiencies in care and cost savings (Kaiser Family Foundation, 2009), a claim that is echoed by several NGOs advocating for minority health and hopeful that HIT implementation, if appropriately distributed, will bring about greater health care equity (California Pan-Ethnic Health Network, 2013). Yet barriers to this potential are likely to pervade a system bedeviled by organizational fragmentation and the absence of clear equity goals, even after major federal health reform, and these barriers are not hard to identify, imagine, or predict.

For instance, a patient with employer-sponsored insurance with a Smart Card and her own EHR to carry around may be able to visit one provider one day, but not the following day, if the provider were no longer in her plan's network, if the patient's employer changed insurers, or if the patient lost her job, thus also her employer-sponsored health plan. Even despite an employer mandate, that compels some (but not all) employers to make available affordable health care benefits or pay a fine, there is the question of which employees qualify as "full-time" under ACA to be eligible for employer-sponsored insurance. A recent analysis suggested that many individuals employed full time yet only part of the year, such as seasonal workers, would see their eligibility compromised (Jost, 2012).

Then there is the question of churning, that is, the phenomenon whereby individuals who qualify for Medicaid plans will go in and out of these plans as their incomes increase or decrease, even if slightly, a very concrete possibility in an era of precarious employment and fluctuating incomes, with the subsequent fluctuation of eligibility for public insurance (Medicaid) or subsidies (Buettgens, Nichols et al., 2012). Also, the range of actuarial values and benefit packages allowable under ACA will vary widely such that even in the best case scenario it will be very difficult for patients to estimate their out-of-pocket expenses when they actually need care, and for providers to know which interventions they can prescribe that their patients can realistically afford. A recent analysis by The Commonwealth Fund showed that plans with identical actuarial values may result in widely different out-of-pocket expenses depending on patients' medical conditions (Ryan Lore, Gabel et al., 2012), not easy to predict when shopping for policies. Last, it is not clear that whichever greater productivity is accrued by HIT implementation at the level of individual health care workers or establishments will be necessarily passed on to users (Sidorov, 2006), who are already seeing their medical bills increase, particularly if employed in small (under 200 employees) firms (Claxton, Rae et al., 2012), even as the amount of care (and quality, if this amount is inadequate) they may receive becomes increasingly small, exactly the opposite of what the concept of productivity entails, and counter to equity goals.

Recently, Kellerman et al. attributed the "disappointing performance of health IT" (p. 63) – that is, its failure to lower costs and increase access to care – to the slow adoption of HIT systems, the choice of IT systems that are neither interoperable nor easy to use, and the medical profession's resistance to let go of fee-for-service and embrace instead payment models that favor value over volume (Kellermann & Jones, 2013) – a popular argument that proposes that fee-for-service, by encouraging greater volume of care, is a key driver of US health care costs.[1]

The authors assert that if "market forces were allowed to work" (p. 65), doctors might, for instance, "drive vendors to produce more usable products" (p.65). In their view, it is also insufficient market forces that are responsible for the fact that the information stored at, say, the Department of Veterans Affairs or Kaiser Permanente, is useless when the patient seeks out-of-network care, as a result of which, conclude the authors, "the current generation of IT records functions less as ATM cards, allowing a patient or provider to access … health information anywhere at any time, than as 'frequent flyer cards' intended to enforce brand loyalty to a particular health care system."

The authors fail to notice that it is precisely these "market forces" that have produced a system of multiple health plans that encourage such "brand loyalty," as they compete for better customers (i.e., less costly patients) and offer a dizzying array of "health insurance products" that impose on health providers alone a burden estimated in three weeks of work per year, or an aggregate annual cost of 23–31 billion (Casalino, Nicholson et al., 2009).

They also fail to mention one critical reason why, as they themselves point out, adoption of HIT in the United States lags that of other wealthy, industrialized nations – Canada, the United Kingdom (UK), Germany, the Netherlands, Australia, and New Zealand (Jha, Doolan et al., 2008). All these countries have universal and publicly financed, or even delivered, systems, with price controls, uniform fee schedules, clear rules governing the adoption of HIT, and a generous package of well-defined medically necessary services guaranteed to all the population, in stark contrast with the "competitive marketplace" that the authors appear to recommend to address the unfilled promises of HIT.

Inscrutable "benefit packages," varying actuarial values, ever narrowing provider networks, changes in coverage with changes in employment status or income level, and increasing prices of policies and out-of-pocket costs are only a handful of the problems created by the commodification of health insurance, that users of US health care will face and that HIT has no ability to address. When debating this ability, US health care policy makers should seek inspiration in the commitment to health care equity that informed the design of Taiwan's health care system. They should also heed the warning that HIT, as other potentially useful modifications in health care at the micro and mezzo levels (e.g., chronic disease management, medical homes), merely provides enabling tools that are of limited value without major systemic changes (Shumaker, 2006).

NOTE

1. This meme is clearly at odds with the intensive, even if undesirable, use of fee-for-service in publicly financed systems such as Taiwan's, Canada's, Germany's, or France's. All these are vastly more efficient and equitable than the US healthcare system even after major federal reform even if all of them include fee for service as a form of payment to varying degrees.

ACKNOWLEDGMENTS

The authors thank Professor Cheming Yang, Professor Tzay-Jinn Chen, and Professor Patrick Fox for their careful reading of drafts and useful feedback. They also thank the faculty at Taipei Medical University and officials at the Bureau of National Health Insurance for sharing their knowledge and experience. Lastly, they thank the staff at the Institute for Health & Aging for their continuing, invaluable support.

REFERENCES

Abelson, R., Creswell, J., & Palmer, G. J. (2012). Medicare bills rise as records turn electronic. *The New York Times*. Retrieved from http://www.nytimes.com/2012/09/22/business/medicare-billing-rises-at-hospitals-with-electronic-records.html?emc=eta1&_r=0. Accessed on September 24, 2012.

Brailer, D. J. (2010). Guiding the health information technology Agenda. *Health Affairs, 29*(4), 586–595.

Brynjolfsson, E., & Hitt, L. M. (2003). Computing productivity: Firm-level evidence. *The Review of Economics and Statistics, 85*(4), 793–808.

Buettgens, M., & Nichols, A. et al. (2012). *Churning under the ACA and state policy options for mitigation*. Urban Institute, Robert Wood Johnson Foundation. Retrieved from http://www.rwjf.org/content/dam/farm/reports/issue_briefs/2012/rwjf73183. Accessed on August 24.

Buntin, M. B., & Burke, M. F. et al. (2011). The benefits of health information technology: A review of the recent literature shows predominantly positive results. *Health Affairs, 30*(3), 464–471.

Bureau of National Health Insurance – Department of Health – Executive Yuan. (2011). *National health insurance in Taiwan 2011 annual report*. Taipei, Bureau of National Health Insurance, Department of Health, Executive Yuan, pp. 1–72.

California Pan-Ethnic Health Network. (2013, February 24). *Equity in the digital age: How health information technology can reduce disparities*. Retrieved from http://www.cpehn.org/pdfs/EquityInTheDigitalAge2013.pdf. Accessed on February 26.

Casalino, L. P., & Nicholson, S. et al. (2009). What does it cost physician practices to interact with health insurance plans? *Health Affairs, 28*(4), w533–w543.

Chan, Y. E. (2007). IT value: The great divide between qualitative and quantitative and individual and organizational measures. In R. Galliers, L. M. Markus, & S. Newell (Eds.), *Exploring information systems research approaches*. London: Routledge.

Chang, S.-J., & Hsiao, H.-C. et al. (2011). Taiwan quality indicator project and hospital productivity growth. *Omega, 39*(1), 14–22.

Chaufan, C. (2011). Influences of policy on health care of families. In M. J. Craft-Rosenberg (Ed.), *Encyclopedia of family health* (pp. 650–658). Newbury Park, CA: SAGE Publications.

Chen, L., & Yip, W. et al. (2007). The effects of Taiwan's national health insurance on access and health status of the elderly. *Health Economics, 16*(3), 223–242.

Cheng, S.-H., & Chen, C.-C. et al. (2012). The impacts of DRG-based payments on health care provider behaviors under a universal coverage system: A population-based study. *Health Policy, 107*(2–3), 202–208.

Cheng, S.-H., & Chiang, T.-L. (1997). The effect of universal health insurance on health care utilization in Taiwan: Results from a natural experiment. *JAMA: The Journal of the American Medical Association, 278*(2), 89–93.

Cheng, T.-M. (2003). Taiwan's new national health insurance program: Genesis and experience so far. *Health Affairs, 22*(3), 61–76.

Cheng, T.-M. (2009). Lessons from Taiwan's universal national health insurance: A conversation with Taiwan's health minister Ching-Chuan Yeh. *Health Affairs, 28*(4), 1035–1044.

Claxton, G., & Rae, M. et al. (2012). Health benefits in 2012: Moderate premium increases for employer-sponsored plans; young adults gained coverage under ACA. *Health Affairs, 31*(10), 2324–2333.

Congressional Budget Office. (2012, September). Payment penalties for being uninsured under the affordable care act. *Washington, DC.* Retrieved from http://www.cbo.gov/sites/default/files/cbofiles/attachments/09-19-12-Indiv_Mandate_Penalty.pdf

Dranove, D., & Forman, C. et al. (2012). *The trillion dollar conundrum: Complementarities and health information technology.* National Bureau of Economic Research. Retrieved from http://www.nber.org/papers/w18281. Accessed on August 24.

GP recruitment ads at Tainan Municipal Hospital. Retrieved from http://www.tmh.org.tw/. Accessed on August 24, 2012 (in Chinese).

Hillestad, R., & Bigelow, J. et al. (2005). Can electronic medical record systems transform health care? Potential health benefits, savings, and costs. *Health Affairs, 24*(5), 1103–1117.

Himmelstein, D. U., & Thorne, D. et al. (2009). Medical bankruptcy in the United States, 2007: Results of a national study. *The American Journal of Medicine, 122*(8), 741–746.

Hu, Q., & Quan, J. J. (2005). Evaluating the impact of IT investments on productivity: A causal analysis at industry level. *International Journal of Information Management, 25*(1), 39–53.

Jha, A. K., & Doolan, D. et al. (2008). The use of health information technology in seven nations. *International Journal of Medical Informatics, 77*(12), 848–854.

Jost, T. (2012). Implementing health reform: A summer lull. *Health Affairs Blog.* Retrieved from http://healthaffairs.org/blog/2012/08/31/implementing-health-reform-a-summer-lull/. Accessed on September 10.

Kaiser Family Foundation. (2009). *Federal support for Health Information Technology in Medicaid: Key provisions in the American Recovery and Reinvestment Act.* Retrieved from http://www.kff.org/medicaid/upload/7955.pdf. Accessed on March 10, 2012.

Kellermann, A. L., & Jones, S. S. (2013). What it will take to achieve the as-yet-unfulfilled promises of health information technology. *Health Affairs, 32*(1), 63–68.

Kuo, C. H., & Li, Y.-C. et al. (2009). An interoperability infrastructure with portable prescription for improving patient safety – The framework of a national standard in Taiwan. *IEEE Computer Society: Proceedings of the 2009 WRI World Congress on Computer Science and Information Engineering, 01,* 293–297.

Lee, Y.-C., & Huang, Y.-T. et al. (2010). The impact of universal national health insurance on population health: The experience of Taiwan. *BMC Health Services Research, 10*(1), 1–8.

Liu, C.-T., & Yang, P.-T. et al. (2006). The impacts of smart cards on hospital information systems – An investigation of the first phase of the national health insurance smart card project in Taiwan. *International Journal of Medical Informatics, 75*(2), 173–181.

Lu, J.-F. R., & Hsiao, W. C. (2003). Does universal health insurance make health care unaffordable? Lessons from Taiwan. *Health Affairs, 22*(3), 77–88.

Nardin, R., & Zallman, L. et al. (2013). The uninsured after implementation of the affordable care act: A demographic and geographic analysis. *Health Affairs.* Retrieved from http://healthaffairs.org/blog/2013/06/06/the-uninsured-after-implementation-of-the-affordable-care-act-a-demographic-and-geographic-analysis/. Accessed on June 6.

O'Malley, A. S. (2010, August 5). *Testimony.* Center for Studying Health System Change. Retrieved from http://www.hschange.com/CONTENT/1140/1140.pdf. Accessed on August 28.

Palvia, P., & Lowe, K. et al. (2012). Information technology issues in healthcare: Hospital CEO and CIO perspectives. *Communications of the Association for Information Systems, 30*(19). Retrieved from http://aisel.aisnet.org/cais/vol30/iss1/19

Personnel Administrator of National Taiwan University. (2012). *Salary standard of new professors.* Retrieved from http://www.personnel.ntu.edu.tw/~persadm/table3/33001.xls. Accessed on August 24, 2012 (in Chinese).

Ross, A., & Ernstberge, K. (2006). Benchmarking the IT productivity paradox: Recent evidence from the manufacturing sector. *Mathematical and Computer Modelling, 44*(1), 30–42.

Ryan Lore, R., & Gabel, J. R. et al. (2012). *Choosing the "best" plan in a health insurance exchange: Actuarial value tells only part of the story* (p. 23). Washington, DC: The Commonwealth Fund. Retrieved from http://www.commonwealthfund.org/Publications/Issue-Briefs/2012/Aug/Choosing-the-Best-Plan-in-a-Health-Insurance-Exchange.aspx#citation. Accessed on August 24.

Schoen, C., & Osborn, R. et al. (2012). A survey of primary care doctors in ten countries shows progress in use of health information technology, less in other areas. *Health Affairs, 31*(12), 2805–2816.

Shumaker, P. (2006). System change, then EHRs. *Health Affairs, 25*(6), 1745.

Sidorov, J. (2006). It ain't necessarily so: The electronic health record and the unlikely prospect of reducing health care costs. *Health Affairs, 25*(4), 1079–1085.

Stolberg, S. G., & Pear, R. (2010). Obama signs health care overhaul bill, with a Flourish. *The New York Times*, March 23. Retrieved from http://www.nytimes.com/2010/03/24/health/policy/24health.html?pagewanted=print. Accessed on March 23, 2010.

Strassmann, P. A. (1997). *The squandered computer: Evaluating the business alignment of information technologies.* New Canaan, CT: The Information Economics Press.

Taylor, R., & Bower, A. et al. (2005). Promoting health information technology: Is there a case for more-aggressive government action? *Health Affairs, 24*(5), 1234–1245.

The President's Council of Advisors on Science and Technology. (2010, December). *Realizing the full potential of health information technology to improve healthcare for Americans: The path forward.* Retrieved from http://www.whitehouse.gov/sites/default/files/microsites/ostp/pcast-health-it-report.pdf. Accessed on August 23.

Wen, C. P., & Tsai, S. P. et al. (2008). A 10-year experience with universal health insurance in Taiwan: Measuring changes in health and health disparity. *Annals of Internal Medicine, 148*(4), 258–267.

World Health Organization. (2000). *The world health report 2000 — Health systems: Improving performance.* WHO, Geneva.

PATTERNS OF ONLINE HEALTH SEARCHING 2002–2010: IMPLICATIONS FOR SOCIAL CAPITAL, HEALTH DISPARITIES AND THE DE-PROFESSIONALIZATION OF MEDICAL KNOWLEDGE

Timothy M. Hale, Melinda Goldner,
Mike Stern, Patricia Drentea and Shelia R. Cotten

ABSTRACT

Purpose — *Since 2000, there has been a dramatic increase in the number of individuals using the Internet, including for health purposes. Internet usage has increased from 46% of adults in 2000 to 79% in 2010. The purpose of this chapter is to examine changes in one type of Internet usage: online health searching. We examine the impact of traditional*

Technology, Communication, Disparities and Government Options in Health and
Health Care Services
Research in the Sociology of Health Care, Volume 32, 35–60
Copyright © 2014 by Emerald Group Publishing Limited
All rights of reproduction in any form reserved
ISSN: 0275-4959/doi:10.1108/S0275-495920140000032016

digital inequality factors on online health searching, and whether these patterns have changed over time.

Methodology – *Using data from five surveys ranging from 2002 to 2010 (*n = 5,967 *for all five surveys combined), we examine changing patterns of online health searching over the past decade.*

Findings – *Effects vary by inequality factor and time period examined. Despite the diffusion of the Internet, most of these gaps persist, and even strengthen, over time. Gender, age, and education gaps persist over time and appear to be increasing. An exception to this is the importance of broadband connection.*

Research limitations – *Since these data were collected, the use of mobile devices to access the Internet has increased. Research is needed on types of access and devices used for online health activities.*

Implications – *Larger scale inequalities play important roles in online health searching. Providing access and skills in evaluating online health information is needed for older and less educated groups. The results of this study have implications for the de-professionalization of medical knowledge.*

Originality – *This is the first study to examine digital inequality factors in online health information seeking over the breadth of this time period.*

Keywords: Online health searching; Internet usage; longitudinal analyses; digital inequality; Pew Internet & American Life Project; social inequalities

INTRODUCTION

Over the past 15 years, there has been a dramatic increase in the number of individuals using the Internet, including for health purposes. Pew Internet & American Life (2014) trend data suggest that Internet usage has increased in the past decade from 46% to 79% of adults in the United States. Although usage levels vary depending on the demographic group being examined (e.g., age, socioeconomic status, race, gender, place) and the specific types of online activities, usage levels are at their highest point in this decade. Individuals routinely turn to the Internet for a variety of health-related activities, such as purchasing prescription drugs and engaging with others who may be experiencing similar medical conditions

(Fox & Jones, 2009; Hale, Cotten, Drentea, & Goldner, 2010; Rice, 2006); however, the purpose of this chapter is to examine changes in the most commonly reported online health activity, searching for health or medical information (Fox, 2011).

Using data from five Pew Internet & American Life Project surveys, ranging from 2002 to 2010, we examine how traditional digital inequality factors affect online health searching, and determine how these patterns may have changed in the past decade. For example, have usage differences based on income and education declined? Are men increasingly using the Internet for health purposes? Are there particular age groups that have increased in usage more than others? What is the most persistent digital divide factor in online health searching?

Changing patterns of online health searching affect patients and medical professionals. Resources garnered from Internet websites can be powerful as social capital (Drentea & Moren-Cross, 2005; Stern & Dillman, 2006). This is important given the potential benefits, including the fact that online health information can educate and empower patients, potentially lessening health care disparities. Understanding how particular socio-demographic groups utilize online health searching may reveal information about larger patterns of digital inequality and health disparities, which may translate into larger scale societal inequalities (DiMaggio & Hargittai, 2001). Also, these shifts in how individuals gain knowledge reflect a larger shift in the de-professionalization of medical knowledge (Cotten & Gupta, 2004). As more people access the esoteric knowledge that was once inaccessible in medicine, the power of the public potentially increases in relation to the medical profession. The implications of these findings for the de-professionalization of medical knowledge and for the enhancement of social capital will be discussed.

LITERATURE REVIEW

As Internet use has proliferated, individuals are shifting the way they gain knowledge. Goldsmith (2000) describes the Internet as "a flexible and powerful new nervous system for the economy and society" (p. 148). Traditional methods of gaining knowledge have shifted to the Internet given its accessibility, scope, cost, and anonymity (Rainie & Fox, 2000).

One important shift encompasses health-related activities. Traditional sources of health information include physicians and the mass media

(Brodie, Kjellson, Hoff, & Parker, 1999; Cotten & Gupta, 2004; Goldsmith, 2000). Most patients still turn to medical professionals first for advice (Fox, 2011); however, individuals increasingly seek health information online (Cotten, 2001; Goldsmith, 2000). In 2000, 55% of Internet users reported that at some point they had searched the Internet for health or medical information (Fox & Rainie, 2000) but this increased to 80% of Internet users by 2010 (Fox, 2011). In particular, individuals are motivated to search online due to health concerns (Rice, 2006), thus they are most likely to use the Internet to research a medical condition or treatment, or to a lesser extent, providers (Fox, 2011). Usage varies by demographic characteristics.

Most studies show that women are more likely than men to use the Internet to search for health information (Baker, Wagner, Singer, & Bundorf, 2003; Brodie et al., 2000; Fox, 2005; Fox & Fallows, 2003; Fox & Rainie, 2000; Hale et al., 2010; Hu, 2000). Using Pew data, Rice (2006) found that gender was one of the "strongest and most consistent influences" (p. 8). Women are more likely than men to utilize health care services and care for their family's health, which might explain these differences (Litt, 2000; Stern, Cotten, & Drentea, 2012). For example, Fox and Fallows (2003) found that women were more likely than men to say that their last online health search entailed finding information for another person. Stern et al. (2012) found that while female and male parents were rather similar in online health searches, women were more likely to put the information to use. Women's feelings toward the information were complex too. They felt more reassured than men, felt more confident to bring it to a health care professional, but also felt more afraid of what they found out online (Stern et al., 2012).

Online health searching is typically related to income, education, and race, because these affect computer access and Internet usage (National Telecommunications and Information Administration [NTIA], 2000). Individuals with higher incomes and educational levels are more likely to search for health information online (Cotten & Gupta, 2004; Hale et al., 2010; Taylor, 2002), even in one sample comprised exclusively of women (Pandey, Hart, & Tiwary, 2003). Education seems to be a key predictor. For example, Baker et al. (2003) found that education, but not income, was a statistically significant predictor. Likewise, Pew data show that non-Hispanic whites were more likely to search for health information; however, this is mainly due to educational differences (Fox & Fallows, 2003). In contrast to this pattern, Brodie et al. (2000) did not find variation by income, education, or race once they narrowed their sample to people who had Internet access at home. We will return to this point later.

Younger individuals are more likely to search for health information online. Cotten and Gupta (2004) found that the mean age of online health seekers was 40, compared to a mean age of 52 for individuals who rely on offline sources such as health magazines. Baker et al. (2003) found that those aged 75 and older were significantly less likely to search while Fox and Jones (2009) found that those aged 18–49 searched more frequently than older individuals. Similar to their data on income, education, and race, Brodie et al. (2000) found that age differences disappear once people have Internet access at home. Thus reliable Internet access at home is a potential equalizer in the digital divide and possibly tangentially to health disparities, access to social capital, and information on health issues.

The importance of access is illustrated in the research on place and broadband usage. Rural communities have historically had less access to broadband (Horrigan & Murray, 2006), but "high-speed, always-on connections enable frequent and in-depth information searches, which is particularly attractive if something important is at stake" (Fox, 2008, p. 2). Not surprisingly then, rural individuals are less likely to search online for health information (Flynn, Smith, & Freese, 2006).

A key strength of this study is that we analyze whether these traditional digital inequality factors vary over time, which can speak to changes in social capital, health disparities, and shifts in power between patients and providers. We would expect these patterns to change, because Internet access has increased as the cost of computers has declined and availability of high-speed wireless access on phones and laptops has grown (Smith, 2010). Importantly, access affects proficiency so people become more comfortable using online resources (Stern, Adams, & Elsasser, 2009).

METHODS

Data

We use five data sets drawn from the surveys conducted by the Pew Internet & American Life Project. These single then dual frame telephone surveys were designed to track trends in Internet access and usage in the United States using a nationally representative sample of adults, ages 18 years and older, who have access to either a landline telephone, or in later surveys, a cellular telephone. These data were collected at roughly two-year intervals and cover an eight-year span, starting in December 2002 and ending in September 2010. Table 1 presents details on each of the five data sets. The data, survey questionnaires, and details about the methodology are available online (http://www.pewinternet.org/datasets/).

Four types of sampling methodology were used in data collection. In 2002 and 2006, the samples were drawn using random digit dial sampling of landline telephones. In 2004 a list-assisted random digit dialing method was used to identify active blocks of residential telephone numbers and generate random telephone numbers. In 2008 and 2010 a sample drawn from cellular telephone numbers was added. The 2008 landline sample was drawn using the same method as in 2004. The cellular telephone sample was drawn from dedicated blocks of wireless numbers and from shared service numbers when these did not include any directory-listed landline numbers. The 2010 landline sample used a similar method as the list-assisted random digit dial method in 2004 and 2008, but was designed to oversample Black and Hispanic households by drawing a larger proportion of numbers from telephone exchanges known to have larger than average minority households. The 2010 cellular telephone sample used the same method as in 2008.

Table 1. Pew Internet & American Life Project Survey Data Details.

Year	Sampling Method	Response Rate	Sample Size	Internet Users	Percent Missing on Key Variables	Analytic Sample
2002	Landline, RDD	Landline 32.8%	2,038	1,223	18.11% ($n=221$)	999
2004[a]	Landline, list-assisted RDD	Landline 32.8%	914	537	19.55% ($n=105$)	432
2006	Landline, RDD	Landline 27.1%	2,928	1,990	22.30% ($n=445$)	1,545
2008	Landline, list-assisted RDD	Landline 20.9%	Landline 1,751	1,650	20.73% ($n=342$)	1,308
	Cellular, RDD	Cellular 24.5%	Cellular 502			
2010	Landline, list-assisted RDD, oversample of African-Americans and Hispanics	Landline 13.6%	Landline 2,001	2,065	18.50% ($n=382$)	1,683
	Cellular, RDD	Cellular 17.0%	Cellular 1,000			

Note: Random Digit Dial (RDD).
[a]Measure of self-rated health is not included in these data.

The focus of this chapter is on examining trends in the factors that predict online health information seeking among Internet users. Thus, we restrict our multivariate analyses to Internet users. Listwise deletion of cases with missing data further reduced the size of the Internet sample by about 20%. The size of the analytic samples for each year is presented in Table 1.

Measures

Dependent Variables – Health-Related Internet Use
Our three dependent variables come from a set of questions that ask Internet users if they have ever looked online for information on a variety of specific health or medical issues, to which they responded yes or no. Unfortunately, the number of questions and the specific types of health or medical information issues varies with only two questions asked across all six surveys. In 2002 and 2004 the surveys included 16 questions. In 2006 one question was added about searching for information on dental health. In 2008 there were 13 questions; 5 were drawn from 2002 and 2004 and 8 questions were new. In 2010 there were 15 questions; only 2 were drawn from 2002 and 2004 and 13 questions were new.

Using this changing set of questions we constructed a binary variable indicating whether participants have *ever sought health information on any topic* if they report using one or more of the 13–16 health or medical topics asked in that survey year. Two questions about specific types of health or medical information searches were asked across all six surveys. We use both of these questions as dependent variables. Participants were asked if they have ever looked online for (1) *information about a specific disease or medical problem,* and (2) *information about a certain medical treatment or procedure.*

Independent Variables
Our independent variables include measures of demographics, type of Internet connection, type of community, and health status.

Demographics
Our first demographic variables measured sex, race, and age. Sex is measured using a binary variable coded 1 = "male" and 0 = "female." Race was recoded from six categories to a binary variable 1 = "white" and 0 = "nonwhite." Participant's age in years was recoded as one of six cohorts described in the Pew report *Generations 2010* (Zickuhr, 2010). The cohorts,

based on people's age in 2010, are Millennials (born 1977–1992 and aged 18–33), Generation X (born 1965–1976 and aged 34–45), Young Boomers (born 1955–1964 and aged 46–55), Older Boomers (born in 1946–1954 and aged 56–64), the Silent Generation (born 1937–1948 and aged 65–73), and the GI Generation (born 1936 or earlier and 74 years of age or older). Ages in years before 2010 have been adjusted to account for the difference in age at the time of the survey. A series of binary indicator variables were created for each age cohort with the youngest age cohort (i.e., 18–33 Millennials born in 1977–1992) used as the reference group.

Level of education was measured across years using seven levels: 1 = "none (grades 1–8)," 2 = "high school incomplete (grades 9–11)," 3 = "high school graduate (grade 12) or GED certificate," 4 = "business, technical, or vocational school after high school," 5 = "some college, no four-year degree," 6 = "college graduate (BS, BA, or other four-year degree)," and 7 = "postgraduate training/professional school after college (master's degree/PhD, Law, or Medical school)." There are few cases with the lowest levels of education and the variable was recoded to four levels: 1 = "high school graduate or less," 2 = "some college," 3 = "college graduate," and 4 = "postgraduate." A series of binary indicator variables were created using "high school graduate or less" as the reference group.

Total family income was measured in 2002–2006 using an ordinal variable with eight levels: 1 = "less than $10,000," 2 = "$10,000 to under $20,000," 3 = "$20,000 to under $30,000," 4 = "$30,000 to under $40,000," 5 = "$40,000 to under $50,000," 6 = "$50,000 to under $75,000," 7 = "$75,000 to under $100,000," and 8 = "$100,000 or more." In 2008–2010 the eighth level was changed to "$100,000 to under $150,000" and a ninth level was added, "$150,000 or more." Data from 2008 to 2010 have been recoded as eight levels to match the coding used in earlier surveys. There are few cases in the lowest two levels (i.e., "less than $10,000" and "$10,000 to under $20,000") and these were collapsed into one level. The final variable consists of seven levels (1 = "less than $20,000" to 7 = "$100,000 or more") that are used as a series of binary indicator variables with the lowest level set as the reference group.

Home Internet Connection
One question asked consistently across surveys regarded the type of Internet connection available in the home. This question included five types of Internet connection: dial-up telephone line, digital subscriber line (DSL), cable modem, wireless connection (either "land-based" or "satellite"), and T-1 or fiber optic connection. Broadband is a binary variable created by

recoding DSL, cable modem, and T-1 or fiber optic connection types as 1 = "broadband." Dial-up telephone line, wireless connection, people with no home Internet connection, and cases with missing values are recoded as 0 = "other connection type."

Type of Community

To account for the effect of place, we include a series of indicator variables that represent the community type (i.e., urban, suburban, rural). These variables are derived from a single variable in the data set that classifies community type based on the participants' zip code. In the multivariate models "urban" is used as the reference category.

Self-Rated Health

Poor health status has been found to be an important factor that motivates people to search for health-related information (Rice, 2006). Unfortunately, the Pew surveys do not consistently include questions about health status; however, a question assessing subjective health status was included. Self-rated health was measured by asking participants, "In general, how would you rate your own health – excellent, good, only fair, or poor?" Responses were recoded to 1 = "poor" to 4 = "excellent" so that a higher value represents better subjective health.

Analytic Strategy

We begin by presenting descriptive statistics (Table 2) for each of our dependent and independent variables using the analytic sample of Internet users that is used in the multivariate logistic models. To understand how each of our independent variables contributes to differences in online health seeking across the five survey years, we begin with bivariate descriptive statistics that show the percentage of subjects who have *ever sought health information on any topic* on the Internet. Next, we examine differences in factors associated with trends in online health-seeking behaviors using both Internet users and nonusers (Table 3). In the last bivariate statistical analysis the sample is restricted to Internet users and the analytic sample used in later multivariate logistic models (Table 4). This allows us to focus the analysis on Internet users to examine the changes in the relative effect of each predictor variable over the course of the five surveys. Weighted percentages and the results of Pearson χ^2 tests are presented in both tables.

Table 2. Descriptive Statistics, Analytic Sample of Internet Users.

	2002 %	2004 %	2006 %	2008 %	2010 %
Online health seeking					
Information on any topic	81.6	80.5	82.2	84.8	81.0
Information on specific disease	65.4	67.8	65.5	66.8	67.4
Information on medical treatment	47.7	54.9	53.5	56.2	57.6
Sex					
Male	50.5	47.8	49.0	47.4	48.0
Female	49.5	52.2	51.0	52.6	52.0
Race					
White	83.7	81.9	84.9	78.7	78.8
Non-white	16.3	18.1	15.1	21.3	21.2
Age cohort					
18–33 Millennials	17.2	18.6	23.5	31.7	35.8
34–45 Gen X	26.7	26.4	27.5	24.1	23.8
46–55 Young Boomers	26.4	25.6	23.3	22.3	19.3
56–64 Older Boomers	16.5	18.3	14.1	12.5	12.6
65–73 Silent Gen	8.5	7.5	7.6	6.2	5.9
74+ GI Gen	4.6	3.6	4.0	3.3	2.6
Education level					
HS graduate or less	29.0	31.8	32.4	34.8	34.8
Some college	35.7	32.7	30.6	30.7	29.6
College grad	21.1	21.3	23.2	20.4	20.8
Postgraduate	14.2	14.2	13.9	14.1	14.8
Household income					
Less than $20,000	10.1	11.1	10.4	15.4	17.4
$20,000–29,999	12.1	11.9	11.8	9.8	11.0
$30,000–39,999	13.6	11.5	10.7	10.1	12.5
$40,000–49,999	12.2	10.2	11.2	12.2	10.0
$50,000–74,999	23.1	22.5	20.1	19.0	17.7
$75,000–99,999	14.7	16.7	16.1	14.5	12.9
$100,000 or more	14.3	16.1	19.8	19.1	18.5
Community type					
Urban	27.8	30.7	29.6	18.9	31.4
Suburban	51.5	51.7	54.0	34.5	50.5
Rural	20.7	17.6	16.4	10.1	14.5
Internet connection					
Broadband	21.6	45.2	60.2	61.4	64.2
Other connection type	78.4	54.8	39.8	38.6	35.8
Self-rated health					
Poor	1.5	a	2.2	2.4	2.8
Fair	5.9	a	10.1	10.6	11.1
Good	49.7	a	49.0	53.0	51.9
Excellent	42.9	a	38.7	33.9	34.2
N	999	432	1,545	1,308	1,683

Note: Weighted percentages.
[a]Data on self-rated health was not collected on the 2004 survey.

Table 3. Descriptive Statistics, Having Ever Sought Health Information on Any Topic, among Full Sample.

	2002 %	2004 %	2006 %	2008 %	2010 %
Sex	$N=936$	$N=422$	$N=1,627$	$N=1,375^{**}$	$N=1,759^{***}$
Male	44.5	43.5	54.8	57.3	53.2
Female	47.3	48.8	56.3	64.5	63.7
Race	$N=912^{***}$	$N=413^{*}$	$N=1,595$	$N=1,345^{***}$	$N=1,716^{***}$
White	48.0	48.6	56.8	63.6	62.0
Non-white	36.7	38.8	51.3	52.6	49.9
Age cohort	$N=910^{***}$	$N=409^{***}$	$N=1,590^{***}$	$N=1,345^{***}$	$N=1,732^{***}$
18–33 Millennials	60.3	49.7	66.6	73.6	69.8
34–45 Gen X	55.5	59.7	70.2	68.8	68.4
46–55 Young Boomers	51.8	56.9	64.4	66.2	57.4
56–64 Older Boomers	50.9	54.3	53.4	59.9	58.1
65–73 Silent Gen	37.4	31.5	37.6	42.9	38.2
74+ GI Gen	12.9	13.8	17.0	18.1	18.0
Education level	$N=933^{***}$	$N=416^{***}$	$N=1,615^{***}$	$N=1,364^{***}$	$N=1,748^{***}$
HS graduate or less	27.4	26.8	36.7	41.2	37.7
Some college	58.8	58.3	62.2	72.3	69.2
College grad	65.9	67.8	79.0	85.2	83.3
Postgraduate	68.6	72.8	85.3	85.4	82.9
Household income	$N=801^{***}$	$N=353^{***}$	$N=1,331^{***}$	$N=1,148^{***}$	$N=1,489^{***}$
Less than $20,000	23.1	24.4	28.8	41.3	36.3
$20,000–29,999	33.3	33.5	49.7	49.2	50.6
$30,000–39,999	48.4	49.8	48.5	57.3	63.8
$40,000–49,999	58.4	42.9	66.2	73.9	67.0
$50,000–74,999	65.7	66.0	74.3	79.3	70.6
$75,000–99,999	66.5	75.1	75.2	75.1	82.1
$100,000 or more	76.7	73.3	81.4	87.3	84.0
Community type	$N=936^{***}$	$N=422^{***}$	$N=1,627^{**}$	$N=1,018^{***}$	$N=1,711^{***}$
Urban	49.9	44.2	55.6	58.0	61.6
Suburban	48.3	52.6	57.7	61.7	61.5
Rural	37.1	34.2	49.1	48.3	48.7
Internet connection	$N=847^{**}$	$N=358^{***}$	$N=1,360^{***}$	$N=1,053^{***}$	$N=1,174^{**}$
Broadband	88.9	86.7	86.0	87.3	82.6
Other connection type	80.1	72.1	75.1	71.9	67.1
Self-rated health	$N=931^{***}$	a	$N=1,619^{***}$	$N=1,368^{***}$	$N=1,758^{***}$
Poor	22.1	a	26.8	36.7	24.7
Fair	18.8	a	43.2	42.8	38.1
Good	47.3	a	55.5	63.7	61.8
Excellent	56.6	a	65.5	70.0	69.5

Note: Weighted percentages. Asterisks represent the results of a Pearson χ^2 test.
$^{*}p<0.05,$ $^{**}p<0.01,$ $^{***}p<0.001.$
aData on self-rated health was not collected on the 2004 survey.

Table 4. Descriptive Statistics, Having Ever Sought Health Information on Any Topic, among Internet Users.

	2002 %	2004 %	2006 %	2008 %	2010 %
Sex					
Male	76.9**	76.3*	80.0*	81.9*	74.0***
Female	86.4	84.4	84.4	87.4	87.5
Race					
White	83.4**	80.8	82.6	85.6	83.1**
Non-white	72.3	79.2	79.7	81.9	73.5
Age cohort					
18–33 Millennials	80.4	72.4	82.0**	86.5	81.4
34–45 Gen X	85.2	85.2	87.7	85.4	84.0
46–55 Young Boomers	78.6	82.7	82.3	83.8	79.6
56–64 Older Boomers	84.0	84.8	77.8	87.1	82.7
65–73 Silent Gen	82.7	69.4	77.0	80.3	75.8
74+ GI Gen	71.4	74.2	70.2	69.3	64.5
Education level					
HS graduate or less	74.6**	72.3*	73.7***	79.3***	69.4
Some college	83.0	81.6	80.8	87.4	85.0
College grad	87.1	88.5	90.7	90.8	90.2
Postgraduate	84.4	84.5	90.9	91.3	87.6
Household income					
Less than $20,000	77.1	64.6*	74.9**	77.6***	69.7***
$20,000–29,999	73.5	73.6	79.1	79.1	76.3
$30,000–39,999	83.1	84.7	74.2	81.5	82.6
$40,000–49,999	86.1	72.0	81.9	89.4	82.2
$50,000–74,999	82.0	84.4	88.2	87.8	81.9
$75,000–99,999	79.5	89.8	81.0	81.1	85.7
$100,000 or more	87.9	83.9	87.3	91.9	88.8
Community type					
Urban	82.0	77.2	84.8	85.8	82.9
Suburban	81.3	84.0	81.5	83.5	81.8
Rural	81.8	76.2	79.7	79.6	75.8
Internet connection					
Broadband	90.0**	86.6**	87.5***	89.5***	83.6**
Other connection type	81.8	74.5	78.7	74.1	65.5
Self-rated health					
Poor	94.9	a	83.8	83.8	65.2
Fair	70.9	a	83.5	83.5	75.8
Good	83.0	a	85.9	85.9	83.0
Excellent	81.0	a	83.4	83.4	81.1
N	999	432	1,545	1,308	1,683

Note: Weighted percentages. Asterisks represent the results of a Pearson χ^2 test.
*$p < 0.05$, **$p < 0.01$, ***$p < 0.001$.
[a]Data on self-rated health was not collected on the 2004 survey.

Multivariate logistic regression models are used for each of the three binary dependent variables: ever seek health information on any topic, ever sought information about a specific disease or medical problem, and ever sought information about a specific medical treatment or procedure. Separate models are conducted for each year and are presented as Odds Ratios (OR) (see Tables 5–7). To illustrate potentially narrowing or

Table 5. Odds Ratios from Logistic Regression Models Predicting Having Ever Sought Health Information on Any Topic, Internet Users.

	2002	2004	2006	2008	2010
Male	0.475***	0.470**	0.649**	0.566**	0.338***
White	1.987**	0.861	1.342	1.446	1.701**
Age cohort[a]					
34–45 Gen X	1.082	1.291	1.100	0.613	0.871
46–55 Young Boomers	0.668	1.339	0.739	0.612	0.588*
56–64 Older Boomers	0.862	1.362	0.579*	0.790	0.728
65–73 Silent Gen	0.824	0.660	0.476**	0.473*	0.500*
74+ GI Gen	0.418*	1.073	0.369**	0.263***	0.254**
Education level[b]					
Some college	1.528	1.652	1.368	1.797**	2.219***
College grad	1.933*	2.452*	3.164***	2.257**	3.431***
Postgraduate	1.658	1.799	3.664***	2.673***	2.518**
Household income[c]					
$20,000–29,999	0.776	1.230	1.299	1.107	1.323
$30,000–39,999	1.242	2.544	0.895	1.307	2.053*
$40,000–49,999	1.680	1.040	1.384	2.286*	1.809
$50,000–74,999	1.174	2.237	1.902*	1.976*	1.690
$75,000–99,999	0.966	3.013	0.915	1.049	1.926
$100,000 or more	1.653	1.831	1.358	2.509**	2.341**
Community type[d]					
Suburban	0.876	1.631	0.803	0.699	0.849
Rural	1.054	1.302	0.990	0.615	0.675
Broadband	2.083**	1.785	2.192***	2.173***	1.377
Self-rated health	0.878	e	0.750*	0.747*	0.970
N	999	432	1,545	1,308	1,683
Pseudo R^2	0.072	0.095	0.094	0.101	0.117

Note: Odds ratios estimated using sampling weights.
*p < 0.05, **p < 0.01, ***p < 0.001 (two-tailed tests).
[a]Reference category = 18–33 Millennials.
[b]Reference category = HS graduate or less education.
[c]Reference category = Less than $20,000.
[d]Reference category = Urban.
[e]Data on self-rated health was not collected on the 2004 survey.

Table 6. Odds Ratios from Logistic Regression Models Predicting Having
Ever Sought Information about Specific Disease or Medical Problem,
Internet Users.

	2002	2004	2006	2008	2010
Male	0.424***	0.476**	0.498***	0.549***	0.398***
White	1.718**	1.181	1.970***	1.459*	1.809***
Age cohort[a]					
34–45 Gen X	1.369	1.787	0.993	1.085	0.936
46–55 Young Boomers	1.268	1.989	0.829	0.967	0.818
56–64 Older Boomers	1.559	2.310*	0.679	1.097	0.831
65–73 Silent Gen	1.562	1.047	0.714	1.035	0.852
74+ GI Gen	1.125	1.583	0.454**	0.457*	0.401*
Education level[b]					
Some college	1.585*	1.791*	1.606**	1.975***	1.919***
College grad	1.538*	2.159*	2.238***	2.597***	1.857**
Postgraduate	1.842*	2.189*	2.654***	2.802***	2.353***
Household income[c]					
$20,000–29,999	1.205	0.735	1.273	1.058	1.510
$30,000–39,999	1.731	1.251	1.128	0.941	1.723*
$40,000–49,999	1.683	0.665	1.569	1.218	1.775*
$50,000–74,999	1.393	1.461	2.170**	1.243	1.574
$75,000–99,999	1.491	1.583	1.422	1.044	2.437**
$100,000 or more	1.338	1.396	1.797*	1.664	3.730***
Community type[d]					
Suburban	1.057	1.299	0.751	0.808	0.961
Rural	1.295	0.944	1.028	1.087	0.958
Broadband	1.817**	1.053	1.921***	1.834***	1.506**
Self-rated health	0.842	e	0.817*	0.730**	0.938
N	999	432	1,545	1,308	1,683
Pseudo R^2	0.069	0.083	0.088	0.086	0.108

Note: Odds Ratios estimated using sampling weights.
*$p < 0.05$, **$p < 0.01$, ***$p < 0.001$ (two-tailed tests).
[a]Reference category = 18–33 Millennials.
[b]Reference category = HS graduate or less education.
[c]Reference category = Less than $20,000.
[d]Reference category = Urban.
[e]Data on self-rated health was not collected on the 2004 survey.

widening of gaps in online health-seeking behavior we have estimated predicted probabilities for selected outcomes and predictor variables (see
Figs. 1 and 2).

All analyses were conducted using the sampling weights included in each
of the data sets. Sampling weights are intended to adjust for nonresponse

Table 7. Odds Ratios from Logistic Regression Models Predicting Having Ever Sought Information about Specific Medical Treatment, Internet Users.

	2002	2004	2006	2008	2010
Male	0.549***	0.521**	0.646***	0.620***	0.465***
White	1.316	0.946	1.627**	1.258	1.564**
Age cohort[a]					
34–45 Gen X	1.304	1.657	1.193	0.923	1.032
46–55 Young Boomers	1.393	1.598	1.067	0.886	1.052
56–64 Older Boomers	1.555	2.058*	0.821	0.809	1.029
65–73 Silent Gen	1.951*	1.693	0.777	1.078	0.840
74+ GI Gen	1.716	1.327	0.546*	0.401**	0.656
Education level[b]					
Some college	1.548*	1.676	1.337	1.853***	1.642**
College grad	1.470	2.036*	1.738***	1.788**	2.302***
Postgraduate	1.795*	1.425	2.139***	1.646*	2.119**
Household income[c]					
$20,000-$29,999	1.372	0.747	1.202	0.888	1.597
$30,000–39,999	1.489	1.179	1.118	0.782	1.352
$40,000–49,999	1.839	0.817	1.424	1.446	1.712*
$50,000–74,999	1.803*	1.526	1.757*	1.631	1.483
$75,000–99,999	1.468	0.908	1.463	1.770*	2.100**
$100,000 or more	1.550	0.947	1.878*	2.224**	2.309**
Community type[d]					
Suburban	0.892	1.443	0.934	0.766	0.884
Rural	1.297	1.016	1.068	0.796	0.778
Broadband	1.641**	1.458	1.435**	1.708***	1.176
Self-rated health	0.853	e	0.814*	0.730**	0.935
N	999	432	1,545	1,308	1,683
Pseudo R^2	0.051	0.061	0.051	0.073	0.076

Note: Odds Ratios estimated using sampling weights.
*$p < 0.05$, **$p < 0.01$, ***$p < 0.001$ (two-tailed tests).
[a]Reference category = 18–33 Millennials.
[b]Reference category = HS graduate or less education.
[c]Reference category = Less than $20,000.
[d]Reference category = Urban.
[e]Data on self-rated health was not collected on the 2004 survey.

bias and create estimates that more closely match known population parameters for sex, age, education, race, Hispanic origin, and region. Population parameters used to construct the weights come from the Census Bureau's Annual Social and Economic Supplement at the time of the survey.

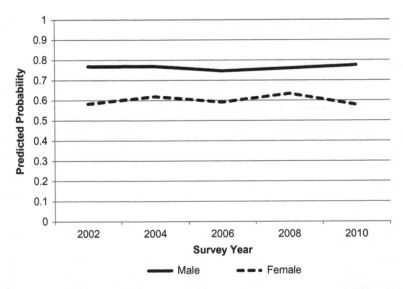

Fig. 1. Predicted Probability of Seeking Information about a Specific Disease or Medical Problem among Internet Users by Sex, Controlling for Socio-Demographics, Community Type, Internet Connection, and Self-Rated Health.

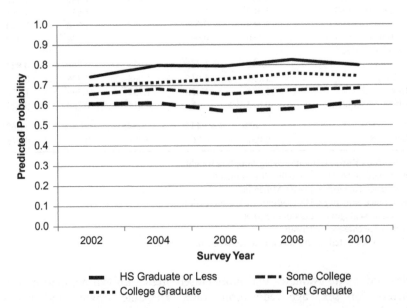

Fig. 2. Predicted Probability of Seeking Information about a Specific Disease or Medical Problem among Internet Users by Education Level, Controlling for Socio-Demographics, Community Type, Internet Connection, and Self-Rated Health.

RESULTS

Descriptives

Table 2 presents weighted percentages for each of our dependent and independent variables among the analytic sample of Internet users. The percentage of people seeking health information about any topic or information about a specific disease or medical condition has remained relatively stable across years. However, the percentage of people who have ever sought information about a specific medical treatment has increased from about 48% in 2002 to 58% in 2010. One interesting trend is the increase in the percentage of people with a broadband Internet connection. In 2002 only 22% connected via broadband; in 2010 64% used a broadband connection.

We next examine simple bivariate descriptive statistics examining socio-demographics, community type, Internet connection, and self-rated health by ever seeking health information on any topic for the years 2002, 2004, 2006, 2008, and 2010 among the full sample. It is important to note that the table includes five separate data collections, which varied by method of collection and by sample size. Thus, when describing these data, we will discuss general trends, and not focus on anomalies, as they are more likely to be the result of a statistical artifact, rather than an actual trend. We feel most confident when we see general trends indicated across the five surveys. Overwhelmingly, the percentages are stable and show gradual increases in expected directions.

Table 3 shows that across all years, whites are more likely than non-whites to have any online health-seeking behavior. From 2002 through 2010, both whites and non-whites have increased health-seeking behavior; however, the percentage of whites increased somewhat more than non-whites over that time. By 2010, 62% of whites and 50% of non-whites had health-seeking behavior.

What is clear is the solid pattern with both education and income. The table shows that within each year, usage increases by level of education, and the more highly educated (i.e., college graduates or postgraduate education) are the most likely to use the Internet for any health-seeking behavior. Still, as one looks across the years, every educational group increases its health-seeking behavior over time. By 2010, about 38% of those with less than a high school degree engage in health-seeking behavior online, but 83% of postgraduates do. A similar pattern emerges with income, both between and among groups; there is an increase in health-seeking behavior over time and as income increases. In 2010, about 36% of those with incomes less than $20,000 engage in health-seeking behavior; however, 84% in the highest income group use the Internet for health-seeking. Both education and income are good examples of the lingering digital divide – despite increases in usage across groups, the divide remains profound.

Regarding sex and age, women appear slightly more likely than men to engage in online health-seeking behavior, and over the years women experienced a greater increase in usage than men. In 2010 about 64% of women and 53% of men used the Internet for health information. As expected, age shows the expected inverse relationship with the oldest age groups being the least likely to seek for information.

Community type shows that urban and suburban inhabitants are more likely to seek health information online, as compared to their rural counterparts. Each group increased over time, with about 62% of both urban and suburban inhabitants, and 49% of rural inhabitants, engaged in any health-seeking behavior.

In sum, we found expected patterns of Internet usage with general rates of increase over this eight-year period, and whites, higher education and income, younger, urban and suburban people being the most active in having any health-seeking behavior. The sex difference was small in 2002, but increased to a 10 percentage point difference in 2010, with women being a bit higher.

Turning to the bivariate descriptive statistics restricted to our analytic sample of Internet users (Table 4), we see some similarities to the results in Table 3, but also some striking differences. Similar to Table 3, we find that females and whites are more likely to engage in any type of health-seeking behavior compared to males or non-whites. Age has the expected inverse relationship to seeking information online. We also see that higher levels of education and household income are associated with a greater likelihood of seeking any type of health information online. Type of Internet connection also matters. People with broadband are more likely to have sought health information on any topic across all five surveys than people with another type of connection. Urban and suburban dwellers are also more likely to search online, although this does not reach statistical significance.

What is different, however, is that across years the likelihood of seeking any type of health information online remains relatively stable for many variables. The exceptions are education level, household income, and self-rated health. Each of these has a marked decline in the percentage of people who have sought information on any topic in 2010. For example, high school graduates or less dropped by 10% points between 2008 and 2010 (from 79% to 69%, respectively). A similar decline is seen for the lowest income level (78–70%), and poor self-rated health (84–65%). The reasons for this decline are not clear, but may be due to the economic crisis of 2008 and the increased number of people unemployed, which peaked in late 2009. The poorest people in the United States may have been forced to forgo their Internet connection services and thus limited their ability to search online.

In sum, when we look at trends among the entire sample (Internet users and nonusers) we see that nearly all groups are increasingly making use of the Internet to seek health information on any topic. In addition, younger adults and the most advantaged consistently make greater use of the Internet to seek health information. When we restrict our analysis to Internet users we see a similar pattern. However, we also see that across years the percentages have remained relatively stable, with little indication of the gap narrowing by various digital divide factors. In fact, in 2010 there is some evidence that the gap might be increasing for those with the lowest levels of education, income, and in poor health. We now turn to our multivariate models.

Multivariate Models

Table 5 reports the results from our logistic regression analysis of whether a respondent *had ever sought health information on any topic*. Men are less likely than women to search for any topics in each of our years. Regarding age cohorts, in 2002 and 2004 there are few statistically significant findings with the exception that people over 65 years of age are less likely to search for health-related topics than younger adults.

Interestingly, there are significant findings for race with this dependent variable. In 2002 and 2010, white respondents were more likely to search for health-related information than others at statistically significant levels (OR 1.987, $p < 0.01$ and OR 1,701, $p < 0.01$, respectively). Education is also more variable by year than one might expect. Although in 2002 and 2004 college graduates were more likely to search for information than less educated respondents, in those same years we find the results for people with some college and postgraduate degrees to be statistically nonsignificant. However, by 2006, higher levels of education have a nearly universal positive effect on searching for health information at statistically significant levels. Again, the results for income are suggestive that greater household income is positively related to searching for health information, yet the coefficients are not consistently significant for income groups net of the influence of other variables across or within years. Broadband access is significant in three out of our five years and, again, it does not reach statistical significance in 2010 at conventionally accepted levels. Finally, and intriguingly, self-rated health status is not significantly associated with searching for health information in two out of the four years.

Having examined whether people have searched online for any health topic, we now move to specific types of health-related searches. Starting with seeking information about a *specific disease or medical problem* (see Table 6), we see that men are less likely to engage in this specific type of searching than are women in every year, at statistically significant levels. White respondents were significantly more likely to search for information on a specific disease or medical problem in four out of the five years. Race is not significant in 2004; however, the number of respondents in 2004 was quite low, thus decreasing the statistical power. As a result, the lack of statistical significance could speak more to an artifact of the data than the uniqueness of that year. Regarding age cohorts, there are few consistent or noteworthy results with the exception that individuals 74 years of age and older were less likely to search for a specific disease or medical problem relative to respondents in younger cohorts at statistically significant levels in 2006, 2008, and 2010.

Educational attainment clearly plays a role in this specific type of health searching. Almost every educational category above a high school degree is significantly associated with our dependent variable at conventionally accepted levels of statistical significance net of other variables across years. In terms of income, there is only one significant finding before 2010 ($50,000−74,999 in 2006). However, in 2010 four of our six income groups were more likely to search for a specific disease or medical problem than lower income groups at statistically significant levels and net of other variables. Broadband access is associated with the likelihood of searching for a specific disease or medical problem in four out of five years, including 2010. Finally, self-rated health is related to this specific type of searching in two out of the four years, thus providing inconsistent results.

Searching for a *specific medical treatment* is our second type of specific type of health searching (see Table 7). Similar to all of our previous analyses, men are less likely than women to engage in this activity than men in every year at statistically significant levels. The results for race are less consistent than with our previous specific type of searching. Whites were more likely than other groups to search for specific medical treatments in 2006 and 2010 at statistically significant levels (OR 1.627, $p < 0.01$ and OR 1.564, $p < 0.01$, respectively). As in previous analyses, age cohorts did not provide consistent results with the exception of the oldest cohort being significantly less likely to search for information compared to other groups in two years. In general, education has a robust, positive effect on specific medical treatments across years; however, the results are most robust in 2008 and 2010. Broadband access is significantly related to this specific type of searching in three out of the five years. The variable approaches significance in 2004 ($p < 0.10$), but is not significant in 2010. Similar to searching for a specific disease or medical problem, self-rated health is significantly related to searching for specific medical treatments in 2006 and 2008, but not in the other two years for which we have data. Interestingly, income has inconsistent findings in the years before 2008. In 2008 and 2010, individuals making over $75,000 annually are significantly more likely to search for a specific medical treatment.

DISCUSSION

This study provides a longitudinal analysis of the impact of a variety of factors on online health searching, including demographics, type of Internet connection, and health status. Our results suggest that the effect varies by the specific factor and time period studied. Despite the diffusion of the Internet, most of these gaps persist, and even strengthen, over time. This has important implications for patients and providers, as well as doctor–patient interactions.

The main objective of this study was to examine the impact of traditional digital inequality factors over time. First, community type was not significant in any of the models. This may be due to the small number of subjects living in rural communities versus urban and suburban areas. Second, two variables, race and self-reported health status, were not always statistically significant. When they were significant, they were in the expected direction with non-Hispanic whites and those who rate their health lower being more likely to search for some types of health information. Third, in most cases, socio-demographic gaps persist and strengthen. To illustrate, women are significantly more likely than men to search for health information online based on all five surveys from the past decade, and this gender gap appears to be increasing in recent years. The persistence of this gap is illustrated in Fig. 1, showing that the probability of women to seek information about a specific disease or medical condition is consistently greater than the probability men will do so. This confirms previous research showing that women are more active in online searching for health information because they tend to search for other individuals, such as children, as well (Fox & Fallows, 2003; Fox & Rainie, 2000; Stern et al., 2012). In addition, variation by age increased from 2002 to 2010, especially since 2006, with younger people consistently being more likely than older cohorts to search. Though older Americans have more reason to search on average, and are doing so more and more, young people still have the advantage of using their technological skills to find information. Thus, doctors may be more likely to have their doctor–patient communication influenced, and even challenged, by Internet research when they interact with younger generations as compared to older generations. Likewise, those with the lowest level of education are the least likely to have ever sought health information online, and this gap is slightly increasing (see Fig. 2). Household income only becomes a stronger predictor in the later surveys, and was not significantly related to health information seeking until 2010. Thus, health disparities may occur from differences in socioeconomic status that are also manifested through Internet access and usage. Assuming knowledge is power, those with the most knowledge are those who use health Internet seeking. The exception to this pattern regards the type of Internet connection at home. Even though individuals with broadband access are significantly more likely than those with other types of connection to search online for health or medical information, the type of Internet connection at home is becoming *less* important in differentiating health information seeking online, especially in 2010 as compared to earlier. The effect of broadband access at home is diminishing, possibly due to greater use of wireless connections outside the home and use of mobile devices (Duggan & Smith, 2013).

Given that many of these digital inequalities have been sustained or increased, social capital is more readily available to those who are more advantaged and to women. Providers have been the major source of medical knowledge for patients (Cotten & Gupta, 2004). As the Internet has expanded, individuals are gathering information, resources, and support from a variety of online sources, including health organizations, professionals, and lay people. Fox and Jones (2009) argue that "technology is not an end, but a means to accelerate the pace of discovery, widen social networks, and sharpen the questions someone might ask when they do get to talk to a health professional. Technology can help to enable the human connection in health care" (p. 7). Enlarging one's network of knowledge and support builds social capital, which refers to these "resources embedded in a social structure that are accessed and/or mobilized in purposive actions" (Lin, 2001, p. 29). Knowledge about health gleaned from multiple sources on the Internet can then translate into social capital when patients are in dialogue with their doctor. Social capital can potentially translate into benefits, such as better health (Drentea & Moren-Cross, 2005). Of course, online health information can be dated, incomplete, or false (Berland et al., 2001), so physicians must help patients decipher and evaluate this information; however, the de-professionalization of medical knowledge changes the balance of power and provides more opportunities for collaboration. The National Research Council (2005) notes:

> The health care sector is undergoing a critical transition from a delivery system aimed at providing episodic institutional care for the treatment of illnesses to an emphasis on information systems that support community-based care, with greater consumer involvement in the prevention and management of illness across the life span. The development of an information and communications technology (ICT) infrastructure is a critical element of this transition. (p. 147)

Our study shows that these potential benefits are not available to everyone equally.

Scholars note the importance of both agency and structure in health. While one's health is impacted by individual choices, and is thus seen as an achievement, it is also dependent on macro-level structures, which limit the choices one can make. Cockerham (2005) identifies a healthy lifestyle then as "collective patterns of health-related behavior based on choices from options available to people according to their life chances" (p. 55). Structural factors, such as socioeconomic status, are linked to health disparities. For example, older adults and those with less education and income have worse health (Link & Phelan, 1995; Schoenborn, Vickerie, & Powell-Griner, 2006). Our results show that these groups are less likely to search for health information online, and thus less likely to tap into that potential social capital. Thus, health disparities may continue and even grow based on who uses the Internet. Policies designed to increase Internet access and proficiency may ameliorate some inequalities.

We expected to see more dramatic changes in usage over time. The Pew Internet & American Life trend data are the most comprehensive data for this type of research question even though there were changes in how the samples were drawn and questions asked over time. Future research should continue tracking these data, and data on other types of online health activities, as we may see more dramatic changes as we expand the years of study. Yet, qualitative interviews would augment this research, because they could examine how the Internet is used as social capital, and how this affects doctor–patient interactions. Further research could examine how power differentials between doctor and patient have been minimized by health knowledge from the Internet. Interviews with physicians could illuminate the degree to which this health information has been helpful in their practice, and or harmful, and whether they feel their professional knowledge has been undermined or minimized by the mass sharing of health information. An in-depth look at individuals and online health activities could provide insight into potential advantages, as well as disadvantages, of Internet use for health purposes. We need more research to devise appropriate policies to improve the health of all groups of people.

REFERENCES

Baker, L., Wagner, T. H., Singer, S., & Bundorf, M. K. (2003). Use of the Internet and e-mail for health care information: Results from a national survey. *The Journal of the American Medical Association, 289,* 2400–2406.

Berland, G. K., Elliott, M. N., Morales, L. S., Kravitz, R. L., Broder, M. S., Kanouse, D. E. ... McGlynn, E. A. (2001). Health information on the internet: Accessibility, quality, and readability in English and Spanish. *Journal of the American Medical Association, 285,* 2612–2621.

Brodie, M., Flournoy, R. E., Altman, D. E., Blendon, R. J., Benson, J. M., & Rosenbaum, M. D. (2000). Health information, the Internet, and the digital divide. *Health Affairs, 19,* 255–265.

Brodie, M., Kjellson, N., Hoff, T., & Parker, M. (1999). Perceptions of Latinos, African Americans, and whites on media as a health information source. *Howard Journal of Communications, 10*(3), 147–167.

Cockerham, W. C. (2005). Health lifestyle theory and the convergence of agency and structure. *Journal of Health and Social Behavior, 46*(1), 51–67.

Cotten, S. R. (2001). Implications of the Internet for medical sociology in the new millennium. *Sociological Spectrum, 21*(3), 319–340.

Cotten, S. R., & Gupta, S. S. (2004). Characteristics of online and offline health information seekers and factors that discriminate between them. *Social Science & Medicine, 59,* 1795–1806.

DiMaggio, P., & Hargittai, E. (2001). *From the "Digital Divide" to "Digital Inequality": Studying Internet use as penetration increases.* Working Paper No. 15. Retrieved from http://www.maximise-ict.co.uk/WP15_DiMaggioHargittai.pdf

Drentea, P., & Moren-Cross, J. (2005). Social capital and social support on the web: The case of an internet mother site. *Sociology of Health and Illness, 27,* 957–967.

Duggan, M., & Smith, A. (2013). *Cell Internet use 2013.* Retrieved from http://www.pewinternet. org/Reports/2013/Cell-Internet.aspx

Flynn, K. E., Smith, M. A., & Freese, J. (2006). When do older adults turn to the internet for health information? Findings from the Wisconsin longitudinal study. *Journal of General Internal Medicine, 21*, 1295–1301.

Fox, S. (2005). *Health information online.* Pew Internet & American Life Project. Retrieved from http://www.pewinternet.org/2005/05/17/health-information-online/

Fox, S. (2008). *The engaged e-patient population.* Washington, DC: Pew Internet & American Life Project. Retrieved from http://www.pewinternet.org/~/media//Files/Reports/2008/PIP_Health_Aug08.pdf.pdf

Fox, S. (2011). *The social life of health information, 2011.* Retrieved from http://www.pewinternet.org/2011/05/12/the-social-life-of-health-information-2011/

Fox, S., & Fallows, D. (2003). *Health searches and email have become more commonplace, but there is room for improvement in searches and overall Internet access.* Retrieved from http://www.pewinternet.org/2003/07/16/internet-health-resources/

Fox, S., & Jones, S. (2009). *The social life of health information.* Washington, DC: The Pew Internet & American Life Project. Retrieved from http://www.pewinternet.org/files/old-media//Files/Reports/2009/PIP_Health_2009.pdf

Fox, S., & Rainie, L. (2000). *The online health care revolution: How the Web helps Americans take better care of themselves.* Retrieved from http://www.pewinternet.org/2000/11/26/the-online-health-care-revolution/

Goldsmith, J. (2000). How will the Internet change our health system? *Health Affairs, 19*(1), 148–156.

Hale, T. M., Cotten, S. R., Drentea, P., & Goldner, M. (2010). Rural-urban differences in general and health-related Internet use. *American Behavioral Sciences, 20*, 1–22.

Horrigan, J., & Murray, K. (2006). *Home broadband adoption in rural America.* Retrieved from http://www.pewinternet.org/2006/02/26/home-broadband-adoption-in-rural-america/

Hu, J. (2000). *Study: Net's gender gap narrows.* Retrieved from http://news.cnet.com/2100-1023-235932.html

Lin, N. (2001). *Social capital.* Cambridge: Cambridge University Press.

Link, B. G., & Phelan, J. (1995). Social conditions as fundamental causes of disease. *Journal of Health and Social Behavior, 35*, 80–94.

Litt, J. S. (2000). *Medicalized motherhood: Perspectives from the lives of African-American and Jewish women.* New Brunswick, NJ: Rutgers University Press.

National Research Council. (2005). *Quality through collaboration: The future of rural health care.* Washington, DC: The National Academies Press.

National Telecommunications and Information Administration. (2000). *Falling through the net: Toward digital inclusion.* Retrieved from http://www.ntia.doc.gov/files/ntia/publications/fttn00.pdf

Pandey, S. K., Hart, J. J., & Tiwary, S. (2003). Women's health and the Internet: Understanding emerging trends and implications. *Social Science & Medicine, 56*, 179–191.

Pew Internet & American Life. (2014). *Internet use over time.* Retrieved from http://www.pewinternet.org/data-trend/internet-use/internet-use-over-time/

Rainie, L., & Fox, S. (2000). *The online health care revolution.* Pew Internet & American Life Project. Retrieved from http://www.pewinternet.org/2000/11/26/the-online-health-care-revolution/

Rice, R. (2006). Influences, usage, and outcomes of Internet health information searching: Multivariate results from the pew surveys. *International Journal of Medical Informatics, 75*, 8–28.

Schoenborn, C. A., Vickerie, J. L., & Powell-Griner, E. (2006). Health characteristics of adults 55 years of age and over. *Advance Data from Vital and Health Statistics*, No. 370. National Center for Health Statistics, Hyattsville, MD. Retrieved from http://www.cdc. gov/nchs/data/ad/ad370.pdf

Smith, A. (2010). *Mobile access 2010*. Pew Internet & American Life Project. Retrieved from http://www.pewinternet.org/files/old-media//Files/Reports/2010/PIP_Mobile_Access_ 2010.pdf

Stern, M. J., Adams, A., & Elsasser, S. (2009). How levels of internet proficiency affect usefulness of access across rural, suburban, and urban communities. *Sociological Inquiry*, *79*, 391−417.

Stern, M. J., Cotten, S. R., & Drentea, P. (2012). The separate spheres on online health: Gender, parenting, and online health information searching in the information age. *Journal of Family Issues*, *33*(10), 1324−1350.

Stern, M. J., & Dillman, D. A. (2006). Community participation, social ties, and use of the internet. *City and Community*, *5*(4), 409−424.

Taylor, H. (2002). *Cyberchondriacs update*. The Harris Poll #21, May 1. Retrieved from http:// www.harrisinteractive.com

Zickuhr, K. (2010). *Generations 2010*. Retrieved from http://www.pewinternet.org/files/old-media//Files/Reports/2010/PIP_Generations_and_Tech10.pdf

PART III
COMMUNICATION

PART III
COMMUNICATION

THE IMPLEMENTATION OF PUBLIC HEALTH COMMUNICATION MESSAGES TO PROMOTE TEENAGE MOTHERS' SENSE OF SELF AND AVERT STIGMA

Neale R. Chumbler, Helen Sanetmatsu and John Parrish-Sprowl

ABSTRACT

Purpose — *Improvements to supportive services targeting pregnant and parenting adolescents can enhance maternal and child outcomes (e.g., repeat pregnancy and child well-being). The purpose of this chapter is to advance the medical sociological literature by implementing multifaceted approaches including developing evidence-based media messaging device modalities as a forum to engage pregnant and parenting adolescents in social normative communication, self-reflection, and self-expression so that they can develop a tailored health prototype service model to accommodate their health and social needs.*

Technology, Communication, Disparities and Government Options in Health and Health Care Services
Research in the Sociology of Health Care, Volume 32, 63–91
Copyright © 2014 by Emerald Group Publishing Limited
All rights of reproduction in any form reserved
ISSN: 0275-4959/doi:10.1108/S0275-495920140000032015

Methodology — *We utilized a purposeful sample of pregnant adolescents or parenting adolescents (of an infant or toddler) ages 15–19 in a large Metropolitan Area in the Midwest. We employed a qualitative research design using two focus groups (n = 15) and participant observation (n = 8) to identify themes. Content analysis was performed to better understand the study participants' experiences and perceptions.*

Findings — *Based on the focus group results, the custom journal was found to be the most popular outlet to offer self-expression and social support. Four main themes emerged from the data, including teen pregnancy overall is a problem, but having their own baby was not; strong desire for more health information and health education; perceived stigma from their teachers and parents; and frustration with the existing service programs.*

Research implications — *The implications of the chapter are that the teen pregnancy norms fostered stigma and "social disgrace" that the pregnant and parenting adolescents experienced and ultimately thwarted their perceived and actual receipt of services. Future research should better understand the potential influences of internal and external pressures brought on by stigmatization as a contributing barrier to communicating social and health needs by pregnant and parenting adolescents.*

Value of chapter — *This chapter developed, implemented, and evaluated media communication and found that it could structure social relations between pregnant and parenting adolescents and service providers. This chapter also extends development communication techniques, with its intellectual roots in rural sociology, by focusing on communication-oriented solutions and the development of new technologies to provide medical information with greater social equality and integrated support services for pregnant and parenting adolescents.*

Keywords: Adolescents; parenting; stigma; communication; journaling

INTRODUCTION

Teenage parenthood is considered a key US social and public health problem and has been a central policy concern for many decades (Furstenberg, 2003; Mollborn & Jacobs, 2011). Approximately 80% of adults in a national poll indicated that teen pregnancy is an "important" or "very serious problem" in the United States (Science and Integrity Survey, 2004). Despite substantial variation in norms and behaviors in the United States, teen pregnancy and childbearing is remarkably prevalent in the general US population. For instance, the United States has the highest rate of teen pregnancy among the fully industrialized countries with about one-in-five of all teenage girls expected to have a child prior to age 20 (Mollborn & Jacobs, 2011). Teenage mothers disproportionately identify themselves as African American and Latina as compared to their non-Latina White or Asian American counterparts (Holcombe, Peterson, & Manlove, 2009). The high prevalence of teen parenthood in these socioeconomically marginalized groups is a principal contributing factor of public concern regarding teen childbearing (Mollborn & Jacobs, 2011). These public health concerns have led to the call for improvements to supportive services targeting pregnant and parenting adolescents and a better understanding of social norms. Such improvements can enhance maternal and child outcomes, including repeat pregnancy, educational attainment, and child well-being.

Social norms, a fundamental sociological concept, has had a long history in the literature, and dating back to the work of Durkheim (1951/1897). Social norms regarding the appropriateness of teen pregnancy underlie many of these public health and social health concerns. Similar to other sociologists, the present study defines social norms as group-level expectations of proper behavior that lead to negative penalties when dishonored (Mollborn & Jacobs, 2011; Settersten, 2004). Norms are theorized as common expectations which emerge about how individuals should act, all of which develop from social interaction with reference groups such as a family (Eitzen & Zinn, 2007). Social norms regarding the appropriate timing and ordering of transitions are projected to regulate whether such outcomes are deleterious or not for the actor (Mollborn & Morningstar, 2009; Neugarten, Moore, & Lowe, 1965). Irrespective of the sanctions experienced, pregnant and parenting adolescents who violate social norms about appropriate transitions to parenthood may experience stigma and shame (Mollborn & Morningstar, 2009). Therefore, a better understanding of the extent to which teenage mothers communicate with their peers and social network and the extent to which they receive communication from other is warranted. This phenomenon has rich sociological theoretical underpinnings from at least two sociologists. First, according to Blau (1964/1992), all social relations and transactions involve communication and social communication is necessary to sustain the structure of social relations. As Blau indicated (1964/1992), media communication is such a mechanism that can provide the mediating links between distant communicators. Second,

Janowitz (1952) identified communication as playing a key role in integrating individuals into their communities and by sustaining their community ties and in fostering interpersonal trust (see also Viswanath, 2008). The primary premise underlying Janowitz's book, *The Community Press in an Urban Setting*, was that any communication system not only shapes but is a byproduct of its social environment, and thus a factor of social interaction. The development by these theorists dovetail with development communication.

Development communication is an area of study that focuses on communication-oriented solutions to problems such as population management, disease prevention and control, and other basic life issues, usually, but not always in less developed countries (Kincaid & Figueroa, 2009). This area of study, established in the 1950s and 1960s, arose from the field of rural sociology, mass communication, journalism, and education (Kincaid & Figueroa, 2009; Moemeka, 1993). As an applied area, it has been studied on such diverse issues as economic development (Parrish-Sprowl, 2000), disease prevention and control (Obregon & Waisbord, 2012), and teen pregnancy (Moemeka, 1993) among other issues. While the early history of development communication was primarily one of engaging mass media to effect solutions to problems, the area has evolved into one that focuses on participatory models that seek to at the least engage, perhaps partner, and at the most simply turn over development to the community (Kincaid & Figueroa, 2009; Moemeka, 2000).

More specifically, in a World Bank report, Inagaki (2007) posits that development communication has evolved in three phases. The first is modernization. In this approach, primarily developers relied on mass media to move countries toward western standards for a modern society (Inagaki, 2007). This approach had limited success for a number of reasons, including limited resources for sustainability, and the limits of a mass media only approach to effect behavioral change (Inagaki, 2007; Obregon & Waisbord, 2012). From this framework evolved the diffusion of innovations model develop by Rogers and colleagues (Inagaki, 2007; Obregon & Waisbord, 2012). This improved development, but still relied primarily on mass media approaches to create behavioral change. Two different meta-analysis of the effects of media campaigns for improved health practices show that at best the effects are modest (Noar, 2006).

Within the past few years, development is increasing moving toward participatory models (Inagaki, 2007; Obregon & Waisbord, 2012). Greater success grows out of the engagement of the people among whom change must occur to improve health outcomes. One example is that of women's NGOs in Africa that train women in the use of communication media so that they can use it to improve health in their communities (Pillsbury & Mayer, 2005). Multiple projects have demonstrated that increasing the capacity of women to use media to provide information in their own language in a way that fits their communities is an effective way to improve health practices related to teen pregnancy, condom use, and other healthy reproductive and sexual behaviors (Pillsbury & Mayer, 2005). That participatory models of intervention tend to be more effective makes sense if one considers the perspective of Giddens' structuration theory (1984). When interventions focus more on the linkages and the reflexive actions of agents and structure rather than one or the other, they are trained on the locus of structuring action that creates both extant conditions and the potential for change. As Giddens (1991) points out, it is in the person's ability to sustain the narrative in which they are situated that we find their identity.

Although most development communication projects are conducted in low- and middle-income nations, this is not exclusively the case. Given some of the intractable problems in the United States of a similar nature, it is reasonable to employ similar participatory approaches to apply the research and models engaged in development projects to issues in the United States. One such area is teen parenting and pregnancy. Although one project in a single community was conducted, it primarily relied on mass media aimed at the audience rather than engaging the members of the community in the creating of the media itself (Moemeka, 1993). Given the evolution of development communication in general, and examples such as those detailed in *Women Connect!* (2005) in particular, research should focus projects that move toward more participatory models when addressing such issues. The present study explores two projects aimed at pregnant and parenting teens in a Midwestern city that utilize participatory models of engagement, with the community involved in the development of the media as a the form of intervention. The present study explores how teenage parenthood influences the lives of pregnant and parenting adolescents and investigates how their perceptions, goals, and challenges were experienced. Our primary intent is to generate a common understanding of pregnant and parenting adolescents' lived experience. This knowledge, in turn, was used to guide the development and implementation of communication modalities to convey communication about pregnancy and to foster self-expression, self-consciousness, and greater development of social life.

METHODS

We employed a descriptive qualitative approach to investigate pregnant and parenting adolescents' perceptions, experiences, goals, and struggles, among others. Because this is a *descriptive* study, the purpose was not to generate theory, as in other qualitative approaches (e.g., grounded theory), but rather to identify and describe the needs and experiences of the pregnant and parenting teens (Sandelowski, 2000). More specifically, qualitative descriptive studies focus on generating a comprehensive summary of practices, experiences, needs, and events as they occur in individuals' everyday contexts (Pashley et al., 2010; Sandelowski, 2000).

We utilized a purposeful sample of pregnant adolescents or parenting adolescents (of an infant or toddler) ages 15–19 in a large Metropolitan Area in the Midwest. We employed a qualitative research design using two focus groups ($n = 15$) and participant observation ($n = 8$) to identify themes.

We used focus groups because they accentuate social interaction among study participants and data can be examined to recognize how participants co-construct their perspectives by sharing knowledge (Lehoux, Poland, & Daudelin, 2006). Facilitators used a flexible interview guide (e.g., "what one thing did you like the best about developing the video?"; "if you could change one thing about the experience developing the video, what would it be?") and encouraged interaction and facilitated a discussion of similarities and differences among the study participants (Kitzinger, 1995). Each focus group was performed by a facilitator and a co-facilitator. The co-facilitator recorded observations of group interactions and the order of those who spoke during the focus groups (Pashley et al., 2010). Sessions began with the same broad question used in the interviews, then more detailed questions followed. Participants were queried about the pregnant and parenting adolescents' experiences working in a small group developing a video with their peers, about the ease of use of working the artifact, and whether they believed the video would enhance their peers' knowledge of pregnancy and maternal health.

We also used the qualitative methods of participant observations. Participant observation consists of monitoring and natural conversations through which researchers integrate themselves with study participants. Through this observation, the researcher talks with study participants as she or he comprehends their perspective of reality. Participant observation enables researchers both an intuitive and intellectual understanding of the way ideas are organized and prioritized; it further enables one to better understand how social and physical boundaries are circumscribed (Burke,

Villero, & Guerra, 2012; LeCompte, 1999). Observations focused on the verbal communication between the respondents while they were working in groups developing the videos; the observations also focused on the facial expressions and dialogue that ensued based on questions or other issues discussed during the development of the videos. Ethics approval for this study was obtained from the Indiana University Institutional Review Board (IRB).

Study Participants

To be eligible to be included in the study, participants had to be pregnant adolescents or parenting adolescents (of an infant or toddler) ages 15–19. Participant recruitment was limited to one large Midwestern city. Signed informed consent forms were obtained from study participants prior to beginning the study. Potential participants were identified through flyers posted at health and community centers, schools, high traffic public places, and were also distributed via service provider email networks. These IRB-approved flyers asked potential participants to call a central number and were explained information about the study and enrollment procedures. We also used a snowball technique as a second strategy to obtain prospective study participants. Once study participants signed informed consent forms and enrolled, they were individually asked if they knew anyone who might be eligible. This enrolled study participants were then asked to notify those individuals about the study opportunity and the contact number. Participants were compensated with gift cards after participating in the sessions and in the focus groups.

DATA COLLECTION

Data collection took place in three phases. In Phase 1, a total of eight study participants took part in the 3-day video development process and all eight participated in the focus group at the end of Day 3. All of the participants were female with an average age of 18.4 years (range, 17–19). At the time of the study, six of the study participants were pregnant. Two of the study participants were still currently enrolled in high school (HS), whereas four of the pregnant study respondents had completed HS. Two were parents of infants or toddlers and not in school, without completed HS or equivalent diplomas. All of the study participants were African Americans from various parts of a large metropolitan area of the Midwest – from suburbs to the west and northeast, from the city center, and from east of the downtown area.

The participants were divided into three groups and each produced a video with the exception of one group that produced two. Each day they were provided lunch and snacks. The participants were informed about the intent of the project, led through creativity exercises, taught the concept of storyboarding, and creating scripts. They learned to use the cameras and the editing software. They edited their videos and created final products. While they were provided all necessary instruction to complete their projects, they were encouraged to create the content with little input from any of the staff. The intended process was designed to enable them to tell their stories in their own way, both visually and in scripted content. They were allowed to work at their own pace and provided the opportunity to use the full range of facilities at the location of the project. At the end of the three days, all of the participants were brought to a table for a debriefing discussion regarding their impression of the project and their thoughts about the future of such a project for other pregnant and parenting adolescents.

In Phase 2, the first of two focus groups were conducted from a sample of the target population. This information set the stage for the rest of the project by uncovering what needed to be addressed in the media messaging prototypes. This focus group took place on a Saturday morning in a secluded large room at a local church. There were a total of five study participants, all of whom were female and African American ranging from 17 to 19 years of age. Two of the five were pregnant at the time of the study, while the other three were not pregnant, but were parents to a child under the age of one. One of the five participants was still enrolled in HS. Two of the participants were life-long friends while the remaining participants were not previously acquainted with each other. Childcare was provided to those who brought their children to the venue. One mother chose to keep her child with her during the discussion; one study participant brought two young children that she was babysitting and utilized childcare. After this focus group concluded, for the next seven days, the research team carefully analyzed the data to identify key themes, insights, and opportunities. With these key ideas in mind, another week was spent on brainstorming prototype ideas and creating the final prototypes.

Once the prototypes were finished, a new group of pregnant and parenting adolescents took part in a second focus group (Phase 3). The study participants were all female ranging in age from 17 to 19. Seven of the 10 were African American and three were Non-White Hispanic. Seven of the 10 were pregnant at the time of the study. Three of the participants had their children with them during the focus group session. Two of the study participants were both a parent and pregnant. To prevent possible biases, all of these study participants did not participate in previous focus groups.

This second focus group consisted of an interactive session that tested the usability of the final prototypes (component 1), followed by a more formal in-depth assessment of the experiences and perceptions related to the interactive session (component 2). The appendix provides an interview guide with the focus group questions and probes for Project B. Individuals desiring more details regarding the interview guide, please notify the first author.

The first component was a usability testing session where the 10 study participants were divided into two groups of five and were presented with various prototypes. The study participants were queried about the pregnant and parenting adolescents' perceptions and observations of the three prototypes created by the design team. The room was divided into three stations, each housing one prototype. The journal prototype was a customizable book that could function as a two-way communication device as well as a space for participants to vent and share insights into their lives. The kiosk prototype is a large interactive station that could function as both an awareness campaign and a tool for connecting young parents to resources and mentoring. The bus prototype would be a traveling classroom, day care, and exhibit that would allow young parents to escape their usual environment and spend time learning and socializing. Some installation was necessary for the projected demo of the kiosk prototype. The other two prototypes − the journal and bus − could be moved easily from one place to another and, in the end, these two stations were combined as it was simpler to move the prototypes to the participants rather than move the participants to the third station. The participants were separated into two groups and rotated to the two stations where each prototype was presented. Members of the research team talked about the features of the prototypes and objects were passed around the group if possible.

The second component involved a focus group session to gauge more in-depth the level of interest of participants toward the prototypes. In addition, the participants inquired further about the prototypes to get a better understanding of how they might work. Many of the questions asked were about practicality, usability, overall user-friendliness, and potential venues for placement and distribution.

DATA MANAGEMENT AND ANALYSIS

All qualitative data was transcribed. Qualitative content analysis (Corbin & Strauss, 2008) was performed on all of the qualitative data collected (i.e., the field notes, audiotapes from the focus groups, observations, and other documented material). It was also conducted on verbatim transcripts of the focus groups to better understand the study participants' experiences and perceptions. The content analysis was performed to better understand the study participants' experiences and perceptions. Concepts were derived inductively from the data using open coding and were integrated into a catalog of main themes (Corbin & Strauss, 2008; Kavanaugh, Stevens, Seers, Sidani, & Watt-Watson, 2010; Ritchie, Spencer, & O'Conn, 2007). Memos were generated to sustain a record of concept development and analytic results. A second analyst independently coded transcripts and comparisons were made before finalizing the codes. When discrepancies occurred one of the following three procedures was performed: (1) retain the original language and meaning of the concept; (2) modify the concept to more accurately signify the meaning of the phenomenon; or (3) add a brand new concept to better represent the content of the data (Kavanaugh et al., 2010).

Several procedures were employed to ensure a reliable account of the findings. We used multiple coders to achieve analytical rigor with ongoing discussion of emerging results at multiple team meetings (Pashley et al., 2010). The investigative team verified the generated themes and reconciled any differences. These deliberations were based profoundly in the data and were concentrated on establishing the best possible representation of the accounts (Pashley et al., 2010). The team also examined the possible meanings of outliers and rival explanations were discussed (Kvale, 1996; Pashley et al., 2010). To ensure logistical consistency in the interpretations of the data, we reviewed notes, project team meeting minutes, and other materials (Pashley et al., 2010; Patton, 1999).

RESULTS

Participant Observation Results: Themes Generated from
Participant Observation

As noted in the description above, the participants produced a total of four videos. While creating these videos, three program facilitators who had extensive experience in project-based learning theory observed the process. Based on the data collected from the participant observation (Phase 1), four themes emerged.

Project-Based Learning
First, the participants evidenced progress in learning how to complete video projects. Working with facilitators, they brainstormed ideas for content, narrowed the ideas into stories with an introduction, body, and conclusion; created storyboards to plan the video shooting, created video content; and finally edited the content into a finished product. The product was impressive given that, as one 19-year-old pregnant participant remarked, "we have never done anything like this before." Participants began developing a sense of criteria regarding the assessment of the quality of work and what might make work better. Regarding the quality (and some limitations) a different study participant (19-year-old parent) observed: "'Cause we probably really could have acted out well with the males here too. It probably would have been a better video, but I think we made a really good one." In total, participants produced four video. In addition, in the debriefing discussion, a 17-year-old pregnant respondent noted and three additional respondents (one being a 17-year-old pregnant and in school and one 18-year-old pregnant respondent and one 19-year-old pregnant respondent) agreed that given more time and opportunity they believed that they could make better videos than the ones they created in the brief time frame allowed.

Self-Reflection
A second key theme emerged from the observations of the participants regarding their self-reflection spurred on by engaging in the process of creating the videos. This outcome is consistent with previous research (Murphy et al., 2007) and illustrates the potential for such projects to make a difference in the future of those who participate in such projects. During the course of the project, one 17-year-old respondent said to the others that she was "scared" of being a mother, and in response another 19-year-old respondent said that it (being a mother) was "scary." Over the three day process of the development of the videos, the participants made a number of these types of comments. More specifically (and expansively) in the debriefing interview one person stated:

> It [making the video] made me think outside of the box more, you know, 'cause, like I used to kind of wonder why my mom or whatever would always have an attitude, but

getting ready to parent myself kind of made me realize that I'm having some days where I'm have that attitude too, because I'ma frustrated with the baby cryin' all the time and me not getting as much sleep and so, it kinda made me see where she was comin from. (Age 17, pregnant)

Another participant, in reflecting on things that were not anticipated, made a strong statement regarding the impact of having a child:

You can't give 'em back. You know how like you babysit somebody's child and you give 'em back, you're always gonna have your child. No matter what, no matter what, you're gonna get annoyed at times, irritated at times, and somehow you just have to like calm yourself down because you can't, your baby can feel like negative vibes or positive vibes and you know, they can see like if you're sad or happy or whatever. Like it's just, you have to, you have to have a strong head on your shoulders in order to take care of a baby, because if you don't then your baby is not gonna make it. (Age 19, parent of a toddler)

Both in observation and in discussion, evidence suggests that the participants gave serious thought to the impact of being pregnant or parenting and the consequences of the choices they had made thus far in life. One 19-year-old pregnant study participant agreed with a facilitator comment that "it helps you to watch yourself."

Video Development Relevant for Peers
A third and related theme is the awareness that such videos could have an impact on others if they were to either view ones like they made or make them themselves. When the question was posed regarding whether watching such videos made by peers might have helped them, two participants responded:

It would have helped me. Like if I didn't have a baby, and wasn't expecting, it would have helped me. (Pregnant 17-year-old)

It's helped me. And it'd still help me now because I see myself talkin' about it. I would never, like, talk about stuff like this. (19-year-old parent to a toddler)

Despite the difficulty to provide a definitive outcome given the low number of participants and the short time frame of the project, the preliminary observational and interview content suggests that the project had a positive impact on the participants and could well have a larger impact in the community if the process and product were used in schools and other community outlets.

Importance of School

A fourth theme was the affirmation of the need to stay in school. This belief was accentuated profoundly during the development of the videos. As one participant stated:

> I think we proved a point like for havin' a baby, you can still go back to school and ... (another participant finishes the statement by saying) still follow your dreams! (Unidentifiable participant and age 17, pregnant, in school)

Two others (one a 19-year-old pregnant respondent and one an 18-year-old respondent) in unison said:

> It's gonna be harder ... but you can do it.

The content of the videos and the discussion by the participants over the course of the project are reflected in the above statements. All of them believe that they need to stay committed to school and that others, even if pregnant, or maybe especially of they are so, need to go to school and build a career.

FOCUS GROUP RESULTS: THEMES GENERATED FROM ALL FOCUS GROUPS

Theme 1: Teen Pregnancy Is a Problem, but My Baby Isn't

Participants were quick to identify the specific characteristics that they liked the most about being a parent. Two 19-year-old respondents, one a parent and one pregnant, considered being a parent: "a blessing." A 19-year-old parent explained, "What I like about being a parent is when my son wakes up in the morning, he still smells like a baby and skin be all soft and hot." She smiled an enticing smile and all of the participants laughed.

Virtually all of the participants acknowledged that spacing children a few years apart was the most ideal situation. But, they also cited benefits of taking time to have a child when they still had perceived instrumental support from family members (e.g., mothers; grandmothers). In the view of a 19-year-old parent, "At least we got the kids, at least we got them out of the way." A particular 19-year-old participant (a parent) graduated at 16. She's now 18 and a sophomore in college. She's certified in billing and coding, and she's working downtown. From one participant's

(17, pregnant, in HS) perspective, "It's not the part of being young. As long as you got yourself together financially, mentally, and emotionally, have a baby."

Several of the study participants made it clear that their child was not a mistake. Their attitude was solidly, "No excuses," and "No regrets." They tended to regret their circumstances, but not their child. At the same time, participants seemed to share the view (or at least recognize the societal view) that teen pregnancy is a problem/mistake. In speaking of her baby daughter, one participant explained:

> But you know, I'm sayin', the only mistake I made was I'm sayin', not usin' the proper protection not to get pregnant at an early age. But I mean if it do happen, I'm still gonna be there for my child [when she's a teen]. This same teen even showed an understanding of the need for teens to plan to space their births. "My baby gotta be walkin', talkin', and in school before I can have another baby ... That's how everybody sometimes do they kids, space 'em out." (Age 19, parent)

These ideas were echoed in another conversation among participants. As another study participant described:

> They have kids just to be havin' 'em ... This girl at my school, she's a Mexican, and she's uhm seventeen, and she's on her third child. As they remarked, "Mm mmm," and "I couldn't do it." (Age 17, pregnant and in HS)

Participants indicated their disapproval and verbally indicated their concern for the parent. Taken as a whole, several participants expressed the idea that teen pregnancy and multiple births was a problem, but their individual child was not.

Theme 2: "Thirsty for Information," but More Importantly, Education

The teens showed an impressive knowledge of family planning and spacing of children. However, they also identified areas where they lack other salient information. Some of these areas related to logistical information about resources and services. However, although they requested some applied information, their comments and discussions had a larger focus on structured, general education. Participants demonstrated a real, pressing interest in applied information at several points in the study. First, when one of the study participants (19-year-old parent) described the fact that she had graduated from HS at 16, then attended college, received a level of certification in billing and coding, and secured a job, several of the participants were intrigued from the information. Detecting that this participant really had her life in order, a 19-year-old parent asked, "How did you do that (i.e., certification in billing and coding) at sixteen?" Then, the 19-year-old parent replied, "I went to Job Corps." Then, at least two other participants responded affirmatively:

> OK, Mmm! and You go girl. (17-year-old pregnant in HS)

> I'm gonna have to go to Job Corps today. (19-year-old parent)

However, participants also — and more often — expressed a desire for general, holistic education. As part of the media messaging initial focus group, participants were asked to imagine an object or device that would help them in their role as a pregnant or parent adolescent. One study participant suggested a novel type of book:

> For me, it would have to be a book about life and like all the stuff that can go bad. You know, like basically what to expect out of life, you know. Even though you want the best out of life, but any guidelines that can help me with parenting, just basically get through my life. So that's what I want, a book that knows about everything. (19-year-old parent)

Although one study participant (age 17, pregnant, in HS) had some concerns over the size of the book and her ability to locate what she needed in it, she and others agreed that it would be a good idea. This same participant had her own idea on how to access the information:

> I come up with like a drink that keep me energized and focused a lot and make me real smart so I could just push through school, like probably just do the work with my eyes closed, get so many diplomas. (Age 17, pregnant, in HS)

All of the participants seemed to value general education and knew that staying in school was important, especially for their children: One study participant underscored this sentiment:

> Regardless of whether I finish school or not, my child is gonna finish school, regardless if you know she did make the mistake I did ... I'm gonna try to push her to give her all the drive and motivation to finish school. (Age 19, parent)

The media messaging group discussed different intervention prototype that can be used to provide tailored information for the study participants. Seven of the 10 participants in the media messaging evaluative focus group rated all three prototypes (journal, bus, and kiosk) very high for their ability to communicate information about programs, pregnancy, and parenting to teens. Participants appreciated the Internet access and library functions of the bus (one of the prototype artifacts developed), the informational section of the journal, and the programmatic element of the kiosk. When indicating which prototypes the participants preferred, one study participant indicated:

> But I would want that too [points to column/kiosk] because people don't know that there's programs that help people. A lot of people don't know that. So they can, not strugglin' for nothin', but they could have had some help ... 'Cause a lot of people don't know about stuff that can help you out, to go to school and daycare and all that stuff like that that you are strugglin' with. Like you can't go to school 'cause you don't have somebody to babysit and the programs tell you, can help you go to school. So it'd be helpin' people get successful. (Age 18, parent and pregnant)

One important element of the kiosk for the participants was that it provided the capability of another study participant to have two-way interaction

> It being a touch screen instead of it just being a television that talks to you, you can actually control what you want to hear and stuff. (Age 19, parent)

> Facilitator: You like that you can interact with it and it's just ...

> 'Cause if it's just talkin', then nobody's gonna just sit there and listen to it, but if you can like push buttons and pick what you want to know and stuff then people gonna listen. (Age 19, parent)

Overall, the examples demonstrate an unmistakable desire for information that does not directly regard pregnancy and parenting practices, but allows teens to fulfill the parenting role. Without direct prompting, the participants requested information on schools, job training, and housing; and the participant requested this information from each other. They also showed an undeniable value for general education and the type of advantages individuals obtain from staying in school.

Theme 3: "You Might as Well Drop Out"

Even though they seemed to value staying in school and maintain a formal education, several of the study participants reported feeling stigmatized. The term "stigma" has been defined as an "attribute that is deeply discrediting" (Goffman, 1963, p. 3) and is typically referred to as a categorization of "social disgrace" (Eitzen & Zinn, 2007, p. 480) and has been characterized as "the perception of difference associated with undesirable traits" (O'Mahen, Henshaw, Jones, & Flynn, 2011). The experience of stigma in an individual's life has been associated with numerous deleterious health outcomes including the prevalence of and seeking treatment for depression

(Given, Katz, Bellamy, & Holmes, 2007). Similarly, stigmatization makes it extremely difficult for pregnant adolescents to finish school. This stigmatization came in various forms ranging from direct statements (e.g., "Well, you might as well drop out") to the more common, indirect stigma and shaming that is woven into everyday experiences. There were several examples of everyday exchanges that served to shame and stigmatize participants. One study participant described an exchange with a school security guard:

> I couldn't do the exercises and the security guard was just walkin around and patrolling the area and whatever. And I'm standin' there and he like, "[Well, what's wrong with you? Why can't you get out there and do what they're doin'?" And I wasn't showin' yet and I'm like, "I'm pregnant." "How old are you?" And I'm like, "I'm eighteen." "That's a shame, you pregnant. Why are you even here?" Come on now, you need to be out there tryin' to find out who your baby's daddy is. I bet you don't even know who your baby's daddy is." I'm like, "Really?" ... 'You don't even need to be here. Why are you here? Go find the daddy?' That's really too much for me. That made me want to, boy, I just try to stay sane. (Age 19, parent)

These comments are genuine-though-awkward attempts to be helpful to pregnant and parenting adolescents. However, they may be interpreted as genuine attempts to encourage pregnant and parenting adolescents to drop out of school before graduating. Again, if pregnant and parenting adolescents perceive the discouragement as real, it is likely real in the consequences. At the time of the study, the aforementioned 19-year-old study participant had not completed her HS education. A different respondent described a similar interaction with this same 19-year-old study participant with reference to one of the coaches of her basketball team:

> They'll tell the other students, "Why you hang around her?" (Age 17, pregnant in HS)

> You gonna be just like her. (Age 19, parent)

> You gonna be the type of person, if that's your friend, she was just like, "You can hang out with better people that will guide you into a better life instead of something negative. When you in something negative, your result is gonna be negative," or something she said like that ... (Age 17, pregnant in HS)

> It discourages you sometimes, 'cause what people be sayin' to you, like, it make you don't even want to be there, 'cause people talk so much stuff, and then you gotta go to school the next day and see the same person that was just talkin' bad about you, like make you want to not even be around them people. (Age 19, parent)

This 17-year-old pregnant study participant's experience took on an additional characteristic. She indicated that these few powerful negative incidents "balanced out" by mentioning the same incident twice in the same focus group:

> Well, it [pregnancy] didn't stop me, because I'm still in school. But like uhm, I was on the cheerleading squad and my cheerleading coach, she would down me and she would talk about me to the cheerleaders, the kids' parents. She'd talk about me in front of my face and everything. And then I just, I don't know, just feeling like what I'm doing is wrong, what I'm doing. I just feel like, I don't know ... (Age 17, pregnant in HS)

> That would stop somebody. (Age 19, parent)

> Participants in Unison: Yeah. That's what made my mother stop going to school. (Age 19, pregnant)

A pregnant 17-year-old respondent proved to be particularly resilient in the face of being "admonished" by authority figures. During the project-based learning phase of Project B, she described a situation she was currently dealing with at church. When her pastor became aware of her pregnancy, he confronted her and explained to her that he wanted her to go before the entire congregation and apologize for the "sin" she had committed by getting pregnant. As a religious person, she was troubled by this requirement and explained that Jesus personified forgiveness.

Still yet, further evidence was apparent of stigmatization. The following passage presents an example of the teens' pressure to embrace their stigmatized identity:

> Yeah, we're both from [Springfield] and we know how people are and it's just, it's just sad and like when you hear so much stuff, you know, and you start to kind of believe it. (Age 19, pregnant)

> Yeah, it's like frustrating because you know who you are, but then you start to hear so much, like you get to school first period and you hear one thing. By the time you get to seventh period at the end of the day, you done heard thirteen things about yourself you didn't even know. (Age 17, pregnant, in school)

> It's like, it's frustrating 'cause you don't know who you are anymore. (Age 19, pregnant)

Although both participants asserted their intentions not to quit school, conditions are already in place that could potentially lead to a much less desirable outcome. The conventional wisdom among the teen participants was that it would not be easy. Many of the study participants considered avoiding the most severely stigmatizing situations by attending alternative schools or leaving school altogether. It was clear that several study participants felt pressure to leave the stigmatized situations, not necessarily because of their discomfort, but because of other people's (primarily administrators') discomfort in interacting with them. The following interactions supported this notion of stigmatization:

> I heard that in these schools, they kick you out if you're pregnant. (Age 18, parent and pregnant)
>
> Participants in Unison: Yes [emphatic].
>
> There are some schools. (Age 19, pregnant)
>
> They don't call it kickin' out. Like at my school, they have an alternative school in out of town. It's called [Smith]. I go to [Springfield High School]. They call me in the office and they say, "Well, we think it's best for you and your baby to go to [Smith]." "No, it's best for you, not me." (Age 17, pregnant, in school)
>
> They push you into an alternative school. (Age 19, parent)
>
> So, do they make you go? (Age 18, parent and pregnant)
>
> They say they're not going to make you go. They say they give you a choice, but in all reality, they're pressuring you, saying, "Oh, but if you go here, you know you have full daycare. And if you go here, you can stay longer." And it's like, "No." (Age 17, pregnant, in school)
>
> I wasn't even pregnant and they were pressuring me into it and they made it sound like it was so great. I hated it. I absolutely hated it. (Age 19, pregnant)

Theme 4: Frustration with Existing Programs

Many of the study participants were frustrated with existing services and service agents. One study participant commented directly on the frustration:

> When I really, like when I'm to the point when I'm like really crying and I done went to all them people, and it's like nothing's working, I just pray. How often? Man! A lot! (Age 17, pregnant in HS)

Although the participants stated that help was not available, the context of their statements made it clear that the problem was not the availability of programs, but rather the structure and climate of the programs that made them less effective. Reflecting on what form the "alien object" prototype should take to help meet the needs of pregnant and parenting teens, one study participant indicated that she needed more help and not necessarily more programs. Indeed, she needed the programs to be tailored for her life and her unique situation:

> Just throw more help out there, not just let them be straining ... I think just the state in general should of just had a little more help like, *another way to come out to people.* Just put a little more help out there. 'Cause it is people who need help and half of the

programs don't even help people with the things they say they need help with [emphasis added]. (Age 19, parent)

The frustration with existing services originated from three sources. First, there is a clear lack of trust between participants and programming. Three study participants supported this notion:

There's always a catch to something. (Age 17, pregnant in HS)

They ain't even givin' you all the information you need to know. There's always holdin' back on somethin'. (Age 19, parent)

Second, it is clear that participants are exposed to a considerable volume of one-way communication. Participants were disappointed in programs and people who offered no opportunity for reciprocal exchange of communication. The participants who were parents indicated that they were often confronted with rhetorical questions from providers who did not expect or want an answer. Different sources of assistance asked the teens questions related to why they were not getting a job or finishing school. The teens cited these as an example of the barrage of unanswerable questions pregnant and parenting adolescents encounter in their interactions with institutional personnel. They also indicated that attempts to continue and complete education often began with derogatory statements that restricted any opportunity for didactic learning:

You should have finished school. (Age 19, parent)

You don't teach your baby nothing'. (Age 19, pregnant)

They try to tell you how you should raise your baby when they don't even know the half. (Age 17, pregnant in HS)

Some people out there just don't really care, because they feel like we're not trying to help ourselves, which we are. (Age 18, parent and pregnant)

Or you go to people with the attitude like you should never got pregnant and maybe you wouldn't be in the situation you're in. (Age 19, pregnant)

In this way, lack of two-way communication and negative experiences with frontline personnel at mainstream service providers could have similar sweeping effects. Third, the teens reported that the narrow focus of programs and personnel kept them from seeing and addressing the holistic reality of parenting. One of the study participants made a point of questioning the researchers:

Do you all see what people go through, young people go through? Do you understand what we go through? (Age 19, parent)

Assistant Facilitator: I don't think we can. I don't think we can understand, but ...

Facilitator: We try to, we definitely try to empathize and that's, I think [AF] is right, that's as much as we can do.

Y'all can relate, but y'all don't understand. (Age 19, parent)

It is not clear, however, that the participants were able to articulate those assertive remarks when dealing with institutional personnel. As such, it is vitally important for participants that institutional representatives understand just how difficult raising a child was from their perspective. The following exchange demonstrated the social environment and living conditions of the study participants and describes the barriers that are in place that thwarts timely access to services. In particular, some of the participants described their apartment complex:

I'm scared for myself and my child. (Age 19, parent)

Me too. (Age 19, parent)

You wouldn't want to be there no way ... . People get shot right in front of your building, right where you're stayin'. (Age 19, parent)

Two people got shot in front of our building the other day. (Age 19, parent)

Dang, you saw their bodies? (Age 17, pregnant in HS)

Yeah. (Age 19, pregnant)

They was still alive. (Age 19, parent)

We actually knew who they were though. (Age 19, pregnant)

Yeah, it's so dangerous ... you can't even stand outside on your porch if you want to ... you can't even walk around to get some warm air. (Age 19, parent)

I can't, like I can't even like, my brother and them want to go outside. "Y'all can't go outside. No. Y'all not fixin' to go outside. Y'all want to go outside and play. Y'all want to go outside and do this. Y'all can't do none of that." You know what I'm sayin? 'Cause I'm scared for them. "Y'all go outside and say y'all mess with somebody else's child or whatever and then they want to come back and shoot up you place. No." (Age 19, parent)

Yeah, and see people come over to my house, everybody that comes over there brings a gun, shotguns, choppers. I'm like don't bring all that over here. (Age 19, parent)

In my house, with my child. It's crazy. (Age 19, parent)

You gotta be on your toes at all times out there. Your baby could be one month old, years old, and you still gotta be on your toes. You could be pregnant and still have to go through all that. (Age 19, parent)

Although the degree to which the living conditions of participants varied, the social phenomena was the same. The incongruence between the
unanswerable questions and what pregnant and parenting adolescents perceived as realistic constituted a barrier between the supply of and demand
for information.

DISCUSSION

The present study explored how teenage parenthood influenced the lives of
pregnant and parenting adolescents and investigated how their perceptions,
goals, and challenges were experienced. Our primary intent is to generate a
common understanding of pregnant and parenting adolescents' lived
experience. This knowledge, in turn, was used to guide the development
and implementation of communication modalities to convey communication about pregnancy and to foster self-expression, self-consciousness, and
greater development of social life.

As Blau (1964/1992) indicated, media communication is such a
mechanism that can provide the mediating links between distant communicators. Consistent with Blau's (1964/1992) perspective, this chapter
developed, implemented, and evaluated media communication and found
that it could structure social relations between pregnant and parenting
adolescents and service providers. Results from our study are more in
line with the work of Giddens' *theory of structuration*. As Giddens suggests, the interaction between these groups reflexively structures each
party in the interaction (Giddens, 1984, 1991). And, as Giddens articu-
lated, structure entails of "rules and resources recursively implicated in
the reproduction of social systems" (1979, p. 64). Our study involved adolescents in the development of media as a mechanism to structure interaction. This activity illuminated the influences of these linkages in both
creating and facilitating this relationship. This chapter also extended
development communication techniques, with its intellectual roots in rural
sociology, by focusing on communication-oriented solutions and the
development of new technologies to provide medical information with
greater social equality and integrated support services for pregnant and
parenting adolescents. These communication-oriented solutions further
bolster teenage mothers' sense of self and can avert the unfortunate
stigma that many of the study participants experienced after experiencing
a pregnancy.

We employed visual media to engage pregnant and parenting adolescents in communication and self-reflection. The participants in this study were universally positive about the experience developing the videos and indicated that they would like to do it again. In addition, the study participants felt that it had benefited them and believed that such videos could have a positive impact on peers. Findings from this study have implications for the field of visual sociology. Our findings are in keeping with the trend toward camera (still and video images) ownership by more individual adolescents via camera phones. According to Sarvas and Frohlich (2011), there is a growing generation of young people who are media-savvy and have had access to cameras of their own rather than a shared camera belonging to the family. Adolescent parents, in particular, may want to learn how to take, edit, and produce images of their lives and their children that can be shared in person or via photo-sharing software and the Internet. There have been several studies that have assessed the outcomes among pregnant and parenting adolescents when they are involved in self-expression through still photography. By using visual sociological components, Blinn (1985) suggested an eight-step weekly process of phototherapeutic activities to improve the self-concept and prevent repeat pregnancies among adolescents. The activities included bringing five photos to the group: that show you as you would like to be, that you are proud of, and that show how you want to feel about yourself in two years. Future research should incorporate future visual sociological components to create an environment more conducive to producing greater reflection, more learning, and better final videos. In addition, the data generated will create not only more input for future efforts, but also provide information for the creation of training materials for others who want to do such projects.

The implications of the chapter are that the stigma and "social disgrace" that the pregnant and parenting adolescents experienced thwarted their perceived and actual receipt of services. Stigmatization acts internally to confuse individual identity, encourage avoidance, and potentially produce self-fulfilling prophecy (Goffman, 1963). On the other hand, stigmatization acts externally to produce levels of discomfort in adults relative to the presence of pregnant and parenting adolescents in their communities and institutions that potentially cause adults to encourage pregnant and parenting adolescents out of school. It is imperative to understand the potential influences of internal and external pressures brought on by stigmatization as a contributing factor in the overwhelming of existing participant values to stay in school. Not only are pregnant and parenting adolescents told directly to leave, but others encourage them to leave because they do not want to have a blemish on their organization. In other words, As Giddens suggests, the stigma and the problems it creates, are a function of structuration born out of linkages between all involved (Giddens, 1984, 1991).

Findings from our study add to the growing body of literature of social science research on stigma. Link and Phelan (2001), in their formative review on the conceptualization and implementation of stigma in social science research, argued that stigma has multifactorial components including status loss, an area that has had less information reported. That is, an individual is "connected to undesirable characteristics that reduce his or her status in the eyes of the stigmatizer" (Link & Phelan, 2001, p. 371). Our findings as it relate to stigma and status loss for pregnant and parenting adolescents dovetail and are congruent with a strand of sociological research on social hierarchies. This perspective posits that external statuses (e.g., race) shape status hierarchies within small groups (Cohen, 1982; also see Link & Phelan, 2001). It is imperative to recognize that future research should better understand the potential influences of internal and external pressures brought on by stigmatization as a contributing barrier to communicating social and health needs by pregnant and parenting adolescents. Future research should also implement this custom journal in a different sample to explore more deeply the construction of the communication between service providers and adolescent parents and enable insight into how it might avert stigma-related barriers (i.e., feeling prejudged and marginalized) to receiving the support and services needed for prenatal care. An important extension of this concept of stigmatization that the study participants reported to feel regarding the need to drop out of school seems to indicate that people are encouraging pregnant and parenting adolescents out to avoid dealing with the damage. It appears that adults are more uncomfortable with the pregnancy than the teens, thus creating their own stigmatizing framing of the event (Giddens, 1984). It is important to make the following distinction − discomfort among adults is entirely external to a pregnant and parenting adolescent's locus of control. In other words, pregnant and parenting adolescents could potentially be armed with coping mechanisms to resist these influences, but remediation of the specific counterproductive behaviors would require intervention by adults.

There are various ways individuals can and do react to stigma. The following examples are particularly relevant and should be considered in future implementation efforts when offering pregnant and parenting adolescents with relevant health information to avert stigma: (1) mastering the activities thought to be closed off to them and employing resilient efforts to remain in school despite the negative influences of authority figures; (2) embracing their new identities as parents and concomitantly developing the means to manage the stigma issues associated with the role (e.g., assuming the corresponding expected behaviors of those identities, including dropping out as means of the fulfillment of role expectations); and (3) avoiding situations in which the mismatch between virtual and real identity is likely to be exposed (perhaps including dropping out as a means of self-isolation). Future research with implementing these types of communication modalities should strive to structure programs to decrease stigmatization from teenage mothers' authority figures.

Future research should also strive to increase opportunities for communication practices that arise from an understanding that linkages between people reflexively structure identities and institutions (Giddens, 1991; Link & Phelan, 2001). Pregnant and parenting adolescents desperately wanted access to information; institutions desperately wanted to get their information disseminated, yet it appeared that very little exchange of information actually took place. Replacing the presumption that communication is one-way with reciprocal systems that facilitate pregnant and parenting adolescents expressing their needs and situations, and, in turn, for institutions to listen, acknowledge, and provide information and services within this relational framework, could improve the apparent gap that presently exists between the two. Furthermore, our data indicated that goals to break down silos of care were on the right track. It may even be worth considering integrating non-health services into considerations of structures of care to more holistically address teens' social experiences.

For pregnant and parenting adolescents, it is vital that institutional representatives be able to understand, if not relate, to their life circumstances in order to recognize what normative expectations for mothers are and are not feasible. Making this effort will facilitate communication and increase the possibility of establishing mutual trust and respect. It appeared that many of the study participants knew about the public health importance of refraining from drinking alcohol, smoking cigarettes, dropping out of school prior to graduation, and increasing the spacing of subsequent pregnancies. However, several of them received strong messages to the contrary. Institutional representatives, for example, are, sometimes literally, telling them "Well, you might as well drop out." These institutional messages are counterproductive to the teenage mothers in their self-development and are a devastating form of stigmatization. As Link and

Phelan (2001, p. 375) pointed out, "stigma is entirely dependent on social, economic, and political power – it takes power to stigmatize."

Even though our study offered several insightful findings, there were a few limitations that need some attention. The primary limitations of this study center on challenges associated with the recruitment of the unique target population. Specific recruitment limitations relate to issues of access and temporal factors. Snowball recruitment, which we employed by gaining referrals from existing participants, was found to be a successful recruitment strategy. Pregnant and parenting adolescents often know other pregnant and parenting adolescents. It should not be assumed, however, that they know more than one or two whom they would be willing to call to refer to recruiters. Snowballing with pregnant and parenting adolescents should be considered as many small, individual branches of two or three potential participants rather than the large tree-like structure researchers imagine. As such, snowballing should be considered a supplement to rather than replacement for recruitment-by-flyer or recruitment by IRB-approved program partners.

Overall, pregnant and parenting adolescents were a group as a whole that was challenging to recruit. Temporally, they may have less hours of availability than other similar populations. They may also have a reluctance to receive and to respond to recruitment messages for many of the reasons discussed in this report. And, they may face communication hurdles (e.g., the lack of a consistently available cell phone to facilitate the sustained interactions that recruitment and research require). Any effort to conduct research with pregnant and parenting adolescents should plan considerable time for successful recruitment of large numbers of diverse study participants. Policy makers may want to take this view into consideration when crafting programs and information. It is important to distinguish teen pregnancy as a social issue from the individual teens and children that programs serve.

ACKNOWLEDGMENTS

This research was conducted with support from a grant funded by the Indiana State Department of Health and the Pregnant and Parenting Supports Services Adolescent Program (Chumbler, Principal Investigator). The authors wish to acknowledge the diligent assistance and impeccable contributions from Barry Barker, Anne Mitchell, Tamara Leech, Lynn Pike, and others of the PPASS program and team.

REFERENCES

Blau, P. M. (1964/1992). *Exchange and power in social life*. New Brunswick, NJ: Transaction.

Blinn, L. (1985). Phototherapeutic intervention to improve self-concept and prevent repeat pregnancies among adolescents. *Family Relations, 36*, 252–257.

Burke, N. J., Villero, O., & Guerra, C. (2012). Passing through: Meanings of survivorship and support among Filipinas with breast cancer. *Qualitative Health Research, 22*, 189–198.

Cohen, E. G. (1982). Expectations states and interracial interaction in school settings. *Annual Review of Sociology, 8*, 209–235.

Corbin, J., & Strauss, A. (2008). *Basics of qualitative research*. Thousand Oaks, CA: Sage.

Durkheim, E. (1951). *Suicide: A study in sociology*. Glencoe, IL: Free Press (Original work published in 1897).

Eitzen, D. S., & Zinn, M. B. (2007). *In conflict and order: Understanding society* (11th ed.). Boston, MA: Allyn & Bacon.

Furstenberg, F. F., Jr. (2003). Teenage childbearing as a public issue and private concern. *Annual Review of Sociology, 29*, 23–39.

Giddens, A. (1979). *Central problems in social theory: Action, structure and contradiction in social analysis*. London: Macmillan Press.

Giddens, A. (1984). *The constitution of society: Outline of the theory of structuration*. Cambridge: Polity Press.

Giddens, A. (1991). *Modernity and self-identity. Self and society in the late modern age*. Cambridge: Polity Press.

Given, J. L., Katz, I. R., Bellamy, S., & Holmes, W. C. (2007). Stigma and the acceptability of depression treatments among African Americans and Whites. *Journal of General Internal Medicine, 22*, 1292–1297.

Goffman, E. (1963). *Stigma: Notes on the management of spoiled identity*. New York, NY: Simon & Schuster.

Holcombe, E., Peterson, K., & Manlove, J. (2009). *Ten reasons to still keep the focus on child-bearing*. Retrieved from http://www.childtrends.org/Files/Child_Trends-2009_04_01_RB_KeepingFocus.pdf. Accessed on January 30, 2013.

Inagaki, N. (2007). *Communicating the impact of communication for development: Recent trends in empirical research*. World Bank Working Paper No. 120. World Bank, Washington, DC.

Janowitz, M. (1952). *The community press in an urban setting*. Chicago, IL: University of Chicago Press.

Kavanaugh, T., Stevens, B., Seers, K., Sidani, S., & Watt-Watson, J. (2010). Process evaluation of appreciative inquiry to translate pain management evidence into pediatric nursing practice. *Implementation Science, 5*, 90.

Kincaid, D. L., & Figueroa, M. E. (2009). Communication for participatory development: Dialogue, action and change. In L. R. Frey & K. N. Cissna (Eds.), *Routledge handbook of applied communication*. New York, NY: Routledge.

Kitzinger, J. (1995). Qualitative research: Introducing focus groups. *British Medical Journal, 311*, 299–302.

Kvale, S. (1996). *The social construction of validity* (pp. 229–252). Thousand Oaks, CA: Sage.

LeCompte, M. D. (1999). *Essential ethnographic methods: Observations, interviews, and questionnaires*. Walnut Creek, CA: AltaMira Press.

Lehoux, P., Poland, B., & Daudelin, G. (2006). Focus group research and "the patients view". *Social Science and Medicine, 63*, 2091–2104.

Link, B. G., & Phelan, J. C. (2001). Conceptualizing stigma. *Annual Review of Sociology, 27*, 363–385.

Moemeka, A. (1993). *Development (social change) communication: Building understanding and creating participation.* New York, NY: McGraw Hill.

Moemeka, A. A. (2000). *Development communication in action: Building understanding and creating participation.* Lanham, MD: University Press of America.

Mollborn, S., & Jacobs, J. (2011). We'll figure a way: Teenage mothers' experiences in shifting social and economic contexts. *Qualitative Sociology, 35*, 23–46.

Mollborn, S., & Morningstar, E. (2009). Investigating the relationship between teenage child-bearing and psychological distress using longitudinal evidence. *Journal of Health and Social Behavior, 50*, 310–326.

Murphy, D., Balka, E., Poureslami, I. L., Diana, E., Nicol, A.-M., & Cruz, T. (2007). Communicating health information: The community engagement model for video production. *Canadian Journal of Communication, 32*(3&4), 383–400.

Neugarten, B. L., Moore, J. W., & Lowe, J. C. (1965). Age norms, age constraints, and adult socialization. *American Journal of Sociology, 70*, 71–717.

Noar, S. (2006). A 10-year retrospective of research in health mass media campaigns: Where do we go from here? *Journal of Health Communication, 11*, 206–221.

Obregon, R., & Waisbord, S. (2012). Theoretical divides and convergence in global health communication. In R. Obregon & S. Waisbord (Eds.), *The handbook of global health communication.* New York, NY: Wiley-Blackwell.

O'Mahen, H. A., Henshaw, E., Jones, J. M., & Flynn, H. A. (2011).Stigma and depression during pregnancy: Does race matter? *Journal of Nervous and Mental Disease, 199*, 257–262.

Parrish-Sprowl, J. (2000). Organizational communication: Linking key processes to effective development. In A. Moemeka (Ed.), *Development communication in action: Building understanding and creating participation* (pp. 179–202). New York, NY: University Press of America.

Pashley, E., Powers, A., McNamee, N., Buivids, R., Piccinin, J., & Gibson, B. E. (2010). Discharge from outpatient orthopaedic physiotherapy: A qualitative descriptive study of physiotherapists' practices. *Physiotherapy Canada, 62*, 224–234.

Patton, M. Q. (1999). Enhancing the quality and credibility of qualitative analysis. *Health Services Research, 34*, 1189–1208.

Pillsbury, B., & Mayer, D. (2005). Women connect! Strengthening communications to meet sexual and reproductive health challenges. *Journal of Health communication, 10*, 361–371.

Ritchie, J., Spencer, L., & O'Connor, W. (2007). Carrying out qualitative analysis. In J. Ritchie & J. Lewis (Eds.), *Qualitative research practice: A guide for social science students and researchers* (pp. 219–262). London: Sage.

Sandelowski, M. (2000). Whatever happened to qualitative description? *Research in Nursing and Health, 23*, 334–340.

Sarvas, R., & Frohlich, D. M. (2011). *From snapshots to social media – The changing picture of domestic photography.* London: Springer.

Science and Integrity Survey. (2004). Science and integrity survey. *iPOLL Databank*, The Roper Center for Public Opinion Research, University of Connecticut, Storrs, CT.

Settersten, R. A., Jr. (2004). Age structuring and the rhythm of the life course. In J. T. Mortimer & M. J. Shanahan (Eds.), *Handbook of the life course* (pp. 81–98). New York, NY: Kluwer Academic.

Viswanath, K. (2008). Social capital and health communications. In K. Viswanath, S. V. Subramanian, & K. Daniel (Eds.), *Social capital and health* (pp. 259–271). New York, NY: Springer.

APPENDIX: INTERVIEW GUIDE FOR FOCUS GROUPS

This focus group began with one of the research team members serving as a facilitator who used a flexible interview guide and included probes to encourage interaction and facilitate a discussion of similarities and differences among participants.

Project B: Focus Group

Following the study participants breaking up into small groups, brief semi-structured interviews were conducted with the study participants at the end of the community-based video development. The interviews were employed with use of an interview guide that will facilitate collection of information about the pregnant and parenting adolescents' experience of working in a small group in developing a video with their peers, about the ease of use of working the artifact, and whether they believed the video would enhance their peers' knowledge of pregnancy and maternal health. The interviews were sufficiently open-ended to enable participants to discuss they considered to be relevant to the development of the video.

Questions

"What one thing did you like the best about developing the video?"

"What one thing did you like the least about developing the video?"

"Were there any parts of the video that seemed inappropriate?"

"Were there any parts of the video that your peers would not like?"

"Do you believe the video will increase knowledge about pregnancy and/or parenting?"

"Do you feel as though this video would help adolescents feel prepared for having children?"

"If you could change one thing about the experience developing the video, what would it be?"

"Do you have any other advice for us as we introduce these videos to other agencies?"

VIRTUAL HEALTH: THE IMPACT OF HEALTH-RELATED WEBSITES ON PATIENT-DOCTOR INTERACTIONS[☆]

Scott V. Savage, Samantha Kwan and Kelly Bergstrand

ABSTRACT

Purpose — *This study illustrates that differences across health-related websites, as well as different Internet usage patterns, have significant implications for how individuals view and interact with their health care providers.*

Methodology/approach — *We rely on a qualitative study of three health-related websites and an ordinary least squares regression analysis of survey data to explore how websites with different organizational*

[☆]Portions of this chapter were presented at the 2009 annual meeting of the American Sociological Association.

Technology, Communication, Disparities and Government Options in Health and Health Care Services
Research in the Sociology of Health Care, Volume 32, 93–116
Copyright © 2014 by Emerald Group Publishing Limited
All rights of reproduction in any form reserved
ISSN: 0275-4959/doi:10.1108/S0275-495920140000032017

motives frame health-related issues and how variations in Internet usage patterns affect patients' perceptions of the patient-doctor interaction.

Findings — *Results reveal differences across three health-related websites and show that both the number and the type of websites patients visit affect their perceptions of physicians' responses. Specifically, visiting multiple websites decreased perceptions of how well doctors listened to or answered patients' questions, whereas using nonprofit or government health-related websites increased evaluations of how well doctors listened to and answered questions.*

Research limitations/implications — *This study suggests that practitioners and scholars should look more closely at how patients use the Internet to understand how it affects doctor-patient interactions. Future research could expand the analysis of website framing or use methods such as in-depth interviewing to more fully understand on-the-ground processes and mechanisms.*

Originality/value of chapter — *This study highlights the importance of fleshing out nuances about what it means to be an Internet-informed patient given that varying patterns of Internet use may affect how patients perceive their physicians.*

Keywords: Patient-doctor interactions; health websites; Internet; consumerism; organizational sector

The proliferation of health-related websites has made it easy for individuals to access health information, and about 113 million Americans rely on the Internet for this purpose (Fox, 2006). People use the Internet to research specific diseases and treatments (Kivits, 2009), learn about clinical trials (Anderson, Rainy, & Eysenbach, 2003), and participate in electronic support groups (Barker, 2008).

The information on the Internet, however, does not come from one unified and consistent body, but rather from a host of self-interested parties. Internet websites act as virtual spaces where various groups can and do lobby for public support as they compete for control over the jurisdiction of health (Barker, 2008; Kroll-Smith, 2003). Such groups are manifold and include professional organizations such as the American Medical Association (AMA), for-profit health information providers such as WebMD, and not-for-profit medical practices such as the Mayo Clinic.

These groups rely on their respective websites to shape public perception by framing the information they present (Anderson, 2002). Their ensuing framing contests reflect the social construction of disease and framing struggles over the production of meanings (Benford & Snow, 2000; Conrad, 1992; Hilgartner & Bosk, 1988).

The Internet, then, is an arena in which groups compete for jurisdictional control (Abbott, 1988) over health and illness by lobbying the public to accept their particular knowledge systems concerning health problems and to select the appropriate means for solving those problems (see, e.g., Kroll-Smith, 2003). In this chapter, we use a mixed-method design to examine how these virtual contests shape how patients perceive and experience the patient-doctor interaction. Specifically, we ask: How do various health-related websites frame health care, and what is the impact of website usage for patient-doctor interactions?

To address these research questions, we begin with an analysis of three health information websites with distinct organizational motives. We turn to archived pages of the online portals of the AMA, WebMD, and the Mayo Clinic (AMA-assn.org, WebMD.com, and MayoClinic.com) to discern the competing meanings promulgated by these groups about health and also about what it means to be a patient. We then turn to the *Impact of the Internet and Advertising on Patients and Physicians* survey (Lo, 2004) to examine how Internet usage actually affects patient-physician encounters. Our qualitative analysis of the three websites suggests that they present different messages about what it means to be a patient and that these messages potentially vary along sector lines, while our quantitative analysis suggests that patients' perceptions of recent encounters with their doctors vary across different patterns of health-related Internet use. Together, these findings help us better explain why browsing the Internet for health information can produce varying effects on the patient-doctor interaction.

HEALTH WEBSITES AND PATIENT-DOCTOR INTERACTIONS

Research on the relationship between the Internet and health care flourished after Hardey (1999) wrote that as a "site of a new struggle over expertise in health … [the Internet] will transform the relationship between the health professionals and their clients" (1999, p. 820). Relying on qualitative data from households that use the Internet to identify health information,

Hardey speculated that individuals use the Internet to free themselves of dependence on the medical professional for health knowledge, thereby eroding the medical profession's control over medical knowledge. This observation initiated a surge in research on how patient consumption of web-based health information might transform the doctor-patient relationship by empowering patients to more readily challenge professional dominance. Much of this work has yielded inconclusive or seemingly contradictory results about whether Internet-provided health information adversely affects this relationship (Broom, 2005b; Kivits, 2004). For instance, Broom (2005a) finds that while some physicians openly embrace Internet-informed patients, others view them negatively as unnecessarily complicating the medical consultation. These tenuous findings have prompted scholars to call for more research on the actual dynamics of patients' Internet use and the doctor-patient encounter (see, e.g., Broom, 2005a).

New research that arises from this call to study the dynamics of patients' Internet use and the doctor-patient encounter, however, must begin with an examination of the websites themselves. Despite political and commercial forces that operate to bring conventional health perspectives to the Internet's foreground (Seale, 2005), it is an overstatement to claim that Internet information is uniform and consistent. Internet websites are virtual spaces where actors present and rally support for their particular interests and vantage points; they are sites where battles of jurisdictional control take place (Abbott, 1988). These include promoting their conceptions of health, what it means to be a patient, and what is deemed an appropriate avenue for solving health-related problems (Kroll-Smith, 2003). For example, Barker's (2008) study of an electronic support group for those affected by the controversial illness fibromyalgia syndrome highlights how the Internet provides a place where lay experts are able to coalesce in an effort to influence what does and does not fall under the jurisdiction of medicine.

In these web competitions to define health and related meanings, each of these actors brings to the metaphorical table different goals and objectives, which result in different claims about what constitutes health care and who should have rights to oversee it. Patient awareness of such contradictions is thought to make evident the subjective qualities of medicine, thereby demystifying medical expertise and awakening patients to the notion that abstract knowledge does not necessarily mean effective professional labor (Haug, 1976). The Internet increases the likelihood of patients finding such discrepant information to the extent that patients access information from multiple and competing sources. So even though there is evidence to suggest that the Internet is converging in such a way as to become a tool of the existing power brokers in health (Seale, 2005), perusing health-related information from multiple websites nevertheless increases the likelihood of patients being exposed to different ideas about medicine and to medical disagreements about how to treat specific health problems. This, in turn, casts doubt on the sanctity of medical expertise (Hardey, 1999).

Patients who rely on multiple websites to access health-related knowledge are also likely to bring more information to the patient-doctor encounter. While theoretically this could generate a more in-depth discussion of patient health, the corporatist model that now pervades modern medicine creates disincentives for doctors to engage in lengthy discussions with patients about health information; third-party payer organizations now have greater say over what medical procedures or opinions are reimbursed and reward physicians for seeing more patients (Potter & McKinlay, 2005). Consequently, patients who access more information by combing through multiple websites might feel as though doctors give short shrift to the information they bring to the office visit. They might also uncover information that on its face disagrees with advice provided by their doctors. Such discrepancies, to the extent that they occur, might erode patient confidence in physicians.

Yet considering only the number of health-related websites an individual visits ignores where individuals actually go to access Internet-provided health information. The Internet dispenses health information from a host of self-interested actors, and these actors have different motivations for doing so. Some, like the mothers studied by Schaffer, Kuczynski, and Skinner (2007), use the Internet and health-related websites to learn and teach others about particular medical conditions. Others, like the consumer groups investigated by Jones (2008), rely on websites to promote and represent the interests of various parties such as patients, users, and caregivers. Pharmaceutical companies, health care providers, and government agencies also use websites to disseminate their respective health messages. Such diversity across health-related websites suggests the need to consider which websites people use when trying to predict how visiting health-related websites might affect the patient-doctor interaction.

One way to classify health-related websites is by examining whether websites belong to the for-profit, nonprofit, or governmental sectors. For-profit entities are driven by financial yield, while government and nonprofit organizations are not. Moreover, government and nonprofit organizations are supposed to provide or work for the public benefit (Weisbrod, 1988). Although competition for resources has driven both nonprofits and government organizations to seek out new markets and, at times, to become more commercial, the public continue to see them as more trustworthy and as having distributional goals inconsistent with the private market (Weisbrod, 1997).

This view is in part a byproduct of variation in actual organizational behavior across sectors. For example, WebMD, a for-profit website, actively advertises pharmaceuticals to consumers, while the AMA, a nonprofit entity, prohibits pharmaceutical advertisements directed toward patients on their website (AMA, 2012b). Such distinctions are interesting given that advertising has been linked to consumerism (Brody, Stoneman, Lane, & Sanders, 1981). A consumerist mentality could contribute to a worldview where doctors are expected to cater to patients as consumers and where health care is a good to be purchased, leading to less reliance on, or personal investment in, a relationship with one's own doctor.

Moreover, there is evidence to suggest that commercial for-profit websites tend to have lower information quality (Hanif et al., 2006). Accessing and bringing lower quality information to doctors might adversely affect patients' views of their interactions with doctors for several reasons. First, if the patient accesses information that counters something the doctor says, then the patient might be more likely to doubt the physician. Second, if the patient presents faulty information to the doctor, the doctor might be less receptive to that information.

In sum, extant research indicates that websites might differ in the messages that they present about what it means to be a patient. We posit that such differences in health-related web content have the potential to ultimately affect the doctor-patient encounter. To gain a more detailed understanding of how websites might differ in framing what it means to be a patient, we now examine the content of three health websites.

AN EXPLORATORY ANALYSIS OF THREE HEALTH WEBSITES

In order to understand how the Internet serves as a platform for the presentation of potentially different frames regarding health care, we examined the archived web pages of three distinct health-related websites: (1) AMA-assn.org, (2) WebMD.com, and (3) MayoClinic.com. We selected these three websites in light of their high cultural resonance and sector differences. The AMA differs from the latter two organizations in that, as a professional organization, its ultimate objective is not to serve the public but rather the physicians who serve that public. Formed in 1847, the AMA has played an instrumental role in shaping the organization of health care (Hacker, 2002). It is this history that has made the AMA a relatively pervasive symbol and a powerful and influential force in the American health care system (Starr, 1982). WebMD.com, a for-profit organization is now one of the most popular sources for health information and actively promotes its services through various television commercials and print advertisements. According to a press release by comScore (2008), a leader in measuring the digital world, WebMD is the most visited site with approximately 17.3 million visitors per month. The Mayo Clinic, a not-for-profit medical practice that is internationally renowned as a pioneer in medicine, is made up of physicians, scientists, medical students, and a host of other medical professionals, such as nurses and medical technicians. WebMD. com and MayoClinic.com were the two most common websites visited by respondents to the survey used in the quantitative portion of this chapter. The three organizations and websites we examine thus can be considered leaders in the field of health care.

Our case study of these three websites involved a discourse analysis, and an analysis of cultural objects aimed at discerning their meanings, particularly those meanings associated with the production and distribution of social knowledge (Blommaert, 2005). Because the data for the quantitative portion of this analysis comes from a survey conducted during 2000 and 2001, we relied on the Internet Archive to analyze pages from these websites during the 2000–2001 time period. The Internet Archive is a nonprofit organization that seeks to preserve Internet records for future generations (http://archive.org/web/web.php), and its Wayback Machine tool allows users to enter web addresses to view archived pages. For each organization, we used this tool to examine their respective websites, paying particular attention to the homepage or main page; the page "about" the organizational entity or website; the page describing the advertising policy; and the "terms and conditions" page. We also focused on select pages that were specifically directed to patients. Finally, where appropriate, we considered additional pages that described in greater detail the missions of these three sites. These pages comprise only a fraction of the pages on each site. Still, we believe they offer important insights into how each conceptualizes health care and the patient. Unlike previous research on the accuracy or quality of health-related information (see, e.g., Seale, 2005), we focused our analytic gaze on the messages these websites used to shape individuals' understandings of what it means to be a patient.

The websites serve different ends for each of these three organizations. For WebMD, the website is a central component to its organizational existence as it provides an opportunity to market WebMD products and services to health care professionals and to collect revenue from advertising. The AMA and the Mayo Clinic do not depend on their respective websites in this way. The AMA uses its website as a tool for assisting in advancing the medical profession through the dissemination of health and medical practice information to physicians and the public, the provisioning of information to physicians about medical ethics and education, the promotion of the Association and its advocacy activities, and the creation of a forum for members to communicate (AMA, 2001c). For the Mayo Clinic, the website is a way to advance their consumer health publishing history by providing "access to the experience and knowledge of the more than 2,000 physicians and scientists of the Mayo Clinic" (Mayo Clinic, 2001a). So, even though both of these organizations recognize the value of these websites for recruiting patients, they do not depend on them to survive and use them as tools for promoting their greater missions. In this respect, these three websites are analytically valuable because they provide venues for a host of relatively powerful actors to strategically present their messages about health and health care to the public.

Despite our suspicion that these websites would present different messages about the delivery of health care, we refrained from making any a priori judgments about what the content of each page would be for each website. Instead, each of the pages was read with an eye geared toward the natural emergence of themes and metaphors. Of course, the exploratory and qualitative nature of the study limits its scope, applicability, and potential generalizability. It is likely the case that a more exhaustive examination of these websites yields a more nuanced understanding. We also recognize that websites are dynamic entities, so findings at one point in time, may not translate to other points in time. However, we also visited the current versions of these websites in 2008 and 2012 and came to similar conclusions in regard to the frames and themes of each organization. We therefore believe our findings offer important qualitative insights that help us explain the quantitative findings that we report later.

Complementary and Alternative Messages about Health

Given that each of the websites examined are relatively mainstream websites, it is not surprising that our analysis revealed certain commonalities.

The most obvious commonality across these three websites was the emphasis on individuals taking greater control over their own health, thereby promoting the notion of self-governance (Dean, 1999). For example, the Mayo Clinic website told visitors to "take charge," and offered tools and guides for planning healthy lifestyles and self-managing their diseases (Mayo Clinic, 2001c). WebMD.com echoed this point, stating that its mission was "to help people play an active role in managing their own health" (WebMD, 2001a). In support of this mission, it too provided visitors with tools geared toward finding information on health-related issues. Compared to these two websites, the AMA website offered a more subdued message of self-governance. Still, even it had pages devoted to connecting patients with health information aimed at helping them "become an active participant in their health care" (AMA, 2001a). All of these messages are consistent with the expectation that laypersons will proactively monitor their health. That these websites display representations that align with the public's need to self-monitor is hardly surprising given that the existence of the three websites (especially, WebMD.com which as a for-profit entity relies on revenue from advertisers) depends on people continuing to seek out health information.

These similarities, however, did not conceal real differences in framing and presentation that existed across the three websites. The most noticeable difference was who or what ultimately was privileged with stewardship of care. The AMA website privileged the medical doctor. For example, while the word "physician" appeared multiple times on the site's homepage, the word "patient" only appeared once (AMA, 2001b). While the core purpose of the AMA is "to promote the science and art of medicine and the betterment of public health" (AMA, 2001c), the website tended to emphasize the role of physicians over other actors in the health care arena. In fact, even those pages directed at patients emphasized the important role of physicians, with one page providing users with a tool to find a doctor. Taken as a whole, the AMA website drove home the point that when patients conceptualize health care, they should think of physicians.

Revisiting the AMA website in 2012 showed that this website continues to privilege medical doctors with stewardship of care. For example, the homepage features a link to a letter to the editor of the *New York Times* emphasizing the importance of the role of the physician in delivering health care and advocating for physician-led health care teams (Hoven, 2012). However, more effort was taken to build a relationship between physicians and patients. For instance, on the patient page phrases such as "You and your doctor" subtly attacked the conception of physicians as interchangeable providers in favor of a more permanent relationship between the patient and physician (AMA, 2012a).

In contrast, the Mayo Clinic website promoted the organization over the individual physician. It delivered messages that encouraged patients to think of the Mayo Clinic, rather than a particular physician, as responsible for their health care. The website made clear that the Mayo Clinic provided more than just the expertise of physicians. Dietitians, scientists, and other medical experts also bring their knowledge to bear. As such, the Mayo Clinic is able to provide answers to user questions from a team of Mayo Clinic specialists (Mayo Clinic, 2001c, 2001d). By privileging the organization, this website suggests to the user the importance of getting information from an expert in *this organization*. Implied is that people should shift their thinking from an individual view of expertise to an organizational one.

The Mayo Clinic website, then, questions the ability of the individual practitioner to consistently provide quality health care. Contra the AMA's conceptualization of health care, the Mayo Clinic seems to contend that patients need a team of medical experts, not just one physician. In fact, the Mayo Clinic assured the patient that "the needs of the patient come first" and that the Mayo Clinic will "Practice medicine as an integrated team of compassionate, multidisciplinary physicians, scientists and allied health professionals who are focused on the needs of patients" (Mayo Clinic, 2001b). It can make this claim because as a large organizational entity it brings to bear all of its resources in the pursuit of solving medical problems. Thus, the messages put forth on the Mayo Clinic website contrast the messages presented on the AMA website by creating a representation of health care that privileges a large health care organization (e.g., a team of 2,000 physicians and scientists at the Mayo Clinic) over the individual medical expert. Still, like the AMA, it recognizes the value of authoritative health knowledge and encourages individuals to seek out expert medical professionals when trying to solve their health problems.

WebMD.com differs from the AMA and Mayo Clinic in that its primary interest is not tied to the actual delivery of care. Rather, as a for-profit entity it aims to generates profits, in part by attracting advertisers who seek to market their products to site users. Attracting these advertisers requires WebMD.com to show that a large number of people visit the website. In turn, it must motivate people to use and continue using the site. WebMD. com accomplished this by giving visitors access to "condition-specific centers and support communities, interactive tools and programs, as well as online health and lifestyle product catalogues and ordering services"

(WebMD, 2001a). Visitors were encouraged to participate in a number of interactive ways, such as by taking a variety of online quizzes that not only tested one's health-related knowledge but also encouraged them to think about whether their symptoms were caused by certain disorders (WebMD, 2001c). Also, WebMD provided avenues for people to relay personal experiences and wisdom, such as offering stories from breast cancer survivors or by providing over 80 message boards where one could "Talk with people who understand" (WebMD, 2001b). These activities get people invested in the broader online community where they can contribute their own medical knowledge, and evaluate and receive feedback from other members and experts. Thus, while AMA privileged the doctor, and the Mayo Clinic emphasized the role of the organization, WebMD highlighted the everyday knowledge and expertise of the average individual.

Lastly, both the Mayo Clinic and the AMA strove to prohibit any advertising on their web pages that did not reflect their larger values. For example, the Mayo Clinic stated that they would "refuse any advertisement that we believe is incompatible with our mission" and prohibited advertisements for alcohol, tobacco, life or health insurance, medical products, vitamins, and certain weight loss products (Mayo Clinic, 2001a). Similarly, the AMA only offered advertising when it "does not interfere with the mission or objectives of the AMA or its publications" (AMA, 2001d). While "WebMD does not endorse any product advertised" (WebMD, 2001e) on its site, it was unclear how its mission and values informed its advertisement policy. Moreover, as a for-profit, WebMD was unique among the three organizations in that it emphasized the importance of profits to its activities by including a section directed at investors (WebMD, 2001d).

WEBSITE SELECTION AND THE
PATIENT-DOCTOR INTERACTION

Our analysis of these three websites reveals sector differences in how health organizations construct messages about health care and what it means to be a patient. While all three websites promote the active involvement of patients in health, they offer slightly different messages about who should oversee patients' medical care. The two not-for-profit websites adopt a more conventional message insofar as they encourage patients to rely on medical experts, whether they are individual physicians or an organization's medical experts. Compared to the messages on AMA-assn.org or

MayoClinic.com, the messages on WebMD.com place less emphasis on the bond between a patient and any particular physician or any particular medical provider. Instead, the WebMD website validates the patient experience as a unique form of medical expertise and encourages patients to rely on it (with the assistance of WebMD) to find the best health care possible, thereby suggesting that patients should take on a more consumerist mentality when seeking out medical advice by using their unique experiences to assess what is and is not "good" medical care.

These qualitative findings hint at the idea that organizational sector might affect the messages delivered by various health websites. Moreover, they suggest that these differences may affect how patients view the patient-doctor interaction. Given this, as well as previous research on the relevance of organizational sector (Weisbrod, 1988, 1997), we conclude that individuals who rely on nonprofit or government websites for health information should be less likely to adopt a consumerist mentality and consequently, be happier and more satisfied with the doctor-patient interaction. As such, we put forth the following hypothesis:

> **Hypothesis 1.** Patients who rely on government or nonprofit websites to access information that they later discuss with their doctors will tend to evaluate those physicians with whom they interact as more competent and more concerned about their well-being than those who do not.

In addition to these sector differences, there is also reason to suspect that visiting multiple websites for health information might affect the patient-doctor interaction. The sheer amount of information provided by each of the three websites we explored is evident. If a patient were to access all of this information and bring it to the doctor, it would be very difficult to sift through it in the time typically allotted for medical consultations, and patients who attempt to do so are likely to feel rushed and to view their physicians as dismissive. Furthermore, and as we noted earlier, all of this information increases the possibility of patients discovering discrepant information about medicine and their medical conditions, thereby undermining the sanctity of medical expertise (Hardey, 1999). Following this, we hypothesize the following:

> **Hypothesis 2.** Patients who rely on multiple health-related websites to find information that they later discuss with their doctors will tend to evaluate those physicians with whom they interact as less competent and less concerned about their well-being than patients who frequent only one website.

QUANTITATIVE DATA AND ANALYTIC STRATEGY

These hypotheses suggest that, because different websites promulgate different conceptions of health, patterns of health-related web use matter. To test these hypotheses, we rely on ordinary least squares regression analyses. These analyses were conducted using the appropriate probability weight; excluding the weight produced comparable results. Our data come from the *Impact of the Internet and Advertising on Patients and Physicians Survey* (Lo, 2004). This survey, conducted between 2000 and 2001, relied upon a stratified sampling technique to create a cross-sectional representative sample of adults in the continental United States. From the larger sample, we depend on information from a subsample of 94 adults who had spoken with their doctor about information they gathered from the Internet and which was relevant to their health and who identified the websites they visited. Individuals in this subsample were asked a battery of questions regarding Internet use, including which websites they visited, and the last time they talked with their doctor during an office or clinic visit about information pulled from the Internet.

The subsample was achieved through several steps. First, the 3,209 survey respondents were asked if they had used the Internet to look for health-related information in the past 12 months; 1,077 respondents answered affirmatively to this question. Of these, 572 were asked if they had talked to a doctor during an office clinic visit about information they had seen on the Internet that was relevant to their health; 305 respondents answered yes. These respondents were asked to name the website(s) that provided the information from a list of 32 websites or, if none of the websites applied, to freely name the website(s) they visited. Although 149 of the 305 respondents provided the name of the website(s) they used, 55 cases were unusable as rather than providing the name of the website, the data was simply coded as other. Thus, the final sample consisted of 94 respondents who visited websites from the prompted list. List-wise deletion was used for missing data.

Variables

The two dependent variables for the regression analyses come from survey respondents' answers to the following questions:

- How would you rate how well [your doctor] answered your questions when you brought the information [from the Internet] to the visit?

• How would you rate how well [your doctor] listened when you brought the information [from the Internet] to the visit?

The first question indirectly addresses a patient's evaluation of his or her physician's competence. If a patient does not believe his or her doctor is able to adequately answer his or her questions, then he or she has reason to doubt the doctor's medical knowledge. The second question speaks to patients' perceptions of their doctors' personal concern, because as others have acknowledged (Hawkins-Walsh, 2000), listening is an important means for medical workers to show that they care about the patient and what he or she is going through. Responses to both questions were measured on a 5-point scale where 1 indicates poor, 2 indicates fair, 3 indicates good, 4 indicates very good, and 5 indicates excellent.

Two independent variables enable us to address the hypotheses posed. Whether an individual received information from either a government or a nonprofit website allows us to test Hypothesis 1. To this end, we constructed an independent variable that measures whether or not a patient relied on a government or nonprofit website to access health information by performing an Internet search for each of the 21 websites identified by respondents and evaluating whether each website was for-profit, not-for-profit, or government. A few of the websites were defunct at the time of data collection. For these, we relied on Lexis-Nexis academic universe and Google search engine to find news clippings detailing their sector status. We assigned a code of 1 whenever a respondent accessed a website that was either government or nonprofit, and a code of 0 whenever a respondent only accessed for-profit websites. An individual could access information from both a government or nonprofit website and a for-profit website and still receive a score of 1. For seven cases, we were unable to come to a determination, because the respondent provided a non-listed website in addition to a listed for-profit website. We coded these indeterminate cases as missing.

Our second independent variable is whether a respondent used multiple websites to gain information that he or she later presented to his or her physician for discussion. We created this dichotomous variable by looking across each of the cases to determine if multiple websites were identified. A score of 1 indicates the use of multiple websites, and a score of 0 indicates otherwise. We use this variable to evaluate Hypothesis 2, which states that in comparison to patients who rely on a single website, patients who visit multiple websites will rate their doctors as less competent and concerned about their medical well-being.

In addition to these two primary independent variables, we control for various relevant variables. These include whether a respondent, when assessing the reliability of Internet gathered information, considers if the website was commercially funded. Research finds that individuals vary in terms of being net-savvy and able to critically assess health information (Eysenbach & Köhler, 2002). Controlling for this variable therefore distinguishes between different types of Internet-informed patients. This variable was measured using a four-point scale ("Not at all," "Not much," "Some," and "A great deal") where respondents indicated the extent to which they considered, if at all, the commercial underpinnings of the website.

We also control for whether a respondent told his or her doctor that the information came from the Internet. This variable is important because, as Broom (2005b) suggests, some doctors, upon identifying that a patient is Internet-informed, will engage in strategies to assert their dominant position, such as, ignoring questions, making patients feel disapproved of, and treating patients as problems. Controlling for this variable accounts for these potential differences in physician behaviors. For this measure, a score of 1 indicates that the patient informed his or her doctor, and a 0 indicates he or she did not.

To control for respondents' unique health situations, we include a measure of self-rated health, where 1 represents poor health and 5 represents excellent health. We do not control for whether respondents had health insurance or a regular doctor as these two variables lacked variation, with the gross majority of respondents having both health insurance and a regular doctor. As such, our findings are most applicable to individuals who have both health insurance and a regular doctor.

Finally, we controlled for various socio-demographic variables, including age, income, sex, and race. Age and income are ordinal variables. Age ranges from 1 to 5 (1 = 19 to 29, 2 = 30 to 39, 3 = 40 to 49, 4 = 50 to 59, and 5 = 60 to 69). We worked with six income ranges. These categories respectively represent an annual income of: $24,999 or less, $25,000 to $34,999, $35,000 to $49,999, $50,000 to $74,999, $75,000 to $99,999, and $100,000 or more. Sex and race are dichotomous variables. A score of 1 on sex indicates male, while a score of 1 on race indicates being nonwhite. We present the descriptive statistics for these variables in Table 1.

Table 1. Descriptive Statistics.

	Mean	St. Dev.	Min.	Max.	N
Socio-demographics					
Health of patient (1 = poor, 5 = excellent)	3.59	1.04	1	5	94
Age (1 = 19 to 29, 5 = 60 to 69)	2.70	1.13	1	5	94
Income (1 = 24,999 or less, 5 = 100,000 or more)	3.46	1.53	1	6	89
Sex (0 = female, 1 = male)	0.47		0	1	94
Race (0 = white, 1 = nonwhite)	0.23		0	1	94
Website use					
Multiple websites (0 = No, 1 = Yes)	0.29		0	1	94
Government or not-for-profit website (0 = No, 1 = Yes)	0.22		0	1	87
Considers commercial funding (1 = not at all, 4 = a great deal)	2.71	1.15	1	4	93
Told doctor information came from the Internet (0 = no, 1 = yes)	0.83		0	1	92
Patient evaluations of					
How well doctor listened (1 = poor, 5 = excellent)	3.76	1.14	1	5	93
How well doctor answered questions (1 = poor, 5 = excellent)	3.84	1.07	1	5	93

RESULTS

Visiting multiple websites as well as not-for-profit or government websites should affect how patients perceive their interactions with doctors. Specifically, we hypothesize a relationship between each of these variables and patients' perceptions of their doctors' competence and concern for their health. Two sets of regression analyses test these hypotheses.

The first set of regression analyses presented in Table 2 evaluates perceptions of competence. As hypothesized, individuals who relied on nonprofit or government websites evaluated the answers they received from their doctors more positively. This finding supports past research, which suggests that a consumerist mentality might shape how patients view and interact with doctors (Hardey, 1999), making them more critical of the doctor's performance. It also helps explain why previous research has produced inconclusive results about whether the Internet will change the doctor-patient interaction (Broom, 2005b). Because websites differ in their content and framing of information, this could lead to differential effects in attitudinal stances toward health care providers.

Visiting multiple websites also matters. As posited, patients who visited multiple health-related websites were less satisfied with the answers they

Table 2. Ordinary Least Squares Regression Results: Patient Evaluations of How Well Physician Answered Questions.

Independent Variables	Model 1	Model 2	Model 3
Multiple websites	−0.78*	−0.95**	−1.13**
	(0.31)	(0.32)	(0.37)
Government or not-for-profit website	0.70**	0.77**	0.73**
	(0.25)	(0.25)	(0.27)
Considers commercial funding		−0.16[+]	−0.08
		(0.10)	(0.11)
Told doctor information came from Internet		0.26	0.44
		(0.31)	(0.33)
Health of patient			−0.02
			(0.13)
Age			−0.06
			(0.12)
Income			0.01
			(0.07)
Sex			0.54*
			(0.24)
Race			−0.51*
			(0.24)
Constant	3.93	4.16	3.93
	(0.14)	(0.33)	(0.45)
N	86	84	79
R^2	0.10	0.17	0.24

Notes: All regression coefficients are unstandardized and were obtained using the appropriate probability weight. Standard errors are in parentheses.
[+] < 0.1; * < 0.05; ** < 0.01; two-tailed tests.

received when they asked doctors questions about the information they had gleaned from the Internet. Presumably, visiting multiple websites improves patients' ability to critically evaluate medical advice and increases skepticism of that advice.

In addition to these variables, we found a relationship between two of the control variables and patient evaluations of the answers provided by physicians. Compared to women, men rated answers more positively. Compared to white individuals, nonwhite patients rated answers less positively. These findings confirm past research on the effects of gender and race for the patient-doctor interaction (Malat, 2001; Shi, 1999; Street, Gordon, Ward, Krupat, & Kravitz, 2005) and illustrate how status processes shape these interactions.

A second set of regression analyses examines the impact of health-related website usage on "patient evaluations about how well the doctor listened" when he or she brought Internet-accessed information to the visit (see Table 3). The independent variables yielding statistically significant relationships with the dependent variable include viewing a government or not-for-profit website, visiting multiple websites, and telling one's doctor that the information came from the Internet.

As hypothesized, viewing a government or nonprofit website had a statistically significant positive effect on evaluations of how well the doctor listened. Given our qualitative findings about how these different types of websites frame what it means to be a patient, there is reason to suspect that this finding follows from these discrepant messages. Patients who only visited for-profit websites may have entered into the doctor-patient interaction

Table 3. Ordinary Least Squares Regression Results: Patient Evaluations of How Well Physician Listened.

Independent Variables	Model 1	Model 2	Model 3
Multiple websites	−0.59*	−0.80**	−1.03*
	(0.27)	(0.25)	(0.40)
Government or not-for-profit website	0.78***	0.80***	0.81**
	(0.23)	(0.21)	(0.28)
Considers commercial funding		−0.19+	−0.08
		(0.11)	(0.12)
Told doctor information came from Internet		0.82*	1.13**
		(0.39)	(0.38)
Health of patient			−0.11
			(0.13)
Age			−0.10
			(0.12)
Income			0.07
			(0.07)
Sex			0.35
			(0.28)
Race			−0.10
			(0.25)
Constant	3.83	3.71	3.45
	(0.16)	(0.40)	(0.50)
N	86	84	79
R^2	0.08	0.23	0.28

Notes: All regression coefficients are unstandardized and were obtained using the appropriate probability weight. Standard errors are in parentheses.
+ < 0.1; * < 0.05; ** < 0.01; *** < 0.001, two-tailed tests.

with a more consumerist mentality, which could lead to greater expectations that the doctor should spend more time listening and responding to the concerns of the patient, thus raising the bar for doctors to receive positive ratings. This, however, may not be the only explanation for this effect. It may also have to do with the quality and source of the information, with doctors being more receptive to hearing information pulled from government or nonprofit sites. More research is needed to flesh out this possibility.

Additionally, there was a relationship between visiting multiple websites and patients expressing lower evaluations about how well physicians listened. Given that telling the doctor that the information came from the Internet resulted in patients feeling that doctors were more willing to listen, we suspect that the negative relationship between visiting multiple websites and perceptions of listening is a product of the sheer amount of information the patient is trying to present. Increasingly physicians are pressured to see a certain number of patients (Waitzkin, 2001), reducing the time physicians can spend listening to any one patient. Thus, patients who bring more information to the medical encounter may feel as though physicians listen to them less. Another possibility is that because sources can provide discrepant information, a patient who has visited multiple websites may not be as clear when relaying medical information, potentially presenting contradicting viewpoints. This could lead doctors to dismiss patients as being confused or misinformed and reduce the amount of time they are willing to listen to the patient. Clearly, more research is needed to disentangle the exact mechanisms underlying how visiting multiple websites affects patients' perceptions of physicians or if individuals predisposed to criticize doctors are more likely to visit multiple websites prior to their visits.

The final significant variable was telling the doctor the information came from the Internet. This variable had a positive effect on how well patients perceived their doctors to listen. Contrary to research which suggests that physicians might engage in strategies to reestablish the boundaries of the traditional interaction and dismiss outright the information (Broom, 2005a; Henwood, Wyatt, Hart, & Smith, 2003), this finding suggests that making one's doctor aware of where the information came from might have positive implications for the doctor-patient encounter.

These results yield general support for the two hypotheses. First, they show that visiting government and nonprofit websites results in an increase in evaluations about how well physicians listened and answered Internet-prompted questions. To the degree that these measures reflect competence and concern for patient's well-being, respectively, we find support for Hypothesis 1. Using the same logic, the negative relationship between viewing multiple websites and the two dependent variables implies empirical support for Hypothesis 2. Combined, these findings suggest the importance of considering usage patterns when discussing the effects of the Internet-informed patient on the patient-doctor encounter. They also lend quantitative support to the qualitative evidence that the messages and frames promulgated by various Internet actors differentially affect understandings about what it means to be a patient and patients' understandings of health care.

DISCUSSION AND CONCLUSION

These findings suggest that when investigating the Internet-informed patient, it is important to consider variations in what it means to be Internet-informed. Respondents have varying patterns of Internet use, and these patterns affect how they perceive physicians with whom they interact. In particular, viewing multiple websites leads to decreased evaluations about how well doctors listen and answer questions. This finding lends evidence to current commentary about how the dissemination of more and more health information to patients will generate a growing skepticism in medicine and doctors. It also supports previous research, which finds that greater health knowledge makes patients more likely to challenge physician authority (Haug & Lavin, 1979, 1981).

Our study also reveals that the websites upon which people rely matter. Websites differ in how they frame and present content. We find that accessing either a government or nonprofit website increases evaluations about how well doctors listened and how well they answered questions, suggesting that the type of content presented by these providers might make patients more likely to evaluate doctors positively. In our content analysis, we found some support for this: the two nonprofit websites, the AMA and the Mayo Clinic, tended to prioritize the role of doctors and expert opinion, while the for-profit website, WebMD, provided the most opportunities for users to post and discuss their own experiences with, and opinions about, health care, emphasizing the expertise of the lay individual. Another possible explanation is self-selection, that the types of people who visit nonprofit and government sites are also the types of people who report higher evaluations of their doctors. While more research is needed to see if this is the case, a logistic regression analysis (not shown) regressing the nonprofit/government website variable on the different socio-demographic variables did not produce any significant results, suggesting that there were not notable differences in the characteristics of individuals choosing for-profit versus nonprofit websites. By exploring both the usage of health-related websites by patients and the content of some of those websites, this study begins to speak to the processes and mechanisms underlying differences in Internet use and doctor-patient interactions, while also contributing to the existing research on sector differences in health care (see Schlesinger & Gray, 2006).

A noteworthy point involves the significant positive relationship between telling one's doctor that the information came from the Internet and patient evaluations about how well the doctor listened. This finding runs counter to prior qualitative research which suggests that physicians, upon hearing that a patient is Internet-informed, will reject, dismiss, or discard the information (Broom, 2005a; Henwood et al., 2003). It seems that doctors, as a whole, may not be as hostile to the presentation of this information as some have found. Rather, and in line with other research (Broom, 2005b), doctors might be more inclined to view this information as enhancing the encounter and thus be more open to it.

Despite the merits of this research, we recognize its limitations. The survey data was collected over 10 years ago and Internet usage patterns may have changed in the interim. However, we hold that the logic of our hypotheses is not dependent on a particular time period and that the general conclusions of our research remain valid. Further, while we have posited various mechanisms underlying the results of this study, additional research, such as in-depth interviews with patients and doctors, would be ideal for identifying the exact processes that guide how patients use information from the Internet in their encounters with physicians. Finally, our case study of the three websites was exploratory in nature and only examined three websites. Future research should build on this to more extensively examine and uncover the similarities and differences across health websites and to track whether they systematically vary by sector.

Still, the results from this study are important as they suggest a continuing need to flesh out nuances about what it means to be an Internet-informed patient. Our qualitative investigation indicates that various actors within the health care arena are using the Internet to present different conceptions of health care. The regression analyses extend this by showing that how people use the Internet to access health-related information affects the doctor-patient interaction. Discovering that sector affects patients' perceptions of their interactions with doctors adds to what we know about the effects of health websites for the delivery of health care. Additional scholarship would benefit from more research into the on-the-ground processes and mechanisms by which selecting and reading information on health care websites ultimately affects health care perceptions and decisions. By mapping these processes we better understand how the Internet is transforming personal attitudes and actions in the health care arena.

REFERENCES

Abbott, A. (1988). *The system of professions: An essay on the division of expert labor*. Chicago, IL: The University of Chicago Press.

American Medical Association. (2001a, November 15). *'Patients*. Retrieved from http://web.archive.org/web/20011115081900/http://www.ama-assn.org/ama/pub/category/3158.html

American Medical Association. (2001b, November 15). *Homepage*. Retrieved from http://web.archive.org/web/20011115012357/http://www.ama-assn.org/

American Medical Association. (2001c, November 16). *Mission*. Retrieved from http://web.archive.org/web/20011116093050/http://www.ama-assn.org/ama/pub/category/1913.html

American Medical Association. (2001d, November 16). *Principles for advertising and sponsorship*. Retrieved from http://web.archive.org/web/20011116001837/http://www.ama-assn.org/ama/pub/category/1905.html

American Medical Association. (2012a). *AMA resources for patients*. Retrieved from http://www.ama-assn.org/ama/pub/patients/patients.page? Accessed on December 29, 2012.

American Medical Association. (2012b). *Advertise with us*. Retrieved from http://www.ama-assn.org/ama/pub/category/9609.html. Accessed on December 29, 2012.

Anderson, A. (2002). In search of the Holy Grail: Media discourse and the new human genetics. *New Genetics and Society, 21*, 327–337.

Anderson, J. G., Rainy, M. R., & Eysenbach, G. (2003). The impact of CyberHealthcare on the physician-patient relationship. *Journal of Medical Systems, 27*, 67–84.

Barker, K. K. (2008). Electronic support groups, patient-consumers, and medicalization: The case of contested illness. *Journal of Health and Social Behavior, 49*, 20–36.

Benford, R. D., & Snow, D. A. (2000). Framing processes and social movements: An overview and assessment. *Annual Review of Sociology, 26*, 611–639.

Blommaert, J. (2005). *Discourse: A critical introduction*. Cambridge: Cambridge University Press.

Brody, G. H., Stoneman, Z., Lane, T. S., & Sanders, A. K. (1981). Television food commercials aimed at children, family grocery shopping, and mother-child interactions. *Family Relations, 30*, 435–439.

Broom, A. (2005a). Medical specialists' accounts of the impact of the internet on the doctor/patient relationship. *Health: An Interdisciplinary Journal for the Social Study of Health, Illness, and Medicine, 9*, 319–338.

Broom, A. (2005b). Virtually he@lthy: The impact of internet use on disease experience and doctor-patient relationship. *Qualitative Health Research, 15*, 325–345.

comScore. (2008). *Online health information category grows at a rate four times faster than total internet.* Retrieved from http://www.comscore.com/Press_Events/Press_Releases/2008/09/Top_Internet_Healths_Sites. Accessed on January 21, 2012.

Conrad, P. (1992). Medicalization and social control. *Annual Review of Sociology, 18*, 209–232.

Dean, M. (1999). *Governmentality: Power and rule in modern society.* London: Sage.

Eysenbach, G., & Köhler, C. (2002). How do consumers search for and appraise health information on the world wide web? Qualitative studies using focus groups, usability tests and in-depth interviews. *British Medical Journal, 324*, 573–577.

Fox, S. (2006). *Online health search 2006.* Washington, DC: Pew Internet and American Life Project. Retrieved from http://www.pewinternet.org. Accessed in April 2008.

Hacker, J. S. (2002). *The divided welfare state: The battle over public and private social benefits in the United States.* New York, NY: Cambridge University Press.

Hanif, F., Sivaprakasam, R., Butler, A., Huguet, E., Pettigrew, G. J., Michael, E. D. A., ... Gibbs, P. (2006). Information about liver transplantation on the world wide web. *Medical Informatics and the Internet in Medicine, 31*, 153–160.

Hardey, M. (1999). Doctor in the house: The internet as a source of lay health knowledge and the challenge to expertise. *Sociology of Health and Illness, 21*, 820–835.

Haug, M. R. (1976). The erosion of professional authority: A cross-cultural inquiry in the case of the physician. *The Milbank Memorial Fund Quarterly. Health and Society, 54*, 83–106.

Haug, M. R., & Lavin, B. (1979). Public challenge of physician authority. *Medical Care, 17*, 844–858.

Haug, M. R., & Lavin, B. (1981). Practitioner or patient – Who's in charge? *Journal of Health and Social Behavior, 22*, 212–229.

Hawkins-Walsh, E. (2000). Listening. *The American Journal of Nursing, 100*, 24BBB–24DDD.

Henwood, F., Wyatt, S., Hart, A., & Smith, J. (2003). "Ignorance is bliss sometimes": Constraints on the emergence of the "informed patient" in the changing landscapes of health information. *Sociology of Health and Illness, 25*, 589–607.

Hilgartner, S., & Bosk, C. L. (1988). The rise and fall of social problems: A public arenas model. *American Journal of Sociology, 94*, 53–78.

Hoven, A. D. (2012). Who should provide our medical care? *New York Times*, December 29. Retrieved from http://www.nytimes.com/2012/12/24/opinion/who-should-provide-our-medical-care.html?src=twrhp&_r=0

Jones, K. (2008). In whose interest? Relationships between health consumer groups and the pharmaceutical industry in the UK. *Sociology of Health and Illness, 30*, 929–943.

Kivits, J. (2004). Researching the "informed patient": The case of online health information seekers. *Information, Communication & Society, 7*, 510–530.

Kivits, J. (2009). Everyday health and the internet: A mediated health perspective on health information seeking. *Sociology of Health and Illness, 31*, 673–687.

Kroll-Smith, S. (2003). Popular media and "excessive daytime sleepiness": A study of rhetorical authority in medical sociology. *Sociology of Health and Illness, 25*, 625–643.

Lo, B. (2004). Impact of the internet and advertising on patients and physicians, 2000–2001: [United States] [Computer file]. ICPSR version. Bernard Lo, University of California, San Francisco [producer], CA. Ann Arbor, MI: Inter-university Consortium for Political and Social Research [distributor].

Malat, J. (2001). Social distance and patients' rating of healthcare providers. *Journal of Health and Social Behavior, 42*, 360–372.

Mayo Clinic. (2001a, August 11). *About MayoClinic.com: Welcome and mission.* Retrieved from http://web.archive.org/web/20010811161957/http://www.mayohealth.org/home?id=9.1.1.1

Mayo Clinic. (2001b, December 18). *About Mayo Clinic: Mission and values.* Retrieved from http://web.archive.org/web/20011218174005/http://www.mayoclinic.org/about/mission values.html

Mayo Clinic. (2001c, November 15). *Homepage.* Retrieved from http://web.archive.org/web/20011115013242/http://www.mayoclinic.com/index.cfm?

Mayo Clinic. (2001d, September 17). *Homepage.* Retrieved from http://web.archive.org/web/20010917020051/http://www.mayohealth.org/home

Potter, S. J., & McKinlay, J. B. (2005). From a relationship to encounter: An examination of longitudinal and lateral dimensions in the doctor-patient relationship. *Social Science & Medicine, 61*, 465–479.

Schaffer, R., Kuczynski, K., & Skinner, D. (2007). Producing genetic knowledge and citizenship through the internet: Mothers, pediatric genetics, and cybermedicine. *Sociology of Health and Illness, 30*, 145–159.

Schlesinger, M., & Gray, B. H. (2006). Nonprofit organizations and health care: Some paradoxes of persistent scrutiny. In W. W. Powell & R. Steignberg (Eds.), *The nonprofit sector: A research handbook* (2nd ed.). New Haven, CT: Yale University Press.

Seale, C. (2005). New directions for critical internet health studies: Representing cancer experience on the web. *Sociology of Health and Illness, 27*, 515–540.

Shi, L. (1999). Experience of primary care by racial and ethnic groups in the United States. *Medical Care, 37*, 1068–1077.

Starr, P. (1982). *The social transformation of American medicine.* New York, NY: Basic Books.

Street, R. L., Gordon, H. S., Ward, M. M., Krupat, E., & Kravitz, R. L. (2005). Patient participation in medical consultations: Why some patients are more involved than others. *Medical Care, 43*, 960–969.

Waitzkin, H. (2001). *At the front lines of medicine.* New York, NY: Rowman & Littlefield.

WebMD. (2001a, November 19). *About us.* Retrieved from http://web.archive.org/web/20011118191500/http://www.webmd.com/corporate/index.html

WebMD. (2001b, October 30). *Homepage.* Retrieved from http://web.archive.org/web/20011030193227/http://my.webmd.com/

WebMD. (2001c, November 14). *Health e-tools.* Retrieved from http://web.archive.org/web/20011114220518/http://my.webmd.com/health-e-tools/3838

WebMD. (2001d, November 27). *Investor information.* Retrieved from http://web.archive.org/web/20011127172333/http://www.webmd.com/corporate/content/investor/content.investor.html

WebMD. (2001e, November 15). *Terms and conditions of use.* Retrieved from http://web.archive.org/web/20011115023629/http://my.webmd.com/medcast_channel_toc/1762#adlinks

Weisbrod, B. (1988). *The nonprofit economy.* Cambridge, MA: Harvard University Press.

Weisbrod, B. (1997). The future of the nonprofit sector: Its entwining with private enterprise and government. *Journal of Policy Analysis and Management, 16*, 541–555.

REJECT, DELAY, OR CONSENT? PARENTS' INTERNET DISCUSSIONS OF THE HPV VACCINE FOR CHILDREN AND IMPLICATIONS FOR HPV VACCINE UPTAKE

Kathy Livingston, Kathleen M. Sutherland and Lauren M. Sardi

ABSTRACT

Purpose — *The purpose of this research is to investigate how parents and caregivers describe their concerns about the HPV vaccine for their children on open Internet websites. The study examines what the discourse among parents reveals about their concerns regarding the HPV vaccine.*

Methodology/approach — *Our exploratory study utilized a grounded theory approach as a method of collecting data and simultaneously formulating research questions based on emerging themes from the data.*

Technology, Communication, Disparities and Government Options in Health and Health Care Services
Research in the Sociology of Health Care, Volume 32, 117–139
ISSN: 0275-4959/doi:10.1108/S0275-495920140000032018

We used purposeful sampling to select sets of comments posted on websites that provided news, scientific information, or parental support regarding HPV and its vaccine.

Findings — *Findings suggest support for Bond and Nolan's (2011) theory that familiarity with a disease is central to parents' assessment of risk, and that dread of a serious disease such as cervical cancer is weaker than dread of unknown possible side effects in parents' motivation to give or withhold the vaccine for their children.*

Research limitations/implications — *Research limitations include our usage of a purposeful convenience sample of websites. The limitation of this sampling technique is that the comments made by website "users" and used in the analysis may not be representative of the wider population, and may include Americans as well as non-Americans.*

Originality/value of chapter — *Our research fills an important gap in the literature by looking at the ways in which parents share their concerns about the HPV vaccine on Internet websites as they consider whether to reject, delay, or consent to the vaccine.*

Keywords: Health information seeking; HPV; vaccines; risk assessment

PURPOSE

The Human Papilloma Virus (HPV) is a symptomless, sexually transmitted infection with an incidence rate in the United States of 6.2 million new cases per year (CDC, 2013). Merck & Co., Inc. created the first HPV vaccine called Gardasil, which was initially approved in 2006 by the U.S. Food and Drug Administration for use in females aged 9 through 26 to prevent HPV types 6 and 11, known to cause genital warts, and HPV types 16 and 18, known to cause cervical cancer. More recently, in 2009, the quadrivalent vaccine was approved for use in males aged 9 through 26 (Liddon, Hood, Wynn, & Markowitz, 2010). The vaccine does not treat or cure HPV, however, and can only be preventative if given before the onset of sexual activity. Although the median age of sexual initiation for American children is 17 (Daley et al., 2006) a small proportion of girls — about 4% — initiate sexual activity before age 13, and this data ultimately influenced policy decisions to target 11- and 12-year-old females for immunization

(Daley et al., 2010). Thus, in 2006, The Advisory Committee on Immunization Practices (ACIP) of the Centers for Disease Control recommended that the quadrivalent vaccine be included in the routine immunization of girls aged 11 and 12, and that females between the ages of 13 and 26 who have not yet had the vaccine or completed the vaccine series should get "catch-up" vaccines (CDC, 2013). In 2011, The ACIP recommended the routine vaccination of boys aged 11 and 12, with "catch-up" vaccines to age 21 (Reiter, McRee, Pepper, Chantala, & Brewer, 2012).

Notably, although nearly 70% of cervical cancer cases and 90% of genital warts cases are linked to just four strains of HPV, the vaccine does not protect against all strains of HPV (CDC, 2013). Researchers have found that 70% of untreated HPV infections clear up in one year, and 90% clear up in two years (Committee on Infectious Diseases, 2012; Moscicki et al., 1998). In addition, the vaccine provides protection against HPV in females for only up to four years (National Cancer Institute, 2013). It is no wonder that some have difficulty weighing the short-term efficacy of the HPV vaccine against the possible adverse side effects.

The Internet has become increasingly important for people seeking information regarding their health concerns. Those who search the Internet have been shown to have more knowledge about health issues (Brewer, 2005) and tend to be more health-oriented (Dutta-Bergman, 2004). Health information seeking enables lay people to learn more about their diagnosis and become increasingly knowledgeable about treatment options; thus, this access to information has transformed the doctor–patient relationship to one of greater equality for the patient in terms of shared medical decision making (Hardey, 1999, 2001; Hartzband & Groopman, 2010). As a result, patients can discuss additional information with their doctors in order to make an informed and appropriate decision.

The purpose of this research is to investigate how parents and caregivers describe their concerns about the HPV vaccine for their children on open Internet websites, or websites that are not password protected. The study examines what the discourse among parents reveals about their tacit and explicit concerns regarding the HPV vaccine. We hypothesized that parents' Internet discussions would be more ambiguous and complex, such that it would be difficult to divide their comments into either "pro" or "anti" vaccine camps. We first explain the significance of the Internet to parents seeking health information about the HPV vaccine and then discuss the current literature about parents' attitudes and behaviors regarding the HPV vaccine for their children. We then offer insight into which HPV vaccine-related issues are essential to parents, and provide a more nuanced view of the incentives and disincentives to immunizing one's child in the future against HPV.

The Significance of the Internet for Health and Vaccine Information

Internet use is widespread and growing rapidly. Approximately 71% of adults in the United States have Internet access (Pew Internet & American Life Project, 2008) and, of those, approximately 80% use the Internet to find health information about: a specific illness; diet and exercise; prescription drugs; preparing for a doctor visit; alternative or experimental treatments; mental health issues; sensitive health topics that are difficult to talk about; and information about a particular doctor or hospital (Fox & Rainie, 2002). The Internet has the potential to help health care consumers become better informed (Baker, Wagner, Singer, & Bundorf, 2003; Berger, Wagner, & Baker, 2005) and has emerged as a mechanism for positive health behavior changes (Ayers & Kronenfeld, 2007; Baker et al., 2003).

Despite the Internet's potential for improving overall health, several concerns exist that information seeking on the Internet may lead lay people to self-diagnose, disregard a physician's advice, or refuse treatment altogether; according to Fox and Rainie (2002, p. 4) "... more people go online for medical advice on any given day than actually visit health professionals, according to figures provided by the American Medical Association." In fact, earlier research found no negative effect on health care utilization as a result of Internet searching (Baker et al., 2003). Ybarra and Suman (2006) found that seeking online health information made Internet users feel more comfortable with their health care provider's advice (Ybarra & Suman, 2006), and these results were especially reliable for those with stigmatized illness conditions (Berger et al., 2005). More recent research, however, has noted a link between online health information seeking and noncompliance with professional medical recommendations (Weaver, Thompson, Weaver, & Hopkins, 2009).

Thus, a second concern has emerged in that lay people do not have sufficient medical expertise to evaluate information on the Internet and this lack of knowledge may cause individuals to make bad or inappropriate health decisions (Nettleton, Burrows, & O'Malley, 2005). Concerns that lay knowledge is insufficient are based on the dominant medical paradigm that regards illness as merely biological and sees conventional medical knowledge as uniformly true (Freidson, 1970). In contrast, the sociological perspective holds that illness is not only biological but that the illness experience involves a negotiation between patient and provider (Brown, 1995; Conrad & Barker, 2010). The social construction of illness perspective also suggests that lay people construct meaning and shape ideas about illness through tacit social agreements about what is considered "acceptable" versus "unacceptable" illness behavior. Hence, lay people construct medical knowledge through interaction with or in addition to assistance from medical professionals (Freidson, 1970).

The sociological perspective demonstrates that, along with illness being socially constructed, medical knowledge is socially constructed, as well; while the dominant medical paradigm may be based on a process of deductive scientific experiment and discovery, it is also the result of sociopolitical and economic forces which allow certain scientific ideas to advance or "succeed" while causing other ideas, which may be just as accurate, to recede or "fail" (Latour, 1987). Just as medical professionals or public health officials have legitimate concerns that lay people will access "accurate" knowledge about HPV on the Internet, lay people have legitimate concerns that HPV information from the Internet will be more inclusive than that given to them by their health care providers. When health problems arise, the attitudes, values, and normative expectations will be different for patients than for medical providers because of their different social roles.

For lay people, the Internet has changed the illness experience from a solitary and private experience to one that can be shared with other lay people having similar health problems or illnesses. The sharing of online health information has resulted in the formation of "illness subcultures" and the proliferation of thousands of online support group websites (Conrad & Stults, 2010) and enables lay people to be *producers* as well as consumers of health knowledge (Hardey, 2001). The Internet is a crucial resource for lay people with ongoing medical needs, mobility issues, and permanent disabilities (Braithwaite, Waldron, & Finn, 1999) to seek, share, and assess health information with like-minded others. Online support and sharing of health information has been found to be associated with positive changes in health attitudes and behaviors among those managing chronic illness (Ayers & Kronenfeld, 2007; Baker et al., 2003; Cotten, 2001).

Given the thousands of health information websites available on the Internet, how do users know what health information to trust? Little is known about how health information seekers choose which websites to read; for example, it is unclear how many read Medline for the results of medical research as compared with Blogs and websites that allow users to share anecdotes and health-related experiences. Fox and Rainie (2002) found that online users have a high level of trust to begin with, as 72% of respondents stated that they would trust all or most of the health information found online. Trust in health information found online has been found to be greater: when the source is a known organization rather than a commercial website; when the knowledge is codified more than anecdotal or experiential knowledge such as that found in chat rooms; and when information is found on more than one website (Nettleton et al., 2005; Pew Internet & American Life Project, 2008).

Predicting what online information lay people will trust has implications for the study of parents seeking online information about HPV because discussions about vaccines have become contentious, due in part to the recent controversy over the Measles, Mumps, and Rubella (MMR) vaccine that played out on the Internet and spilled over into daily conversations; such claims revolved around the idea that Thimerosal, which the vaccine initially contained, causes Autism. Although researchers now conclude definitively that there is no causal relationship between the MMR vaccine and Autism, there is some indication that the MMR controversy may have "cried wolf" for future vaccine discussion, causing those who question the safety and efficacy of any vaccine to become stigmatized and labeled with the pejorative term: "anti-vaxx." Parents commonly want information about drugs, vaccines, or medical procedures for their child before consenting to them. However, the HPV vaccine uptake program coming on the heels of the Autism controversy may make it difficult for parents to have their concerns about the HPV vaccine heard or taken seriously. Studies of parents' attitudes toward the HPV vaccine tend to be hortatory; they assume that the dominant medical paradigm is true for both physicians and lay people, and insist that increasing parents' "knowledge" about the HPV vaccine will increase HPV vaccine uptake overall (Perkins, Pierre-Joseph, Marquez, Iloka, & Clark, 2010; Reynolds & O'Connell, 2012). But these studies equate lay knowledge with conventional medical knowledge and undervalue the importance of parents' wisdom in the socially constructed definitions of health and illness. These studies also ignore the complexities inherent in the decision-making process about whether to vaccinate one's child against HPV, including the fact that immunization against a sexually transmitted disease for children is, heretofore, unprecedented for parents.

Zimmerman et al. (2005) warn that "anti-vaccination" websites have the potential to influence parents' refusal of vaccination for their children. To date, however, no empirical studies have measured this. Some websites considered "anti-vaxx" websites might actually contribute to vaccine uptake by allowing parents to consider the information and experiences posted by other parents and then reconsider that information at a later date.

Parents and the HPV Vaccine

Studies of parents indicate that acceptance of the HPV vaccination, at least for daughters, is generally high, with most parents holding positive views about the HPV vaccine (Gerend, Weibley, & Bland, 2009; Marlow, Waller, & Wardle, 2007; Olshen, Woods, Austin, Luskin, & Bauchner, 2005). Epidemiological data show that uptake of the HPV vaccine is increasing; for example, of all girls in the United States, age 13–17, 37% were vaccinated in 2008 and 48% were vaccinated in 2010. However, this rate of uptake is slower than expected by the CDC and other public health officials (Dorell, Yankey, Santibanez, & Markowitz, 2011). And if parents' compliance with other immunization schedules is any harbinger, HPV uptake may continue to be sluggish; a recent study showed that 13% of parents with children age 6 and under alter the vaccination schedule recommended by the CDC or refuse to vaccine their children altogether (Dempsey, Schaffer, Butchart, Davis, & Freed, 2011).

Parental fear that the HPV vaccine will promote sexual activity or promiscuity in daughters is a reality but one which is held by a minority of parents (Constantine & Jerman, 2007; Gerend et al., 2009; Zimet, Liddon, & Rosenthal, 2006). Parental dread about possible adverse side effects from a vaccine is telling; Raithatha, Holland, Gerrard, and Harvey (2003) found that thinking about harmful side effects provoked feelings of dread even when parents realize that such side effects are rare. In particular, parents dreaded the possibility of long-term disability for their very young children. Bond and Nolan (2011) found that parents who dread the unknown or long-term side effects of a vaccine were less likely to immunize their child than parents who merely dreaded the disease in question.

The most important factor influencing parents' approval of the HPV vaccine for daughters is a doctor's recommendation (Brewer & Fazekas, 2007; Dorell et al., 2011; Gerend et al., 2009; Grantham, Ahern, & Connolly-Ahern, 2011; Liddon et al., 2010) but only 53% of parents said their doctor had ever recommended the HPV vaccine. Studies of physicians show that most general practitioners and pediatricians are likely to recommend the HPV vaccine, but they are less likely to recommend it for their 11- and 12-year-old patients than they are for the 13- through 18-year-old group (Daley et al., 2010; Feemster, Winters, Fiks, Kinsman, & Kahn, 2008; Hughes, Jones, Feemster, & Fiks, 2011; Weiss, Zimet, Rosenthal, Brennerman, & Klein, 2010). Hence, the age group for whom physicians are least likely to recommend the HPV vaccine is the age group identified by the CDC as the most important age group to target.

The strongest predictor of the tendency to recommend the HPV vaccine for teens but not preteens is physicians' reluctance to discuss sexuality and the sexual activity of very young children (Daley et al., 2010, 2006; Kahn et al., 2005; Riedesel et al., 2005). This reluctance stems from physicians' apprehension about parents' discomfort in discussing the sexual activity of their children and concerns about the vaccine (Daley et al., 2006; Feemster et al., 2008; Hughes et al., 2011; Kahn et al., 2007).

Hughes et al. (2011) found that some parents delayed, rather than refused, the HPV vaccine for their child, and when these parents expressed their reluctance to vaccinate, clinicians were hesitant to engage them in a discussion about it. Thus, if physicians and parents are reluctant to discuss the vaccine for preteens, how, then, do parents of young children learn about HPV and the HPV vaccine?

In a survey of parents (Hughes et al., 2009) or caregivers of girls between 10 and 18 years of age, most respondents (83%) had heard of the HPV vaccine through pharmaceutical company advertisements, but less than half, or 45%, had heard of the vaccine from health care providers. The Internet was the *least* likely source of having heard about the HPV vaccine (22%) but was the *most* likely source respondents chose when asked about future information seeking about the vaccine (Hughes et al., 2009).

Various studies about use of the Internet to learn about vaccines, in general, found that many websites were "anti-vaccination" in nature, that they were increasing in number, and that the vitriol found there might influence parents to refuse inoculating their children (Zimmerman et al., 2005). Only one study was found regarding parents' use of the Internet to seek information specifically about HPV and the HPV vaccine; McRee, Reiter, and Brewer (2012) found that Internet use was associated with higher levels of knowledge and positive attitudes toward the vaccine for all parents, with parents of daughters more willing to consent to the HPV vaccine than parents of sons. Thus, our research fills an important gap in the literature by looking at the ways in which parents share their concerns about the HPV vaccine on Internet websites as they consider whether to reject, delay, or consent to the vaccine.

METHODOLOGY

This study is based on grounded theory (Glaser & Strauss, 1967) as a method of collecting data and simultaneously formulating research questions based on themes that emerge from the data, with the ultimate goal of developing a theory about the process by which parents converse about the HPV vaccine (Leedy & Ormrod, 2005). This research is exploratory; first, we wanted to explore parents' ideas, attitudes, and beliefs about the vaccine *from their point of view* as both consumers and providers of information. Second, this research uses unobtrusive measures (Webb, Campbell, Schwartz, & Sechrest, 1966) to discover which concerns seemed most relevant to parents; thus we "listened in" on parents' conversations by analyzing their comments on Internet websites. The combination of a grounded theory approach with unobtrusive research measures was particularly useful in looking at ways in which such texts "exist independent of the research process" (Hesse-Biber & Leavy, 2004, p. 303). Rather than interacting with parents, we chose to observe and examine linguistic and thematic patterns that emerged organically from online textual data. Texts are important to study in particular because they reflect current thinking as well as power/knowledge relations that are constantly being (re)shaped over time (see Hall, 1981).

In an attempt to reflect a balance in the websites, we used purposeful sampling to select sets of comments posted on 21 websites that provided news, scientific information about HPV, or parent support. (For a more detailed discussion of purposeful sampling through online methods, see Mann & Stewart, 2004.) Approximately one-third of these websites were concerned specifically with the HPV/Gardasil vaccine; these websites appeared as early as 2009. Another third of the websites were online news sources that reported a "breaking" news story about the HPV vaccine on a particular day, which was followed by discussion comments over the days or weeks that followed. About a third of the remaining websites were "science blogger" websites specific to the HPV vaccine which offered conventional biomedical evidentiary information about the vaccine. From the entire set of 21 websites, 15 websites were selected based on two criteria: (1) if the website appealed directly to parents or had the word "parent" or "daughter" or "son" in the banner; and (2) if the website appeared after the Gardasil vaccine was approved for use in both girls and boys (Table 1).

Data analysis relied on the selective coding (Strauss & Corbin, 1998) of ideas that emerged in each set of comments on 15 websites. The repetition of these ideas across websites allowed us to form themes within the data, and we present the interrelationships of these themes as "major concerns" in the discussion and debate among parents (Leedy & Ormrod, 2005, p. 141). We coded data according to common themes that emerged from parents' comments (Hesse-Biber & Leavy, 2004).

Table 1.   List of Websites Utilized in Study.

1.	Grandmother Protests Gardasil Dosed on CA Boy Without Parental Consent Under AB499	http://www.ageofautism.com/2011/10/ grandmother-protests-gardasil-dosed-on-ca-boy.html
2.	Local Woman Questions Grandson's HPV Vaccination	http://www.10news.com/politics/ 29524532/detail.html
3.	Parents Talk: To Give or Not to Give the Gardasil Vaccine?	http://westdesmoines.patch.com/articles/ parents-talk-to-give-or-not-to-give-the-gardasil-vaccine
4.	Are Parents Avoiding the Sex Talk – or Gardasil?	http://mommyish.com/pregnancy-health/ are-parents-avoiding-the-sex-talk-or-gardasil-144/
5.	Gardasil Side Effects: A Public Forum on Gardasil Side Effects	http://www.gardasilhpv.com/
6.	Gardasil: What About the Boys?	http://gerardnadal.com/2011/10/31/ gardasil-what-about-the-boys/
7.	Gardasil – HPV Vaccine	http://www.cbc.ca/news/health/story/ 2009/08/19/gardasil-hpv-vaccine-explainer263.html
8.	HPV Vaccine for Boys Recommended in Canada	http://www.cbc.ca/news/health/story/ 2012/01/25/hpv-vaccine-males-gardasil. html
9.	Surprise, Surprise! CDC Recommends Gardasil for All Young Boys	http://www.thehealthyhomeeconomist. com/surprise-surprise-cdc-recomm ends-gardasil-for-8-year-old-boys/
10.	Gardasil Human Papillomavirus Vaccine	http://www.rateadrug.com/Gardasil-Human-Papillomavirus-Vaccine-user-reviews-and-comments.aspx#
11.	27 Dirty Little Vaccine Secrets Every Parent Needs to Know About	http://vactruth.com/2011/11/04/27-dirty-little-vaccine-secrets/
12.	Christian Parents and the HPV Vaccine	http://www.firstthings.com/onthesquare/ 2011/06/christian-parents-and-the-hpv-vaccine
13.	Parents Delaying, Skipping Recommended Vaccines	http://www.reuters.com/article/2011/10/ 03/us-vaccines-idUSTRE7920HH201 11003
14.	We Need to Talk About HPV – Seriously	http://www.newscientist.com/article/ dn20928-we-need-to-talk-about-hpv-vaccination–seriously.html
15.	Should Boys Be Given the HPV Vaccine?	http://blogs.discovermagazine.com/crux/ 2011/11/14/should-boys-be-given-the-hpv-vaccine-the-science-is-weaker-than-the-marketing/#.UOM1AuTLe4I

We wanted to get parents' ideas and comments from a source that would yield the most uninhibited and uncensored comments as possible. Although our sample is nonrandom and does not represent all parents, the benefits to utilizing textual data from the Internet is due to its nature as a public forum which also allows for anonymity. The reliability of data from focus groups or attitudinal surveys can be compromised by the Hawthorne effect or participants who feel inhibited from expressing their honest opinions. Due to the anonymity of the textual data, we believe this analysis investigates parents' real concerns as they exist in parents' every-day lives. While we have no evidence to prove that those who claim to be parents actually are parents, we are attempting to balance the issue of authenticity and anonymity, in that obtaining further data to verify a user's identity also compromises their anonymity in the first place (Mann & Stewart, 2004). Clearly, the balance of achieving authentic data while protecting anonymity remains a core methodological dilemma in unobtrusive, online data collection. Across these websites, two types of conversational activity are seen: (1) information sharing; and (2) debating the issue. Users share relevant information including "anti-vaccine" as well as "pro-vaccine" information. Some of the information shared by users is inaccurate according to current, conventional medical knowledge about the vaccine and such "wrong" comments invite correction by other discussants. Many users also include links in their post to other websites or to published medical studies for further reading about vaccine risks/benefits and epidemiology.

FINDINGS

Analysis of parents' discourse on HPV vaccine websites showed that controversy does not break down along clear lines. Ostensibly, discussants appeared either "pro-vaccine" or "anti-vaccine," but a deeper analysis indicates that the discussion was more rich and complex. Because websites are places where discussants can post anonymously, many are free to express their feelings, including fears, as well as their thoughts on the issue. Some discussants used screen names and posted numerous times on a site, or on different websites, and we discerned that a discussant's comment could be perceived as "anti-vaxx" in one post yet "pro-vaxx" in another post. These initial findings allowed us to analyze the data in a more detailed and nuanced way, which led to a number of themes which emerged over time.

Themes Reflected in the Data and Data Analysis

Proportionally, the most frequent theme of discussion is the safety (e.g., "Will the vaccine cause adverse side effects for my child?") and efficacy (e.g., "How long would my child be protected from HPV?" and "How complete is the protection?") of the vaccine, with comments about safety being more numerous. The other main themes found in the data include sexuality of the child; age of immunization for HPV; gender issues; and conflict among parents with their process of information seeking. Because many websites reflect parents' concerns about vaccine safety in general and concerns about other vaccines, our research addresses only those concerns specific to the HPV vaccine.

Safety and Efficacy Specific to the HPV Vaccine

Parents use many websites in their quest for health and vaccine information, including the website for Merck & Co., Inc., the manufacturer of Gardasil, which details how the vaccine has been tested and shown to be safe in the general population. The safety concerns mentioned most frequently by parents are about possible side effects, and the idea is bolstered by the fact that, by Merck's own admission, 73% of clinical trial subjects acquired a new medical condition by the end of the trial study. Thus, some parents visit and refer other parents to websites containing anecdotal evidence and stories about young women who experience mild to severe health problems after receiving the first, second, or third dose of the vaccine. Symptoms of these reported health problems included migraine headache, fatigue, missed menstrual periods, seizures, muscle, joint or bone pain, nerve damage, chronic fatigue, chemical sensitivities, and death, as reported to the Vaccine Adverse Event Reporting System (VAERS). Parents also caution other parents to not believe all that they read on these or other "anti-vaxx" websites. No comments favorable to Merck were found, and in general, parents referring specifically to Merck & Co. expressed distrust; for example, some parents noted that Merck rushed the vaccine to market without adequate testing, and that trials of Gardasil on which government approval were based, lacked testing for carcinogeneity and genotoxicity. Parents expressed worry that the way the vaccine works in an individual child is not the same as what is found in the highly controlled and limited world of a clinical trial. Some fear that Gardasil is associated with *more serious* side effects than other vaccine shots given to similar aged children, such as the MMR vaccine. Parents advised one another to delay the vaccine until more information is known about adverse side effects. No comments addressed those cases of delay where a child starts the vaccine and does not follow through with subsequent (second and third) doses. At the same time, many parents argue that the vaccine has been shown to be safe, it is effective, and that the government should pay for it.

Along with the discussion about side effects are comments about vaccine efficacy; for example, some parents stated that the vaccine had not been tested on children, specifically girls under 15 years of age, while other parents argued that this was not worth worrying about. An additional concern is that the prevention of HPV has been shown to last only a few years, so that vaccinating a child at 11 years of age, for example, may not protect her if she becomes sexually active five years later. Some parents also argued that the vaccine does not protect against all types of HPV, and others offered comments to help one another discern which strains of HPV children would be inoculated against. Parents grappled with trying to understand technical medical information, as when a study published by the Committee on Infectious Diseases from the American Academy of Pediatrics reported that "… the body rids itself of HPV infection on its own 95% of the time within 2 years if no vaccine is given" (evidence most recently reported by the Committee on Infectious Diseases, 2012). This concept was difficult for many parents to interpret, and their comments show an attempt to help one another to figure out the "odds" of vaccinating versus not vaccinating against HPV. In their assessment of risk, parents discussed their own risk for "anticipatory regret" if they withhold the vaccine now and later find it was a wrong decision. One parent said: "It's quite possible that in 10, 20, 30 years one of my kids will be one of the tiny minority of women who suffer the effects of a persistent HPV infection, and I'll bitterly regret my choice. It's also quite possible that if I gave it to them I would be one of the tiny minority of parents who bitterly regret saying yes to Gardasil. There's no perfect choice" (Website 5).

This quote makes clear the heavy burden parents carry from having to weigh the benefits of giving versus not giving the vaccine. In effect, parents assess risk by choosing between dread of the possible disease, itself, and dread of the unknown side effects or health hazards that they believe can result from vaccinating their child (Bond & Nolan, 2011).

Age of the Child

When a parent asked, "if my child is not having sex, why do I have to approve the vaccine?" other parents explained that the vaccine can be effective only if given before the child initiates sexual activity, and that the CDC recommends that children age 9 and over be vaccinated. Some parents were appalled by the recommended age for this vaccine because they found it difficult to think about their child's sexuality and the prevention of a sexually transmitted disease when their child is so young. As one parent said: "My son is 8, is home schooled and he focuses on nouns, wanting to be an artist and other non-sexual activity" (Website 9). Other parents warned that preventing disease should be paramount and cautioned one another that thinking one's child is not old enough to be sexual is naïve and potentially dangerous. In fact, some parents equated refusal to vaccinate with bad parenting and admonished one another for doing so. For many parents, however, the question of when to vaccinate presents a real quandary because some feel that giving the vaccine to one's child will give the child license to begin having sex.

Sexual Activity and Talking with Children about HPV

Parents debated the notion that children, if vaccinated against HPV, will start having sex or become "promiscuous" because they will take their parents' approval as tacit endorsement to initiate sex. "Promiscuous" was the buzzword for this notion, and parents debated this idea intellectually rather than expressing fear that their own child would actually do so. Some pointed out that withholding the vaccine will not prevent a child from initiating sexual contact while others said that the HPV vaccine would not promote "promiscuity," since it only protects against one, and not other, sexually transmitted infections. The suggestion was often made to "talk with your child about sex" and this was done in both contexts of approving the vaccine and delaying or withholding the vaccine. For example, some parents were adamant that every attempt should be made to protect one's child, such as getting the HPV vaccine as well as educating one's child about sexual and reproductive health. One parent, for example, said: "I can see why this vaccine is a little scary. But if you're discussing sex with your kids, nothing about this should be controversial."

Others saw educating one's child about sex and urging abstinence as a way to avoid getting the HPV vaccine: "… For now, explaining to them the serious risks of the vaccine and of immoral behavior, not to mention teaching good values, should be sufficient protection from HPV (something that is very unpleasant and can cause but is not guaranteed to cause cancer many years down the road)" (Website 6). Another parent commented: "Let's teach our children it's not okay to sleep around with whoever, whenever rather than that it's okay to sleep around, and if you do, there are drugs that will protect you if you do so" (Website 9).

The topic of discussing sex with one's child brought the act of parenting, as a whole, into question and was a theme that incited angry comments suggesting that parents who withhold the vaccine are irresponsible, or that children are not protected if they feel they can't talk to their parents about sex. For example, one parent noted that: "To imply that people would rather take their chances with their daughters' lives rather than sit down and have an uncomfortable talk with them is not only wrong, it's insulting."

Some parents who expressed strong religious prohibitions against premarital sex also expressed strong views against the HPV vaccine. One parent suggested that parents could vaccinate the child but not tell the child what the vaccine is for, as well as getting the doctors and nurses to "play along," so that the child would be protected against HPV but not know it. Parents with religious views that were central in their decision making about the HPV vaccine brought about responses from others who remarked that children are more sexually savvy than most are willing to admit, and that parents who think their children will delay having sex at an early age or stay celibate are "kidding themselves."

Gender Issues

Use of the HPV vaccine for boys is relatively new and some parents expressed the assumption that boys are the carriers of HPV and that they spread it to girls. Others expressed concern that males are the carriers of HPV but females have a greater disease burden from the risk for cervical cancer. These assumptions may explain why the majority of gender-specific comments referred to girls; discussions about sexual activity or "promiscuity" increased after the HPV vaccine pointed to girls as the target of concern. These comments reflected an awareness of the double standard for girls – that it is acceptable for boys to have many sexual partners, but not for girls – or that young women bear the sole burden in preventing sexually transmitted diseases like HPV: "It's unfair to girls that they are viewed as gatekeepers of teen sexuality and are taught to deny their sexuality and should 'just say no' to boys. But not giving the vaccine isn't going to *stop* them from having sex ....." Thus, this double standard existed solely for girls but was not found to be present when discussing the issue of vaccinating boys.

A combined gender/efficacy concern was found in these discussions, as is illustrated by the following statement from an online user: "The efficacy is different in boys and girls. The efficacy (for HPV 18) is lost in 35% of girls after 5 years. The efficacy for boys (for strains 6 and 11) is lost in 38% of boys after 2 years." This comment is representative of parents' attempts to help one another assess the risks and benefits involved as they grapple with confusion over whether the vaccine's efficacy is different for boys than for girls. Parents' comments reflected a gender difference, albeit slight, in their concerns about vaccinating their child but no parent mentioned an intention to refuse the vaccine based on gender.

Conflict among Discussants in Information Seeking

Previous studies of "anti-vaxx" websites (Davies, Chapman, & Leask, 2002; Nasir, 2000; Zimmerman et al., 2005) make no mention of the effort parents spend trying to learn about vaccines nor do they address the level of technical discussion within parents' vaccine discussions. One parent noted: "I'm impressed at the quality of discussion on this page, given the contentiousness of the issue" (Website 6). Parents are faced with many tough junctures in the decision tree to assess what is best for their child. One physician (Haug, 2009, p. 795) who has critiqued the HPV vaccine movement asked: "So how should a parent ... or anyone else decide whether it is a good thing to give young girls a vaccine that partly prevents infection caused by a sexually transmitted disease, an infection that, in a few cases will cause cancer 20 to 40 years from now?"

As previously mentioned, the overall topic of responsible parenting is hotly contested in these discussions. On one hand, parents who question vaccine safety complain about those parents who follow recommendations for this vaccine, blindly, calling them sheep or "sheeple;" as one parent says "The sheeple must wake up, or they're lambs docilely going to slaughter" (Website 9). On the other hand, there are parents who believe in the concept of herd immunity; that if some but not all children are immunized, the vaccine uptake program will not eliminate HPV from the population. They see those parents who delay or refuse to vaccinate as both ignorant parents and irresponsible citizens. One parent drew this divide, saying: "I'm glad someone has realized that Gardasil has to protect girls AND boys from HPV. The only way to prevent infection is to vaccinate everyone before they're sexually active. I'm sick of the anti-vaccine community scaring parents off decisions that will protect their children's long-term health."

Our data continue to suggest that the issues are far too complex to be easily bifurcated into "pro-vaxx" and "anti-vaxx," as is illustrated by the following quote:

> Please understand that I am not an anti-vaccine vigilante; far from it. This is quite a different sort of vaccine than those which prevent communicable and deadly childhood illnesses. In fact, I spent almost 14 years of my legal practice as a health care lawyer, and most of them at HHS. Many of my family members are physicians. What has concerned me most about this vaccine, is that parents are not being given adequate information about the potential downsides of it. Not because of a conspiracy among doctors of course, but because the primary care docs simply haven't received much information about the negatives – all while their associations, the CDC and State governments are giving it a major push into widespread public use, even to the extent of requiring it for rising middle schoolers in some districts ... The only criticism I would make is of the editor's casual dismissal of self-reported websites ... as being unreliable, compared to peer reviewed studies. While that's generally true, one has to also realize that many of these families do so because they have no other avenue of reporting. (Website 15)

There was both criticism of and support for the use of anecdotal evidence by parents, with one parent stating: "The editor (of this blog) has several times recommended caution in considering anecdotes and VAERS reports of adverse HPV vaccine reactions. Parental anecdotes are also eyewitness accounts, and certainly should not be routinely discounted; the simple fact is, if the vaccine left terrible consequences in its wake for even one girl, it certainly can damage others, and medical science has no way of predicting who will react adversely."

These data suggest that website parents are motivated to learn about the vaccine, and that they do not draw clear lines in the sand about the HPV vaccine when they discuss their numerous concerns.

SOCIAL IMPLICATIONS

There are a number of substantive and theoretical implications of these findings. First, there is support for the "dread" theory about parents' risk assessment of vaccines; Bond and Nolan (2011) suggest that people are "lay epidemiologists" and must make judgments frequently about disease with each new epidemic that emerges. When parents must assess whether to immunize their child against a particular disease, it is not the number of people affected by that disease but the familiarity or unfamiliarity with the disease and characteristics of those who have it that determine whether parents will take preventive action. When parents were familiar with a disease, for example the flu, and knew many people who had it, they were less likely to immunize their child against that disease. But diseases where parents had *less* familiarity were associated with dread of the disease, and these "unfamiliar" parents fell into two groups: "Immunizers" dread that the risk of getting the disease may be small but that the outcome of the disease will be severe and they are unwilling to run that risk. They fear that the worst will happen if their child gets the disease. "Non-immunizers," on the other hand, dread the unknown of long-term effects of a vaccine on their child's overall health; they believe that if their unvaccinated child gets the disease, the complications will be small or manageable compared to the long term and unknown safety risks that can follow vaccination (Bond & Nolan, 2011).

HPV is a disease that parents of young children may be unfamiliar with because they may not know of anyone who has it; first, although estimates suggest that HPV is very common in the population, symptoms are silent and many who have it do not know it and thus cannot talk openly about it. Second, those who do know they have HPV would be unlikely to disclose it to others due to the stigma associated with having a sexually transmitted disease. What is of paramount importance for this study is that HPV is a disease that parents of young children may not be familiar with, and our data suggest that parents are more likely to dread the unknown than to dread a disease they have no experience with. As one parent said:

> When I was very young, polio was an epidemic and moms worried that kids would catch this highly contagious disease and die a very young death – or be paralyzed or disabled if one was lucky enough to catch this disease and still live. So when the polio vaccine came out, everyone got it …. Moms had already known of children in grade school who had died of polio and even IF the polio vaccine had some risk (actually it was quite safe) the risks would have been worth it considering the risk of the illness. But HPV is a different story in many ways. Healthy kids playing on school playgrounds don't get cervical cancer and die – the average age of a cervical cancer patient is 48 years old …. the women at risk are adult women, decades older than the 11 year olds now being vaccinated. And for those 11 year olds, the risks (of adverse effects) are now, and very serious. (Website 6)

Our findings suggest that the parents we studied have high levels of health knowledge in general but, as "lay epidemiologists" (Bond & Nolan,

2011) they do not believe everyone in the population has an equal risk for HPV. They may lack familiarity with HPV if they do not know of or see many people in the population with the disease, and consequently, they may not perceive the disease as a serious or imminent threat for their young children. For example, no comments were made that began with the concept of "I have a friend who has HPV" or "people I know who have HPV disease do this." We suggest that future studies might examine parental perception of HPV as a serious threat along with their knowledge level about HPV and what causes it. In addition, future research should examine the function of dread, as it is described by Bond and Nolan (2011), to examine whether dread of the disease or dread of the unknown is the more important factor in parents' decision-making process about the HPV vaccine for their children, especially very young children.

LIMITATIONS OF THIS STUDY

It is important to note that there are several limitations of our study. For example, hundreds of websites were available but not included in our study; we used a purposeful convenience sample of websites at a time when news stories about the HPV vaccine were ubiquitous. The limitation of this sampling technique is that the comments made by website "users" and used in the analysis may not be representative of the wider population, may include Americans as well as non-Americans, and may overrepresent a particular group. As previously noted, we assumed that a website user was a parent if he or she identified themselves as such. There may be a tendency for particular types of parents to be disproportionately represented on particular Internet websites, so that parents who have negative regard for the vaccine may outnumber those who have a positive one, although our analysis did not find that to be the case.

REFERENCES

Ayers, S., & Kronenfeld, J. (2007). Chronic illness and health-seeking information on the Internet. *Health: An Interdisciplinary Journal for the Social Study of Health, Illness and Medicine, 11*(3), 327–347.

Baker, L., Wagner, T., Singer, S., & Bundorf, M. (2003). Use of the Internet and e-mail for health care information: Results from a national survey. *The Journal of the American Medical Association, 289*(18), 2400–2406.

Berger, M., Wagner, T., & Baker, L. (2005). Internet use and stigmatized illness. *Social Science & Medicine, 61*, 1821–1827.

Bond, L., & Nolan, T. (2011). Making sense of perceptions of risk of diseases and vaccinations: A qualitative study combining models of health beliefs, decision making and risk perception. *BMC Public Health, 11*, 943. Retrieved from http://www.biomedcentral. com/1471-2458/11/943. Accessed on January 20, 2012.

Braithwaite, D., Waldron, V., & Finn, J. (1999). Communication of social support in computer-mediated groups for people with disabilities. *Health Communication, 11*(2), 123–151.

Brewer, N., & Fazekas, K. (2007). Predictors of HPV vaccine acceptability: A theory-informed, systematic review. *Preventive Medicine, 45*, 107–114.

Brewer, N. T. (2005). The impact of Internet use on health cognitions and health behavior. In C. P. Haugtvedt, K. M. Machleit, & R. Yalch (Eds.), *Online consumer psychology: Understanding and influencing consumer behavior in the virtual world*. Mahwah, NJ: Lawrence Erlbaum.

Brown, P. (1995). Naming and framing: The social construction of diagnosis and illness. *Journal of Health and Social Behavior, 36*(Extra Issue), 34–52.

CDC (The Centers for Disease Control and Prevention). (2013). Retrieved from http://www. cdc.gov/std/hpv/STDFact-HPV-vaccine-young-women.htm. Accessed on January 26.

Committee on Infectious Diseases. (2012). HPV vaccine recommendations. *Pediatrics, 129*, 602–605.

Conrad, P., & Barker, K. (2010). The social construction of illness: Key insights and policy implications. *Journal of Health and Social Behavior, 51*(S), S67–S79.

Conrad, P., & Stults, C. (2010). The Internet and the experience of illness. In C. E. Bird, P. Conrad, A. M. Fremont, & S. Timmermans (Eds.), *Handbook of medical sociology* (6th ed., pp. 179–191). Nashville, TN: Vanderbilt University Press.

Constantine, N., & Jerman, P. (2007). Acceptance of human papilloma-virus vaccination among Californian parents of daughters. *Journal of Adolescent Health, 40*, 108–115.

Cotten, S. R. (2001). Implications of Internet technology for medical sociology in the new millennium. *Sociological Spectrum: Mid-South Sociological Association, 21*(3), 319–340.

Daley, M., Crane, L., Markowitz, L., Black, S., Beaty, B., Barrow, J., ... Kempe, A. (2010). Human papillomavirus vaccination practices: A survey of US physicians 18 months after licensure. *Pediatrics, 126*(3), 425–443.

Daley, M., Liddon, N., Crane, L., Beaty, B., Barrow, J., Babbel, C., ... Kempe, A. (2006). A national survey of pediatrician knowledge and attitudes regarding human papilloma-virus vaccination. *Pediatrics, 118*(6), 2280–2289.

Davies, P., Chapman, S., & Leask, J. (2002). Antivaccination activists on the World Wide Web. *Archives of Disease in Childhood, 87*(1), 22–25.

Dempsey, A., Schaffer, D., Butchart, A., Davis, M., & Freed, G. (2011). Alternative vaccination schedule preferences among parents of young children. *Pediatrics, 128*, 848–856.

Dorell, C., Yankey, D., Santibanez, L., & Markowitz, L. (2011). Human papillomavirus vaccination series initiation and completion: 2008–2009. *Pediatrics, 128*, 830–839.

Dutta-Bergman, M. J. (2004). Health attitudes, health cognitions, and health behaviors among Internet health information seekers: Population based survey. *Journal of Medical Internet Research, 6*(2), e15.

Feemster, K., Winters, S., Fiks, A., Kinsman, S., & Kahn, J. (2008). Pediatricians' intention to recommend human papillomavirus (HPV) vaccines to 11- to 12-year-old girls postlicensing. *Journal of Adolescent Health, 43*(4), 408−411.

Fox, S., & Rainie, L. (2002). *Vital decisions: How Internet users decide what information to trust when they or their loved ones are sick.* Pew Internet & American Life Project: Online report. Retrieved from http://www.pewinternet.org

Freidson, E. (1970). *The profession of medicine: A study of the sociology of applied knowledge.* New York, NY: Dodd, Mead & Co.

Gerend, M., Weibley, E., & Bland, H. (2009). Parental response to human papillomavirus vaccine availability: Uptake and intentions. *Journal of Adolescent Health, 45*, 528−531.

Glaser, B. G., & Strauss, A. (1967). *The discovery of grounded theory.* Chicago, IL: Aldine.

Grantham, S., Ahern, L., & Connolly-Ahern, C. (2011). *Merck's one less campaign: Using risk message frames to promote the use of Gardasil in HPV prevention.* Retrieved from http://www.academia.edu/1104233/Mercks_One_Less_Campaign_Using_Risk_Message_Frames_to_Promote_the_Use_of_Gardasil_in_HPV_Prevention. Accessed on July 7, 2012.

Hall, S. (1981). Notes on deconstructing "the popular". In R. Samuel (Ed.), *People's history and socialist theory.* London: Routledge.

Hardey, M. (1999). Doctor in the house: The Internet as a source of health knowledge and a challenge to expertise. *Sociology of Health and Illness, 21*(6), 820−835.

Hardey, M. (2001). "E-health:" The Internet and the transformation of patients into consumers and producers of health knowledge. *Information, Communication & Society, 4*(3), 388−405.

Hartzband, P., & Groopman, G. (2010). Untangling the web: Patients, doctors, and the Internet. *New England Journal of Medicine, 362*(12), 1063−1066.

Haug, C. (2009). The risks and benefits of HPV vaccination. *The Journal of the American Medical Association, 302*(7), 795−796.

Hesse-Biber, S. N., & Leavy, P. (Eds.). (2004). *Approaches to qualitative research.* New York, NY: Oxford.

Hughes, C. C., Jones, A. L., Feemster, K. A., & Fiks, A. G. (2011). HPV vaccine decision making in pediatric primary care: A semi-structured interview study. *BMC Pediatrics, 11*, 74.

Hughes, J., Cates, J., Liddon, N., Smith, J., Gottlieb, S., & Brewer, N. (2009). Disparities in how parents are learning about the human papilloma vaccine. *Cancer Epidemiology Biomarkers Prevention, 18*(2), 363−372.

Kahn, J., Rosenthal, S., Tissot, A., Bernstein, D., Wetzel, C., & Zimet, G. (2007). Factors influencing pediatricians' intention to recommend human papillomavirus vaccines. *Ambulatory Pediatrics, 7*(5), 367−373.

Kahn, J., Zimet, G., Bernstein, D., Riedesel, M., Lan, D., Huang, B., & Rosenthal, S. (2005). Pediatricians' intention to administer human papillomavirus vaccine: The role of practice characteristics, knowledge, and attitudes. *Journal of Adolescent Health, 37*, 502−510.

Latour, B. (1987). *Science in action: How to follow scientists and engineers through society.* Cambridge, MA: Harvard University Press.

Leedy, P., & Ormrod, J. E. (2005). *Practical research.* Upper Saddle River, NJ: Pearson Prentice Hall.

Liddon, N., Hood, J., Wynn, B., & Markowitz, L. (2010). Acceptability of human papillomavirus vaccine for males: A review of the literature. *Journal of Adolescent Health, 46*, 113–123.

Mann, C., & Stewart, F. (2004). Introducing online methods. In S. N. Hesse-Biber & P. Leavy (Eds.), *Approaches to qualitative research*. New York, NY: Oxford.

Marlow, L. A. V., Waller, J., & Wardle, J. (2007). Parental attitudes to pre-pubertal HPV vaccination. *Vaccine, 25*, 1945–1952.

McRee, A., Reiter, P., & Brewer, N. (2012). Parents' Internet use for information about HPV vaccine. *Vaccine, 30*(25), 3757–3762.

Moscicki, A., Shiboski, S., Broering, J., Powell, K., Clayton, L., Jay, N., ... Palefsky, J. (1998). The natural history of human papillomavirus infection as measured by repeated DNA testing in adolescent and young women. *Journal of Pediatrics, 132*(2), 277–284.

Nasir, L. (2000). Reconnoitering the antivaccination web sites: News from the front. *Journal of Family Practice, 49*(8), 731–733.

National Cancer Institute. (2013). *Human papillomavirus (HPV) vaccines*. Retrieved from http://www.cancer.gov/cancertopics/factsheet/prevention/HPV-vaccine. Accessed on January 28, 2013.

Nettleton, S., Burrows, R., & O'Malley, L. (2005). The mundane realities of the everyday lay use of the Internet for health, and their consequences for media convergence. *Sociology of Health & Illness, 27*(7), 972–992.

Olshen, E., Woods, E. R., Austin, S. B., Luskin, M., & Bauchner, H. (2005). Parental acceptance of the human papillomavirus vaccine. *Journal of Adolescent Medicine, 37*, 248–251.

Perkins, R., Pierre-Joseph, N., Marquez, C., Iloka, S., & Clark, J. (2010). Why do low-income minority parents choose human papillomavirus vaccination for their daughters? *The Journal of Pediatrics, 157*(4), 617–622.

Pew Internet & American Life Project. (2008). Retrieved from http://www.pewinternet.org. Accessed on May 30, 2013.

Raithatha, N., Holland, R., Gerrard, S., & Harvey, I. (2003). A qualitative investigation of vaccine risk perception amongst parents who immunize their child: A matter of public health concern. *Journal of Public Health Medicine, 25*(2), 161–164.

Reiter, P., McRee, A. L., Pepper, J., Chantala, K., & Brewer, N. (2012). Improving human papillomavirus vaccine delivery: A national study of parents and their adolescent sons. *Journal of Adolescent Health, 51*(1), 32–37.

Reynolds, D., & O'Connell, K. (2012). Testing a model for parental acceptance of human papillomavirus vaccine in 9-to 18-year-old girls: A theory-guided study. *Journal of Pediatric Nursing, 27*, 614–625.

Riedesel, J., Rosenthal, S., Zimet, G., Bernstein, D., Huang, B., Lan, D., & Kahn, J. (2005). Attitudes about human papillomavirus vaccine among family physicians. *Journal of Pediatric Adolescent Gynecology, 18*(6), 391–398.

Strauss, A., & Corbin, J. (1998). *Basics of qualitative research: Techniques and procedures for developing grounded theory* (2nd ed.). Thousand Oaks, CA: Sage.

Weaver, J., Thompson, N., Weaver, S., & Hopkins, G. (2009). Healthcare non-adherence decisions and Internet health information. *Computers in Human Behavior, 25*, 1373–1380.

Webb, D., Campbell, D., Schwartz, R., & Sechrest, L. (1966). *Unobtrusive measures: Nonreactive research in the social sciences*. Chicago, IL: Rand McNally.

Weiss, T., Zimet, G., Rosenthal, S., Brennerman, S., & Klein, J. (2010). Human papilloma-virus vaccination of males: Attitudes and perceptions of physicians who vaccinate females. *Journal of Adolescent Health, 47*, 3–11.

Ybarra, M., & Suman, M. (2006). Help seeking behavior and the Internet: A national survey. *International Journal of Medical Informatics, 75*, 29–41.

Zimet, G. D., Liddon, N., & Rosenthal, S. L. (2006). Psychosocial aspects of vaccine accept-ability. *Vaccine, 24*(Suppl. 3), S201–S209.

Zimmerman, R. K., Wolfe, R. M., Fox, D. E., Fox, J. R., Nowalk, M. P., Troy, J. A., & Sharp, L. K. (2005). Vaccine criticism on the World Wide Web. *Journal of Medical Internet Research, 7*(2), 1438–8871.

PART IV
GOVERNMENT ROLES AND
LESSONS FROM OTHER
COUNTRIES

DETERMINANTS IN NORWEGIAN LOCAL GOVERNMENT HEALTH PROMOTION – INSTITUTIONAL PERSPECTIVES [☆]

Marit K. Helgesen and Hege Hofstad

ABSTRACT

Purpose – *This chapter analyses and discusses local government health promotion in Norway.*

Approach/methodology – *Institutional theory indicates that political and administrative jurisdictions are path dependent in their policy formation and implementation. By using data from different sources this assumption is analysed and discussed according to health promotion in Norwegian municipalities. The main methodology is cross tabulations,*

[☆]The chapter is written as a part of Norwegian Research Council project no. 806614: *Addressing the Social Determinants of Health. Multilevel Governance of Policies Aimed at Families with Children* and Norwegian Research Council project no. 208276: *Challenges for Governance and Planning in Cities and Municipalities* (Research institution-based strategic project – SIS-miljø).

Technology, Communication, Disparities and Government Options in Health and Health Care Services
Research in the Sociology of Health Care, Volume 32, 143–180
Copyright © 2014 by Emerald Group Publishing Limited
All rights of reproduction in any form reserved
ISSN: 0275-4959/doi:10.1108/S0275-495920140000032019

bivariate correlations and regression is carried out to supplement analyses.

Findings — *Municipalities are path dependent in their health promotion policies. They acknowledge and prioritize health behaviour independent of experienced socio-economic challenges, municipal capacity as size and income, and local government political profile. Competence devoted to health promotion can create changes in policies.*

Limitation/policy implications — *The rhetoric on determinants and social determinants in particular is new in Norway. Rhetoric on, and interventions, that highlight the social determinants of health need to be coordinated.*

Originality — *The chapter presents new knowledge on Norwegian local government health promotion and how this is implemented in relation to the challenges experienced.*

Keywords: Health determinants; path dependency; health behaviour; living conditions; local government; Norway

INTRODUCTION

Environments are structured, as Dahlgren and Whitehead (1991/2007) have so eloquently elaborated, by a first layer of individual lifestyle factors closely related to individual hereditary factors; a second layer of social and community networks; a third layer of living and working conditions; and a fourth layer where the general socio-economic, cultural and environmental factors are found. These are the determinants of health ranged from the individual via the middle level (communities, municipalities and regions) to the macro level of society (Elstad, 2005; Kelly, 2006). Thus, the determinants are grouped into four and each group is accorded to a societal level. We will elaborate on the groups of determinants that are accorded to individuals and their living conditions, which are the social determinants, at the middle level in Norway.

The determinants are structured not only so as they distribute differences between rich and poor, rather they shape a pattern of a gradient through populations: the higher the positions in the social hierarchy, the lower the risk of ill health (Graham, 2002, 2004; Siegrist & Marmont, 2006; Sund, 2010). This social health gradient has received attention in policy documents at the international and national level, and how to act on these differences at the local level where policies are further elaborated and implemented is changing. Hence, the determinants for health are an extremely interesting field of study. In our previous research we have focused upon the interpretation of the call for larger focus on health promotion at the local level. In this chapter, we will contribute to the understanding of what conditions acknowledgement and prioritization of the determinants that creates social health inequalities at the local level.

According to public health and health promotion literature the understanding of causes for ill health over time has varied. Initially, ill health was seen as a result of societal structures: people fell ill because of a lack of material resources and to reduce ill health emanating from infectious diseases societal reforms had to be implemented and infrastructures had to be built for the handling of garbage, sewage, water supplies and the like (Elstad, 2005; Strand & Næss, 2010). Later, this materialist explanation was replaced by a strong focus on non-infectious diseases and epidemiologists delivered results that oriented health promotion towards individual determinants of health and the importance of health behaviour as reasons for ill health (Robertson & Minkler, 1994). The centrality of health behaviour unleashed a series of interventions directed towards the individual level (Report No. 20, 2002–2003). Today, the health promotion agenda combines social epidemiological research and neo-materialist perspectives when explaining ill health (Mackenbach, 2012; Raphael, 2011). Neo-materialist theories argue that health promotion has to be targeted towards the root causes of ill health, the living conditions, and therefore, measures should include making all sectors accountable for health promotion, engaging communities in such work and giving attention to the impact of the socio-ecological environment on health (WHO, 2009; Wilkinson & Pickett, 2010). Thus, focus on individual risk factors, it is argued, is not sufficient to prevent disease and illness (Samdal & Wold, 2012).

Traditionally, local government health promotion in Norway has been assigned with the health sector and it was as well oriented towards the individual (Fosse, 2012; Stenvoll, Elvbakken, & Malterud, 2005). Accordingly it is physical activity and protection of recreational areas that has gained admittance to municipal plans (Hofstad, 2011), and the most frequent participants in health promotion partnerships between local government and private actors are organizations that work with sports and outdoor recreation.

Our source of interest lies in this tension between the individual on the one hand and social determinants of health on the other, not least due to the enhanced focus on social inequalities in health in Norwegian policies in the last couple of years (Fosse, 2009; Vallgårda, 2011). More specifically, we are interested in whether different institutional factors are able to redirect the existing path where individual health behaviour is at the centre of attention to the understanding of social determinants as a health challenge and priority for local health promotion.

The institutional factors to be discussed are broadly divided into three: (1) *the socio-economic challenges* — the number of inhabitants living on social assistance and unemployment benefits; (2) *instrumental or material conditions* — population size, economic manoeuvrability and administrative personnel responsible for coordinating health promotion work that together constitutes local government capacity; and (3) *political factors* — the political profile of local governments. The broad question we ask is how these institutional factors affect the acknowledgement and prioritization of living conditions in local policy-making:

To what extent can institutional factors contribute to direct local government health promotion policies towards the social determinants of health?

This research question will be illuminated by drawing on different forms of quantitative data measuring the influence of institutional factors in Norwegian municipalities (independent variables) on the acknowledgement and prioritization of social determinants of health as health challenges (dependent variable). The chapter proceeds with a presentation of the Norwegian context, and the methods and data used, before presenting theories on institutions and path dependence, hypotheses and our empirical findings. Finally these findings are discussed in relation to our theoretical expectations and implications for future research are drawn.

THE NORWEGIAN CONTEXT

Norway is an interesting case for at least three reasons. Firstly, in 1984 general health and care services were decentralized to municipalities as the law on health services in municipalities was enacted. First and foremost this meant that local governments took on most of the responsibility for employing general practitioners, but the law as well included care and rehabilitation (Heløe, 2010). Development of services followed the path of decentralization and local governments were given the responsibility for new services as the need was acknowledged. This included schools, one of the first services to be decentralized, social services, child services and kindergartens, care for the elderly, handicapped and the mentally ill.

Today most of human services are a responsibility for local governments to provide.

Secondly, Norway is one of the richest and most equal societies in the world and is organized according to the Nordic, social democratic welfare model (Esping-Andersen, 1990; Navarro et al., 2006; Raphael, 2012; Wilkinson & Pickett, 2010, pp. 17–21). This model is demarcated by *high employment* that is a precondition for a broad tax base and a necessity for the comprehensive welfare state (Grøholt, Dahl, & Elstad, 2007). *Egalitarianism* is another trait of the Nordic welfare model. The wage structure is relatively compressed and combined with progressive taxation that results in an egalitarian distribution of economic resources among individuals. *Uniform social protection and a democratic right* to adequate living conditions are yet other core traits. Together, these elements can explain why the arguments to better the social position of disadvantaged groups in the population, was not framed by the rhetoric of health promotion and the reduction of social inequities in health (Raphael, 2012). Thus, the social determinants of health were generally overlooked until around a decade ago as one assumed that the welfare model was based in a political economy that secured small health differences, a conviction that has proved to be wrong (Grøholt et al., 2007).

Thirdly, from being a laggard in its approach to the social determinants of health (Dahl, 2002), Norway has worked to create a knowledge base describing core challenges and tying this knowledge closer to policy-making in order to set the stage for the development of policy entry points (Strand et al., 2010). Norwegian health promotion goals include fairness and social justice embedded in reducing the steepness of the gradient. The argument was first introduced in 'Prescriptions for a Healthier Norway' (Report No. 16, 2002–2003). Later on it was reinforced in the 'National Strategy to Reduce Social Inequalities in Health' (Report No. 20, 2006–2007, p. 44) where it is stated that '*Equity is good public health policy*', as well as in the newly released white paper Report on Public Health: Good Health – A Common Responsibility (2013) which states that '*the efforts should be directed at the early stages in the causal chain of health that impact upon health and social differences in health*' (Report No. 34, 2012–2013, p. 15). The policy presupposes that life expectancy, health and quality of life increases with increasing socio-economic status (Directorate of Health, 2010a; Fosse, 2009). Policies to act on social determinants of health have been integrated in acts and regulations. The Norwegian Health Promotion Act (HPA) stresses that municipalities are important settings for health promotion work. This is the setting in which health is to be attended to. An important policy goal is the reduction of social inequalities in health: '*The municipality shall ... contribute to reduce social health inequalities*' (HPA, 2012 §4). Hence, social inequalities in health are given top priority in governmental policy documents and regulations (Grimm, Helgesen, & Fosse, submitted; Prop 90L, 2010–2011; Report No. 20, 2006–2007; Report No. 34, 2012–2013). Given local government's core role in the implementation of health promotion policies and the combination of institutional abilities and political willingness, Norway and its municipalities should be comparatively well equipped to act on the social determinants of health and are therefore a best case on this matter.

SOCIAL DETERMINANTS OF HEALTH

Health is determined by a complex combination of individual and social factors (Dahlgren & Whitehead, 1991/2007). The determinants at the individual level are partly biological and genealogical factors and partly individual lifestyle factors. The determinants at the societal level consist, broadly speaking, of how we have organized our societies in terms of power and economic redistribution (Navarro, 2009; Navarro et al., 2006). Are there for instance policies to include people in the labour market or to give them coverage in case of ill health? Also how we organize our political institutions and the different social arenas we are a part of are of importance: who takes part in political decisions, how are communities governed, does schools provide education for all, are working places organized to reduce stress, do the physical environments, that is residential areas, offer access to recreational areas? Health determinants are seen as making up a causal chain starting with *material and social resources* as income, work, childhood environments and education, via *risk factors* as health behaviour as well as living and working environment, to *health services* as the curative and preventive work done within the health sector (Directorate of Health, 2010a; Report No. 20, 2006–2007; Report No. 34, 2012–2013). In the political discourse, material and social resources resembles what is often called living conditions, while risk factors correspond to lifestyle factors. Together, these resources, factors and services make up a *causal chain of health* which is shown in Fig. 1.

A recent understanding in health promotion is that policies and interventions should be directed at the social determinants and implemented as early in the causal chain as possible (Marmot, 2007; Navarro, 2009; Wilkinson & Pickett, 2010). In practice, it means to direct health policies

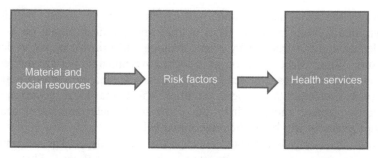

Fig. 1. The Causal Chain of Health. *Source:* Report No. 20 (2006–2007).

and interventions towards communities' and individuals' material and social resources.

However, policies and interventions directed at the other stages in the causal chain of health can contribute to reduced social inequalities in health. For example, interventions aiming at motivating individuals to be physically active, which is associated with risk factors, can be designed as low threshold – low cost interventions, adapted to fit designated groups, and this has been at the core of Norwegian health policy (Report No. 34, 2012–2013). Also health services, as health services for youth, can be arranged as low threshold–low cost interventions. The universal rights and obligations that are at the basis of the Scandinavian welfare states are seen as an important component for equity in health (Marmot, 2007; Raphael, 2012; Wilkinson & Pickett, 2010). However, our main attention will be on the root causes of health, the living conditions.

UNDERSTANDING THE HANDLING OF HEALTH DETERMINANTS AT THE MIDDLE LEVEL: INSTITUTIONAL PERSPECTIVES

The chapter does not intend to measure material changes in Norwegian municipalities in the form of organizational changes or the development and implementation of new interventions. Rather, the centre of attention is the extent to which the municipalities acknowledge and prioritize living conditions in their policies and interventions on health promotion. More specifically, what we base our analyses on is the local chief executives judgment of the municipality's approach to the health determinants and especially the social determinants. As such, this study delves into how local governments create meaning from polities and political debate on health challenges and the gradient by acknowledging and prioritizing social determinants. What affect this process in local governments? We are interested in how the challenges experienced and the institutional conditions making up each municipality's unique abilities affect the local government's acknowledgement and prioritization of the social determinants of health. This proposition will be further elaborated below.

Path dependency is a topical concept for our analysis. The concept of path dependency is closely connected to institutional theory. This theory directs attention to the regulatory, normative and cognitive structures and activities that provide stability and meaning to social behaviour (Scott, 1995, p. 33), that is how decisions, preferences and meanings are artefacts of institutions (Immergut, 1998, p. 10). Path dependency raises attention to institutional conditions that affect the creation of new policies and organizations (Thelen & Steinmo, 1992). The institutional conditions make up a path that is a relatively established way of unifying, organizing and regulating a certain policy field (Torfing, 2001, p. 286). Such paths are by no means perfect responses to social needs and problems (North, 1993), rather they are agglomerations and imprints of previous and existing discourses, norms, organizational forms and coincidental developments. This is not to say that further development of the policy field is inevitable, only that it is conditioned by the regulations, norms and cognitive understandings that have been imputed or selected previously. As Jacob Torfing (2001, p. 277) puts it, '*[T]he cynical wisdom of most social scientists is that despite political attempts to change the world everything tends to stay pretty much the same. In the long run, the world is changing, but the process is slow and incremental*'. New policy paths will be marked by the old path by recycling former rules, norms and understandings. Thus in many instances, new demands and events can be met by stretching the interpretative schemes, modifying operating procedures and/or domesticating new storylines within the realms of existing discourses (Torfing, 2001). Thus, the introduction of new policies is not incidental as the institutional context facilitates some policies and hampers others (Torfing, 2004, p. 58). The mechanism that strengthens existing paths is according to Pierson and Skocpol (2002) self-reinforcing, positive feedback processes that in an economic language are called 'increasing returns processes'. These processes make it difficult to reverse course because power inequalities can be reinforced and embedded in organizations, institutions and dominant modes of political understanding (Pierson & Skocpol, 2002, p. 6).

However, the institutions that the existing path consists of may be weakened, or even punctuated. According to Gains, John, and Stoker (2005, pp. 28–29), the theory of positive feedback processes have trouble of explaining such punctuations. Firstly, they claim that the role of positive feedback is over-exaggerated. Negative feedback situations may just as well prevail. There are always some actors that do not benefit from the existing institutional framework and therefore have an interest in institutional changes. Secondly, they maintain that there are clear incentives to apt for change for actors with a prospect of career movement built on the reputation of being a reformer. Coupled with the short time horizon often existing in political life the gains of a spectacular reform may be greater than the path's corrective mechanisms. Thirdly, they argue that the theory of positive feedback processes in institutional development misunderstand how institutions work. Institutions, they claim, are not designed to be change resistant, but to reproduce themselves in a complex manner. And this reproduction initiates change. Hence, change is an underestimated part of the path dependence concept, '… the forces of increasing returns may at a certain tipping point move from primarily backing the status quo to providing a force behind further change' (Gains et al., 2005, p. 29). Hence, when faced with new problems, problem-understandings and altered power structures with little or no resonance in existing institutional rules, norms and cognitive structures, the coherence of existing paths may crack-up and, thus, create opportunity for change.

Discursive or social constructivist institutionalism pays special attention to how institutional change occurs. More specifically, this strand of the literature is preoccupied with the transformative potential of ideas, discourses and identities (March & Olsen, 1989, 2009; Schmidt, 2008, 2010; Torfing, 2001, 2004). The focus is on how institutions shape the very identity of the actors, their perceptions of themselves, the world and which ideas are legitimate and which actions that is appropriate (Torfing, 2001). According to March and Olsen (1989, 2009, p. 4), to act appropriately is to proceed according to the institutionalized practices of a collective based on mutual, and often tacit, understandings of what is true, reasonable, natural, right and good. This involves matching and changing an ambiguous set of contingent rules to a changing and ambiguous set of situations (March & Olsen, 2009, p. 8). The resulting ideational framework is the structure in which policy makers view the world, understand problems, define what is important and devise what they consider appropriate policy solutions (Torfing, 2001). In contrast to the other new institutionalisms where institutions serve primarily as constraints, discursive/social constructivist institutionalism maintains that institutions are simultaneously constraining structures and enabling constructs of meaning (Schmidt, 2008, 2010). The enabling factor consists of discourses as a transformative force; it is very difficult to explain and know what people are thinking or why they act until they formulate these thoughts (Schmidt, 2010, p. 15). Hence, institutional changes are dependent on the extent to which actors are able to think outside the institutions in which they continue to act (Schmidt, 2010, p. 16). New paths are created by a combination of the part of the former path that still makes up the structural basis for political action and interventions, and new ideas, imaginations and regulative measures aiming to solve the problem (Torfing, 2004, p. 55). Hence, there will be an institutional core that hampers, constrains and directs new policy initiatives (Torfing, 2001). In our case, we argue that this institutional core is attention towards health behaviour in local government health promotion. The question here is if certain institutional factors can facilitate change towards a stronger focus on living conditions that, at the national level, make up a core element of health promotion. In the next section we first present the independent variables and formulate hypothesis of their effect on the dependent variable, then we present relevant data and lastly we discuss major findings according to the institutional theories presented.

DATA AND METHODS

Our data stem from the following sources:

- A survey sent to the chief executive in all Norwegian municipalities in November 2011. The respondents were asked about different aspects of their health promotion work.
- The municipal database administered by Norwegian social scientific data service (NSD), on local authorities' political profile.
- Statistics Norway (SSB) on municipal revenues and number of inhabitants receiving social assistance.
- The Norwegian Labour and Welfare Administration (NAV) on number of inhabitants receiving unemployment benefits.

By connecting these sources of data we are able to address to what extent the independent variables influence the local governments' acknowledgement of living conditions as challenges to be solved and whether or not they prioritize interventions to better them. Firstly we will use *the number of inhabitants on social assistance and unemployment benefits* in the municipalities to spell out some of the socio-economic challenges municipalities encounter. These are variables that measure local characteristics that are results of social and economic conditions created and developed partly on the local level, partly on the regional and national level through economic policies. Secondly we analyse the dependent variables towards municipal *population size*, to find if size affects local government acknowledgement and priority of social health determinant factors. Thereafter we analyse the independent variables of *municipal revenues per capita* and *municipal competence* on health promotion in a similar way to find if relations can be detected. Whether or not municipalities have employed a public health coordinator gives indication to how health promotion is prioritized. The last variable introduced in our chapter is the *political profile* of municipalities that measures a possible effect of the political leadership in municipalities. In Table 1 we have summarized our independent variables.

A quantitative scheme is selected to be able to address the general picture. The downside of such a scheme is a loss of particularities and nuances. However, at this stage, where local implementation of policies to act on social determinants are changing, we find it interesting to establish the broader picture at the middle, municipal level in order to provide a basis for further policy development.

There are two dependent variables in our analysis. The first is constructed the following way: In the questionnaire sent to chief executives we listed 24 items relating to the determinants of health. The list was based in theories on determinants and empirical research according to inclusion, health behaviour, physical traits of place, planning, general service provision and educational services provided in municipalities. The chief executives were asked to mark the items they considered to be the most important health challenges in their municipality. To acknowledge a problem is not the same as prioritizing it. Therefore we have asked chief executives in Norwegian

Table 1.   Independent Variables.

Socio-Economic Challenges (Poverty)	Material/Instrumental	Neo-Institutional/ Normative
Number of inhabitants on social care	Population size	Local government political profile
Number of inhabitants on unemployment benefits	Room of manoeuvre (per capita revenues in municipalities) Competence on public health/health promotion	

municipalities to indicate the municipality's main priority in health promotion. Here the alternatives were already aggregated into 'interventions directed towards living conditions', 'interventions directed towards health behaviour', 'interventions directed towards the environment', 'interventions in the health services', 'population oriented, inter-sectorial interventions that affect larger groups independent of risk vulnerability' (i.e. interventions in schools), 'interventions directed towards vulnerable groups or groups with health risk' and finally 'the municipality do not have a main priority'. Seen through the lenses of the causal chain of health, living conditions indicate prioritization of social determinants, while health behaviour indicates that individual determinants are prioritized. Therefore, our second dependent variable will concentrate on these two categories in our scheme: prioritization of living conditions and prioritization of health behaviour.

DETERMINANTS OF HEALTH IN LOCAL GOVERNMENT POLICIES: CHALLENGES, ABILITIES AND ATTENTION

Before doing cross tabulations and regression analyses, factor analysis to see if the 24 items assessing dependent variable 1 tied to acknowledge of health challenges clustered together in a meaningful way. Not surprisingly, there was a cluster on *health behaviour* consisting of diet, tobacco and physical activity. We expected alcohol and drug abuse also to belong to this cluster, but it did not. Further, we found a cluster *on income and inclusion* that consists of poverty, inclusion on the labour market, housing and the physical item of noise, air, water and radiation. These physical aspects are strongly related to housing (Braubach & Fairburn, 2010). Also, a cluster on *groups at risk* consisting of the challenges of alcohol and drug abuse, child care and mental health were found. Finally, the analysis revealed a cluster on *education* that consists of childhood environments. These clusters harmonize with the outlining of health determinants and the causal chain of health shown in Fig. 1. In Table 2, the first dependent variable clustered in the four groups identified through the factor analysis is presented.

The first dependent variable is thus, parted into four. In sum the three first constitute the *living condition determinants* that during data presentation and discussion will be contrasted with the fourth cluster on *health behaviour determinants* representing the present institutional path in Norwegian health promotion policy.

Table 2.   Dependent Variable 1.

Income and Inclusion	Groups at Risk	Education	Health Behaviour
Poverty	Alcohol and drug abuse	Kindergartens	Diet
Labour market inclusion	Child care	Schools/education	Tobacco
Housing	Mental health	Child environment	Physical activity
Noise, air, water, radiation			

In the following sections we delve into the results from cross tabulations carried out to find differences among groups of municipalities. We argue that five institutional variables are of special interest to understand local government health promotion; these are population size, socio-economic challenges, economic manoeuvrability, competence and capacity, and political profile. The results for each of these variables will be presented sequentially.

Population Size

We know from former research that health challenges according to living conditions are concentrated in the central areas of larger municipalities and in small municipalities in the Northern part of Norway (Barstad, 2011). Hence, there is reason to ask if these types of municipalities acknowledge and prioritize living conditions as health challenges more than other municipalities.

Norwegian municipalities have many mandated welfare tasks. Even though these are similar for all irrespective of their population size and capacity, the regional and local differences in health are striking in Norway. This is especially so in the light of the efforts put into regional policy and welfare state development (Strand & Næss, 2010). Historically, mortality has been higher in urban than in rural areas (Bore, 2010). There is a three-year difference in expected life span between the lowest (Oslo and Finnmark) and the highest life duration (The Western region) (Sund & Jørgensen, 2009, p. 41). But also within cities large gaps in expected life span has been revealed. In Oslo, there is a 12-year difference in expected life duration between the affluent western part of the city and the eastern city districts. However, if one studies different types of diseases, the results go in different directions and counterbalance each other and make it difficult to draw clear conclusions (Sund & Jørgensen, 2009, pp. 43, 47–50). To formulate well-founded hypotheses in relation to the geographical variables is therefore challenging. So rather than operating with urbanity as independent variable, we use municipal *population size* (Barstad, 2011; Dyb, Solheim, & Ytrehus, 2004), and anticipate that larger municipalities, those with the highest number of people living from income support, have greater health challenges than smaller municipalities. In addition, there is reason to believe that the difference in size affects the capacity as income per capita and level of competence, and thereby also the municipalities' ability to acknowledge and prioritize social inequalities in health. Thus, we will measure if municipal size affects the acknowledgement and prioritization of living conditions. We have the following hypothesis:

Hypothesis 1: Large municipalities are more prone to acknowledge and prioritize the social challenges to health than smaller municipalities due to greater health challenges and higher capacity in the organization.

The first independent variable to be analysed is population size. Table 3 shows the relation between size and acknowledgement and prioritization of the four dependent variables.

In total, only 17 of 302 municipalities (6 per cent) prioritize living conditions in their health promotion work and 31 per cent prioritize health behaviour (Helgesen & Hofstad, 2012). Table 3 shows that the municipalities that in fact prioritize living conditions are among the biggest ones. The table further shows that the relation between population size and income and inclusion is almost linear, the bigger the municipalities the more income and inclusion is acknowledged as a challenge to health, and there is a significant correlation. Groups at risk are acknowledged more except by the biggest municipalities while education is the least acknowledged. Small municipalities are the ones that acknowledge them the least, although they as well experience socio-economic challenges to health. The share of municipalities that prioritize interventions to change living conditions is small, but again there is a significant correlation. This indicates that living conditions as a challenge to health is acknowledged. The share that prioritizes interventions to change health behaviour is a lot bigger but correlations are not significant.

Thus, our assumptions gains some support. A plausible understanding of this gap between acknowledgement and prioritization is that the development of policies and interventions to better living conditions still are hampered by central and local government institutions who act to reinforce existing paths. We will return to this in the discussion.

Thus, population size seems to matter. An interesting question is why big municipalities to a larger extent acknowledge social challenges to health

Table 3. Population Size and the Acknowledgement and Prioritization of Living Conditions as Health Challenges, in Per Cent, Numbers in Parenthesis.

Population Size/Health Challenge		<3,000 Inhabitants N=98	3,000–4,999 Inhabitants N=46	5,000–9,999 Inhabitants N=66	10,000–34,999 Inhabitants N=69	35,000< N=18	Correlation
Acknowledge living conditions as challenges	Income and inclusion	36 (35)	54 (25)	62 (41)	61 (42)	83 (15)	P. corr.: 0.305** Sig.: 0.000
	Groups at risk	66 (65)	78 (36)	79 (52)	85.5 (59)	67 (12)	P. corr.: 0.152** Sig.: 0.009
	Education	41 (40)	43 (20)	58 (38)	54 (37)	55.5 (10)	No significant correlation
Acknowledge health behaviour as challenges		63 (62)	54 (25)	62 (41)	54 (37)	72 (15)	No significant correlation
Priority of interventions to change living conditions		1 (1)	2 (1)	5 (3)	11 (8)	18 (4)	P. corr.: 0.288** Sig.: 0.000
Priority of interventions to change health behaviour		36 (35)	30 (14)	45.5 (30)	25 (17)	39 (7)	No significant correlation

**Correlation is significant at the 0.01 level (2 tailed).

and prioritize living conditions. Is it due to differences in local challenges that there are more challenges according to living conditions in larger municipalities? Or is it because they have sufficient slack, in the form of manoeuvrability and competence, in the organization to be able to relate to them? Or is it a combination of the two?

Socio-Economic Challenges to Health

Socio-economic challenges are measured by analysing the number of inhabitants living from social assistance and unemployment benefits in groups of municipalities. Income inequalities are targeted by health promotion policies at all levels of society. While social assistance is a responsibility for municipalities, the unemployment policies and benefits are a central state responsibility. They are, however, administered by the same institution at the local level, the Labour market and Welfare Administration (NAV) (Christensen, Fimreite, & Lægreid, 2007). Municipalities can thus implement policies and interventions to reduce unemployment. If health promotion and interventions to level the gradient succeed, the number of inhabitants on social assistance and unemployment benefits should diminish. When relating these anticipations to our research question we formulate the following hypothesis:

Hypothesis 2: Municipalities with larger number of inhabitants living from income support are more prone to acknowledge and prioritize living conditions as challenges to health than others.

Income disparities among groups of the population enhance inequalities in health and income support schemes are implemented to reduce such inequalities. Nevertheless, receivers of social assistance have worse living conditions and experience poorer self-reported health than other groups (Report No. 34, 2012–2013, p. 53)

The municipalities with most inhabitants living on social assistance are those who to a large extent acknowledge living conditions as challenges to health and prioritize interventions to better them, and there are positive correlations (Table 4). Among the living conditions variables, the determinants according to groups at risk are the most acknowledged while education is the least, income and inclusion is the most acknowledged among the 35 municipalities with 500 people or more living from social assistance. The share of municipalities that acknowledge health behaviour as a challenge to health is high at a stable level irrespective of the number of people living

Table 4. Number of Inhabitants on Social Assistance and the Acknowledgement and Prioritization of Health Challenges, in Per Cent, Numbers in Parenthesis.

Inhabitants on Social Assistance and Municipalities		<15	16–49	50–99	100–199	200–499	500 <	Correlation
		$N=16$	$N=57/56$	$N=63$	$N=56$	$N=70$	$N=35$	
Acknowledge living conditions as challenges	Income and inclusion	19 (3)	30 (17)	48 (30)	73 (41)	54 (38)	83 (29)	P. corr.: 0.337** Sig.: 0.000
	Groups at risk	56 (9)	65 (37)	71 (45)	82 (46)	87 (61)	74 (26)	P. corr.: 0.176** Sig.: 0.002
	Education	25 (4)	42 (24)	44 (28)	58 (29)	60 (42)	51 (18)	No significant correlation
Acknowledge health behaviour challenges		69 (11)	58 (33)	59 (37)	69 (36)	57 (41)	57 (20)	No significant correlation
Priority of interventions to change living condition		4 (1)	2 (1)	3 (2)	2 (1)	1 (5)	20 (7)	P. corr.: 0.202** Sig.: 0.000
Priority of interventions to change health behaviour		24 (5)	36 (20)	38 (24)	39 (22)	34 (24)	26 (9)	No significant correlation

**Correlation is significant at the 0.01 level (2 tailed).

from social assistance. The share prioritizing health behaviour is also high, but there is no significant correlation.

Inclusion into the labour market is the main strategy in the Norwegian government policy to reduce social inequalities in health, and besides being the main source of income for individuals, inclusion into the labour market as well are supposed to create self-respect and possibilities to live a full life (Report No. 34, 2012–2013, p. 54). Table 5 shows the relation between number of inhabitants on unemployment benefits and the acknowledgement and prioritization of health challenges.

Looking at the number of inhabitants living from unemployment benefits we find that the overall pattern is the same as for social assistance: The more people in the municipalities that live from unemployment benefits, the more the municipalities acknowledge living conditions and especially income and inclusion to be a health challenge. Groups at risk are again acknowledged the most and education the least. For income and inclusion and groups at risk there are positive correlations. Health behaviour challenges are highly acknowledged by municipalities covering the whole spectre of number of recipients of unemployment benefits. The number of municipalities prioritizing interventions directed towards living conditions is small, but the share is rising with rising numbers living from unemployment benefits and the correlations are positive.

Our analyses show that all municipalities experience socio-economic challenges to health. To experience such challenges are not confined to the biggest municipalities and those located in specific geographical areas. The analyses also show that the more municipalities experience these challenges to health the more they are willing to prioritize interventions to change them. Our hypothesis: municipalities that have a large number of inhabitants living from income support are more prone to acknowledge and prioritize the living condition challenges than the others, gains support. However, the tendency to prioritize interventions to change health behaviour is stronger than the tendency to prioritize those that change living conditions. This is independent of the number of inhabitants living from income support. This, we argue, is a result of the path-dependent policy and development of interventions to promote health in the municipalities.

In the next paragraph we will look into whether this path dependency and lack of acknowledgement and willingness to prioritize living conditions stems from the material resources making up the administrative capacity of municipalities. These are revenues per capita and the presence of health promotion competence in the municipal organization.

Table 5. Number of Inhabitants on Unemployment Benefits and the Acknowledgement and Prioritization of Health Challenges, in Per Cent, Numbers in Parenthesis.

Inhabitants on Unemployment Benefits and Municipalities		<15 N=45	16–49 N=96	50–99 N=56	100–199 N=52	200–499 N=29	500 < N=19	Correlation
Acknowledge living conditions as challenges	Income and inclusion	24 (11)	51 (49)	52 (29)	60 (31)	69 (20)	84 (16)	P. corr.: 0.343** Sig.: 0.000
	Groups at risk	58 (26)	73 (70)	82 (46)	85 (44)	90 (26)	63 (12)	No significant correlation
	Education	35.5 (16)	44 (42)	52 (29)	65 (34)	48 (14)	53 (10)	No significant correlation
Acknowledge health behaviour as challenge		60 (27)	47 (45)	69 (39)	58 (30)	48 (14)	79 (15)	No significant correlation
Priority of interventions to change living conditions		0	1 (1)	5 (3)	8 (4)	14 (4)	21 (4)	P. corr.: 0.249** Sig.: 0.000
Priority of interventions to change health behaviour		27 (12)	42 (40)	39 (22)	33 (17)	14 (6)	32 (6)	No significant correlation

**Correlation is significant at the 0.01 level (2 tailed).

Manoeuvrability

The neo-materialist explanations to social inequalities in health points to material resources being unequally distributed both at the individual and community level and that this may lead to the accumulation of exposures and experiences that affect health over the life course (Mackenbach, 2012). The tradition of decentralization of policies leaves an option for Norwegian municipalities to develop and implement policies and interventions to influence the distribution of health in their population by changing some of the social health determinants and thereby better their inhabitants' living conditions. Local governments' ability to do so may depend on accessible economic resources (Wilkinson & Pickett, 2010). Thus, we have formulated the following hypothesis:

Hypothesis 3: Municipalities that have the largest revenues/resources are more prone to prioritize interventions aimed at changing living conditions.

We will first, however, look at how the level of manoeuvrability is distributed on municipal size.

Table 6 shows that the small municipalities are richer than the big ones. Fifty-eight per cent of the smallest municipalities can be placed in the group with the highest revenues, while none of the municipalities having more than 5,000 inhabitants are found in this category.

Table 7 shows that the municipalities with the lowest income per capita to a higher degree acknowledge living conditions to be a health challenge than municipalities with the highest income, and there is a negative correlation both according to income and inclusion as well as groups at risk. Groups at risk are also here the most acknowledged while income and inclusion is least acknowledged except for the municipalities with an

Table 6. Municipal Size and Income Per Capita, in Per Cent, Numbers in Parenthesis.

Municipal Size/ Income Per Capita	<3,000 Inhabitants	3,000–4,999 Inhabitants	5,000–9,999 Inhabitants	10,000–34,999 Inhabitants	35,000 <	Total
<40,000	0	0	6 (5)	39 (34)	45 (9)	12 (48)
40,001–55,000	42 (64)	93 (65)	94 (81)	61 (54)	55 (11)	66 (275)
55,100 <	58 (90)	7 (5)	0	0	0	22 (95)
Total	100 (154)	100 (70)	100 (86)	100 (88)	100 (20)	100 (418)

Table 7. Municipal Revenues and the Acknowledgement and Prioritization of Health Challenges, in Per Cent, Numbers in Parenthesis.

Revenues and Number of Municipalities		>40,000 N=39	40,001–55,000 N=196	55,001 < N=59	Correlation
Acknowledge living conditions as challenges	Income and inclusion	67 (26)	57 (111)	32 (19)	P. corr.: −0.207** Sig.: 0.000
	Groups at risk	79 (31)	79 (155)	61 (36)	P. corr.: −0.154** Sig.: 0.008
	Education	46 (18)	47 (92)	37 (22)	No significant correlation
Acknowledge health behaviour as challenges		49 (19)	61 (119)	60 (38)	P. corr.: 0.128* Sig.: 0.028
Priority of interventions to change living conditions		9 (3)	7 (13)	0	No significant correlation
Priority of interventions to change health behaviour		26 (10)	35 (68)	37 (22)	No significant correlation

** Correlation significant at the 0.01 level (2 tailed).
* Correlation significant at the 0.05 level (2 tailed).

income per capita at 55,100 and over who acknowledge education over income and inclusion.

There is a positive relation between municipal revenues per capita and the acknowledgement of health behaviour as a challenge. This is in line with the results of the analyses discussed over in which municipal acknowledgement of living conditions as a health challenge is found to vary positively with municipal size; the bigger the municipality the more living conditions are acknowledged. Small municipalities tend to have higher revenues per capita than the bigger and they to a lesser degree tend to acknowledge living conditions as a challenge to health. This is even more accentuated as no municipality among those with the highest income per capita is among those who do prioritize it. The prioritization of interventions to change health behaviour on the other hand is again high among all groups of municipalities and highest among those with the highest income per capita.

The analysis made in Table 3 on population size showed that municipalities across all size groups tend to act path dependent and both acknowledge and prioritize health behaviour over living conditions as health challenges. The analysis in Table 7 gives reason to believe that small municipalities are more path dependent than bigger, even though their revenues per capita is higher. Higher revenues are although not the only capacity factor. We believe that competence is crucial for acknowledging and prioritizing health challenges.

Competence and Its Capacity

There are reasons to believe that the capacity to implement new policies and interventions does depend on what competence municipalities are in position of. The 'Prescriptions for a Healthier Norway' from 2002 introduced a new (optional) position in the local administration – the public health coordinator that can '... *contribute to release local engagement, support local activities and cross-sector work, and coordinate the effort of various actors. A Public Health Coordinator function as "glue" in local health promotion work*' (Report No. 16, 2002–2003, p. 76). A follow-up from the report was a project that among others enabled county municipalities (elected regional level) to institute a small grant regime for municipalities who wanted to employ public health coordinators. The government urged municipalities that have not already employed a public health coordinator to do so (Prop 90L, 2010–2011; Report No. 34, 2012–2013, p. 152).

Still all municipalities have not employed one and for those who do, they have variegated educational backgrounds. Nevertheless they represent resources as competence and time being devoted to health promotion. Analyses among others show that municipalities who have employed a coordinator to a greater extent than others include health topics in their mandated plans (Helgesen & Hofstad, 2012). The employment of such a coordinator still is optional. Table 8 shows public health coordinators distributed on municipal size.

As the analyses displayed in Table 8 show there is no pattern in the distribution of public health coordinators among municipalities according to population size but the biggest and the lower middle sized (3,000–4,999 inhabitants) municipalities employ coordinators to a lesser extent than the others. Table 9 shows that there is no significant relation between the employment of public health coordinators and any of the dependent variables; neither health behaviour nor living conditions. This highlights that it is not the experienced challenges that is the reasons why municipalities employ public health coordinators and that small municipalities also employ them. This is not surprising as they also have the highest revenues per capita. In Table 9 the effect on the acknowledgement and prioritization of living conditions versus health behaviour from having a public health coordinator is displayed.

To have a public health coordinator has a positive effect on the acknowledgement of living conditions as challenges. However, the employment of public health coordinators in Norwegian municipalities is not enough to make local government prioritize interventions to change living conditions. So, the gap between the acknowledgement of living conditions and the prioritization of interventions to change them exists also in relation

Table 8. The Public Health Coordinator Distributed on Municipal Size, in Per Cent, Numbers in Parenthesis ($N = 346$).

Municipal Size/Public Health Coordinator	<3,000 Inhabitants	3,000–4,999 Inhabitants	5,000–9,999 Inhabitants	10,000–34,999 Inhabitants	35,000<	Total
Yes	73 (86)	69 (36)	76 (55)	80 (65)	65 (15)	74 (257)
No	25 (30)	29 (15)	22 (16)	19 (15)	35 (8)	24 (84)
Do not know	2 (2)	2 (1)	1 (1)	1 (1)	0 (0)	1 (5)
Total	100 (118)	100 (52)	100 (72)	100 (81)	100 (23)	100 (346)

Table 9. Public Health Coordinator and the Acknowledgement and Prioritization of Health Challenges as Living Conditions and Health Behaviour, in Per Cent, Numbers in Parenthesis.

Public Health Coordinator		Yes (N = 231)	No (N = 62)	Correlation
Acknowledge living	Income and inclusion	55 (128)	43.5 (27)	No significant correlation
condition as challenges	Risk	77 (177)	69 (43)	No significant correlation
	Education	53 (122)	37 (23)	No significant correlation
Acknowledge health behaviour challenges		55 (127)	61 (38)	No significant correlation
Priority of interventions to change living conditions		6 (13)	5 (3)	No significant correlation
Priority of interventions to change health behaviour		38 (89)	22 (14)	P. corr.: 0.131 Sig.: 0.025*

*Correlation is significant at the 0.05 level (2 tailed).

to this institutional variable. Neither is there any significant correlation between the acknowledgement of health behaviour as challenges to health and having employed a public health coordinator.

To have a public health coordinator has little effect on the extent to which municipalities acknowledge the dependent variables in health promotion as it gets strong attention also in municipalities without a public health coordinator. As for the acknowledgement and prioritization of living conditions, the shares of municipalities that prioritize interventions to change health behaviour are reduced compared to the shares that acknowledge it as a challenge. However, the reduction is not as radical as for living conditions. In addition, we find that to have a public health coordinator has a positive effect on the ability to prioritize interventions to change health behaviour as 38 per cent of the municipalities with a public health coordinator prioritize them, while only 22 per cent of the municipalities without public health coordinator do the same. These analyses therefore reinforces the previous analyses that municipalities are path dependent in their approach to health promotion as the employment of a public health coordinator do not make them change their acknowledgement and prioritization of living conditions over health behaviour.

It as well reinforces that small municipalities are even more path dependent than the bigger ones.

In municipalities that have a public health coordinator respondents have been asked to mark the percentage of time the coordinator can spend on health promotion. The analyses made in Helgesen and Hofstad (2012) show that public health coordinators often share their time between other forms of health-related work and public health coordination. Small municipalities tend to employ public health coordinators in smaller positions than bigger municipalities. The most regular percentage of combined positions used on health promotion is 10−20 per cent among the smallest municipalities. Respondents commented in the survey among others that '10 per cent is the official time amounted to health promotion while 1−2 per cent is the reality'. Ninety to hundred per cent is most frequent in the medium sized and big municipalities. Hence, the share of time amounted to health promotion is most interesting in relation to municipal size and thus can be a plausible explanation of why larger municipalities acknowledge living conditions to a larger extent than smaller ones.

Thus, the ability to spend a large share of their time resources is equally important to the extent to which the municipalities have a public health coordinator, and can thus be the institutional change that punctuates the positive feedback process and levels the municipalities out of the path-dependent approach to health promotion. Table 10 show that it is the medium sized and big municipalities that most often have employed a full time public health coordinator. However, the differences between the municipalities are not dramatically large.

Table 10. The Public Health Coordinator's Percentage Used on Health Promotion Work Distributed on Municipal Size, in Per Cent, Numbers in Parenthesis (*N* = 257).

Inhabitants/ Percentage Used on Health Promotion	<3,000 Inhabitants	3,000−4,999 Inhabitants	5,000−9,999 Inhabitants	10,000−34,999 Inhabitants	35,000 <	Total
10−20%	49 (41)	42 (15)	36 (20)	27 (18)	20 (3)	38 (97)
30−40%	17 (14)	28 (10)	24 (13)	22 (15)	7 (1)	21 (53)
50−60%	24 (20)	19 (7)	20 (11)	15 (10)	13 (2)	20 (50)
70−80%	1 (1)	6 (2)	4 (2)	3 (2)	7 (1)	3 (8)
90−100%	10 (8)	6 (2)	16 (9)	33 (22)	53 (8)	19 (49)
Total	100 (84)	100 (36)	55 (100)	100 (67)	100 (15)	100 (257)

Political Profile of Local Government

When comparing health promotion policies across nations their political regime – liberal and Christian democratic regimes on the one side and social democratic regimes on the other – are used as an explanation to observed differences. In the literature, it is argued that nations belonging to the social democratic regime tend to implement policies that to a greater extent sustain small socio-economic differences in their populations (Navarro, 2009; Raphael, 2012; Wilkinson & Pickett, 2010). Norway has for long belonged to the groups of countries with a social democratic regime and the Norwegian red–green coalition, The Labour Party, the Socialist Party and the Centre Party (with a strong focus on agricultural and district interests), that has been in charge since 2005 has a strong political attention towards social inequalities in health and the rhetoric is strong in national policies to promote health (Directorate of Health, 2009, 2010b; Elstad, 2005; Report No. 20, 2006–2007). Their receipt emphasize on universal, structural measures to counteract the social gradient, that is the material and social resources in Fig. 1 (Fosse, 2005; Fosse & Strand, 2010a). In contrast, the former non-socialist government to a larger extent focused on vulnerable individuals and groups at risk of developing ill health thereby concentrating on the middle square in the chain of health (Fig. 1) (ibid.). So in a Norwegian setting, and probably also internationally, health promotion is a field of policy where the left–right axis is still active (Vallgårda, 2011). But is this the case also at the local level? Are there political differences in the acknowledgement of living conditions to be a health challenge and the prioritization of interventions to change them? Based on former research, in hypothesis 4 we anticipate that:

Municipalities with a left wing political profile are more prone to prioritize interventions to change living conditions than municipalities with a right wing political profile.

The analysis is shown in Table 11. Municipalities with left wing political profiles have a mayor from one of the parties forming the red–green coalition while the municipalities with a right wing political profile have a mayor from The Christian Democratic Party, The Conservative Party or The Progressive Party.

Table 11 shows that the municipalities with a left wing political profile are more prone to prioritize interventions to change health behaviour while the municipalities with a right wing profile are more prone to prioritize interventions to change living conditions. The number of municipalities that prioritize interventions to change living conditions is very small, nevertheless the share of municipalities with a left wing profile that do so is smaller than for those with a right wing profile. Our hypothesis thus gains little support. One explanation can be found in the consensus-oriented organization of Norwegian local government political institutions; both in decisions and implementations of policies and interventions there is a tradition for collaboration across political divides. There is room for further elaboration and analyses of these results. However, this lies outside the scope of this chapter.

Which of the Independent Variables Explains the Most?

In order to assess which of the independent variables that explains the most, we have carried out a regression analysis of the theoretical-driven independent variables with each of our dependent variables. The results are shown in Table 12.

As shown in Table 12, none of the relations are significant, which is understandable. In Norway, health promotion is changing. Reforms have been launched and implemented as policy guidelines and regulations, but it takes time before these policies are implemented at the local level. In addition, the history of health promotion and health prevention is that ambitions formulated by the government not necessarily are implemented as expected at the local level (Helgesen, 2012). However, there are relations here that show moderate to strong correlation.

Table 12 is complex. We compare independent variables and their impact on the dependent variable.

We will start with *income and inclusion*. This dependent variable consists, as shown in Table 2, of the health challenges poverty, labour market inclusion, housing, as well as noise, air, water and radiation. Overall, income and inclusion are the dependent variable that has the highest correlation with the independent variables. Municipalities that have many inhabitants on social assistance and unemployment benefits tend to acknowledge income and inclusion to a higher extent than municipalities with fewer inhabitants with socio-economic challenges. We find also that municipalities with public health coordinators able to devote most of their time to health promotion are moderately, but positively, correlated with acknowledgement of income and inclusion.

If we turn to *groups at risk*, consisting of the health challenges alcohol and drug abuse, child care and mental health, we find, again, that municipalities with high levels of inhabitants with socio-economic challenges

Table 11. Political Profile and the Acknowledgement and Prioritization of Health Challenges as Living Conditions and Health Behaviour, in Per Cent, Numbers in Parenthesis.

Number of Municipalities and Political Profile		Left Wing (N = 171)	Right Wing (N = 111)
Acknowledge living conditions as challenges	Income and inclusion	32 (54) P. corr.: 0.119* Sig.: 0.041	56 (62) No sig. corr.
	Groups at risk	75 (128) No sig. corr.	77 (86) No sig. corr.
	Education	48 (82) No sig. corr.	53 (59) No sig. corr.
Acknowledge health behaviour as challenges		47 (80) No sig. corr.	60 (67) No sig. corr.
Priority of interventions to change living conditions		5 (8) No sig. corr.	6 (7) No sig. corr.
Priority of interventions to change health behaviour		35 (60) No sig. corr.	31 (35) No sig. corr.

*Correlation is significant at the 0.05 level (2 tailed).

Table 12. Relations between Independent and Dependent Variables, Regression Analyses.

Independent Variables / Dependent Variables		Sos. Ass.	Unemp.	Size	Income	Have PHC	PHC Time to Health Prom	Political Profile
Acknowledge living condition as challenges	Income and inclusion	0.008	0.031	0.111	0.274	0.185	0.127	0.716
	Groups at risk	0.069	0.109	0.811	0.171	0.690	0.318	0.467
	Education	0.961	0.657	0.339	0.913	0.554	0.018	0.946
Acknowledge health behaviour as challenges		0.993	0.422	0.525	0.030	0.732	0.063	0.979
Priority of interventions to change living conditions		0.909	0.047	0.718	0.972	0.914	0.205	0.412
Priority of interventions to change health behaviour		0.860	0.177	0.125	0.162	0.167	0.317	0.732

have a tendency to acknowledge such groups as challenges to health. Interestingly, acknowledgement of groups at risk is moderately related to income. Hence, municipalities with larger economic manoeuvrability have a stronger tendency to focus on groups at risk. Again, the public health coordinators' time to health promotion impact on the acknowledgement of risk groups. However, the relations are weaker than is the case for income and inclusion.

The last variable making up living condition challenges, *education*, is weakly related to the independent variables except for public health coordinators' time devoted to health promotion. Of the dependent variables, education is the one that has the strongest correlation with public health coordinators' time. This indicates that when public health coordinators have time to work with health promotion, they choose to focus on health promotion on the arenas where children and youth spend their time – in kindergartens, schools and in their living environment. This harmonizes with the fact that children and youth are at the centre of attention in local government health promotion (Helgesen & Hofstad, 2012; Hofstad & Vestby, 2009).

Health behaviour – consisting of the health challenges diet, tobacco and physical activity – is pursued most distinctively by municipalities with a high income and a high share of public health coordinators' time devoted to health promotion. However, the correlations are moderate.

When we turn to the *prioritization* of living conditions and health behaviour, we see that in general, prioritization of health behaviour is more strongly correlated to the independent variables than living conditions. We know that health promotion, irrespective of orientation, has a weak anchorage in local government. However, if they prioritize anything, there is a clear tendency towards health behaviour. Nevertheless, the strongest correlation when it comes to prioritization is between living conditions and unemployment. Municipalities with a high number of unemployed citizens have a tendency to prioritize living conditions.

Comparison across the independent variables reveals some interesting patterns that we will comment upon. Firstly, the two measures of *public health coordinators* (to employ a PHC and for the PHC to have high share of the position devoted to health promotion) confirm the results discussed previously: to have a public health coordinator is not enough: How much time the PHCs spend on health promotion work has the strongest effect on acknowledgement and prioritization of health challenges. Hence, this result supports policies aimed at strengthening the public health coordinator position either by merging small positions in neighbouring municipalities or by offering state grants to enhance the positions. Secondly, size does not in itself have a strong effect on acknowledgement and prioritization of health challenges. The exception is in relation to the acknowledgement of income and inclusion and prioritization of health behaviour. Thirdly, political profile is weakly correlated to the dependent variables. This is somewhat surprising in light of the heated debate on welfare issues between the left wing and right wing parties. This may underline an argument proliferating in Norwegian political discourse, that the social democratic welfare regime in Norway is supported across the political spectrum. And additionally, that the political cleavages at the local level are less marked than at the national level where there is a tradition for close collaboration across political divides.

DISCUSSION

Path dependency refers to the regulatory, normative and cognitive structures and activities that designate which ideas and actions that are legitimate and appropriate. Local government and public health coordinators so far have followed the path of individual health behaviour in promoting health. Individual health behaviour has been an important part of the central government policies to promote health since 2003 and the attention by local governments to the individual health behaviour has been strengthened in the aftermath of this report. Positive feedback mechanisms tend to keep their standing because the central governments launches interventions directed at the diets of school children, physical activity and smoke cessation. Especially diets and physical activity also are part of the general debate on health and how to best promote it. Among others there has been a central government action plan to direct local government attention at physical activity; it also suggested concrete interventions municipalities could implement (Norwegian Ministries, 2005). In addition, action plans have been launched according to diet (Directorate of Health, 2011) and tobacco. The last campaign to promote smoke cessation was launched on 3 January 2013 (Directorate of Health (2013)) (http://helsedirektoratet.no/folkehelse/tobakk/tobakkskampanjer/Sider/kampanje-royker-royker-ikke. aspx). According to the Report No. 34 (2012–2013) this line is to be followed also in the future.

Also according to the ongoing Coordination Reform physical activity gains attention as an intervention that will make municipalities able to curb hospital admissions and thus save money they otherwise would have to use to co-fund the admissions; a physically fit population does not need the services of the hospital. As a result municipalities establish healthy living centres as an intervention or enter into agreements with private fitness centres to which doctors and the Norwegian Employment and Welfare Administration (NAV) can refer patients they consider needs to be more physically active. In about 33 per cent of the municipalities that answered our survey the public health coordinator in fact undertakes operative functions at healthy living centres (Helgesen & Hofstad, 2012). Physical activity also came to be at the core of the relations between local governments and civil society organizations, continuing the trend that civil society organizations promoting physical activity cooperate with local governments by entering into public health partnerships with them (Hofstad et al., 2013; Ouff et al., 2010).

The connections made between hospital admissions and the profile of local government health promotion is especially critical for what can be considered appropriate actions and thus interventions. In 50 per cent of the municipalities public health coordinators hold administrative positions in the local government health sector, some even as a chief medical officer or head of department (Helgesen & Hofstad, 2012). To the extent that health promotion has been funded from central government it has as well been directed at the local government health sectors (Fosse, 2012). Both these traits reinforce a positive feedback mechanism interpreting health promotion as health policy by highlighting that health promotion can save money for the health sector. A handbook on physical activity made for health and care personnel serves as illustration: 'Physical activity – a handbook. Physical activity in prevention and treatment' (Directorate of Health, 2009). Other regulatory mechanism in use has been special funding for physical activity directed towards both local governments and civil society organizations.

Mechanisms directed at changing individual health behaviour are mostly uncontroversial, concrete and easy to understand. As our analyses show the big picture is that health behaviour is both acknowledged and prioritized; it is embedded in the local government institutions. This is shown in both the cross tabulation and the correlation that displayed a positive relation between acknowledging health behaviour as challenge to health and per capita revenues. Probably they are as well embedded in the dominant mode of political understanding of health promotion as a difference could not be detected among political profiles to the left or right: Almost independent of political profile municipalities had their attention at and used their abilities on policies and interventions directed at changing individual health behaviour.

Similar suggestions are more difficult to make according to the social determinants of health as they tend to be more abstract. An action plan to combat inequalities in health was launched in 2005. The two main goals listed were to develop knowledge by strengthening the expertise at all levels and develop interventions to reduce social inequalities. These interventions mainly were directed to the municipalities as health impact assessments and a strategy to strengthen inter sectoral perspectives (Directorate of Health, 2005). These interventions have not undergone evaluations of a character that gives them a visible position in the evidence base (Grimm et al., submitted).

It is not likely that the public health coordinators will be the actors promoting any changes in local government health promotion, at least not in the near future. As far as can be seen their career opportunities are connected to the established positive feedback mechanisms of health behaviour and not to reforming local government health promotion. But are there not any possibilities that this picture can change? Are there signs of path punctuation? We will argue that there are. As noted above social determinants were highlighted in a governmental report in 2007 and in the aftermath of this the Directorate of Health was assigned the task of continuously monitoring determinants as among others inclusion on the labour market, childhood environments and education, workplace environments and poverty and the results are published annually in policy reports on public health. The last report covered 2011 (Directorate of Health, 2012). Knowledge reports on municipalities are also made by the Public Health Institute and sent directly to them. Entry points for policy change can be connected to these annual events as they as well will belong to the central government policy initiatives and be part of the institutionalized environments of municipalities. The variance between groups of municipalities will be essential as it is shown according to land use and planning that the use of customized data is dependent on urbanity and revenues (Kartez & Casto, 2008). Urban and large size municipalities have competence that can translate this knowledge meaningfully to the local setting. Those are, among others, to mainstream health in ordinary planning and steering processes and develop interventions. Due to their lower level of competence and capacity, these translation processes will be harder to accomplish in small municipalities.

For big municipalities thus there can be an entry point as they to a greater extent consider challenges to health to be of a social character and to be tied to questions according to income and inclusion.

Municipalities in all size groups acknowledge risk groups to be challenges to health. They even consider them bigger challenges than health behaviour. The attention towards risk groups can function as a bridge between health behaviour and living conditions, and thus put the social determinants in the forefront. This is somewhat more discussed below.

Even though it is not likely that public health coordinators will be actors promoting changes in local government health promotion in the near future, they may do so in the long run. To have a coordinator and especially to have a coordinator in a full time or a near full time position, directs municipal attention at the necessity of having competence present locally. Many coordinators have been employed for a short time period only and when they get to know the organization and the tasks their orientation might be broadened beyond health behaviour. Social determinants belong to central state policy initiatives and thus are part of the institutionalized environments of local government health promotion policies, and can create an atmosphere in which the social determinants to a greater extent than today are acknowledged and prioritized.

We have found that municipalities prioritizing interventions to change living conditions are mostly found among bigger municipalities. This result highlights municipal size as an entry point for policy change. The red−green coalition governing the country today has not institutionalized any incentives for municipal mergers. This have changed after the national referendum fall 2013 which the right wing parties won and a structural reform of municipalities is now launched. As is in line with the above argument, bigger municipalities tend to have more health promotion competence who thus can act as health promotion entrepreneurs. On the other hand, a nonsocialist government will not necessarily think positively about social health determinants, but as local governments are independently elected the policy need not be the same at local and central levels of government. The fact that more municipalities among the richest, and thus smallest, considered groups at risk to be a challenge to health is also an entry point to policy changes. Groups at risk can be a bridge between a strong attention at health behaviour and attention at living conditions because municipalities that have employed a public health coordinator in some substantive position also tend to acknowledge questions according to education as a challenge to health. Central government policy initiatives are made to combat drop-outs among pupils at both lower and upper secondary schools. This can function as a punctuation of the existing positive feedback mechanisms according to health behaviour, or at least it can broaden the existing ones as groups at risk and education are seen in concert and the national policies will enter into the institutionalized environments for both public health coordinators and all size groups of municipalities.

As Norway has many small municipalities, municipal amalgamations often tend to be launched as solutions to different types of challenges. Arguments contend that bigger municipalities have more sustainable political-administrative capacity and competence. Our analyses tend to support such a view. We find that bigger municipalities more often have public health coordinators in bigger shares of positions than smaller. The central government does advice municipalities to employ public health coordinators in at least 20 per cent positions. This will be economically sustainable also for the small ones although it will not result in any immediate bettering of the situation. Nevertheless, over time this can also raise the municipal awareness of the importance to have health promotion competence. There is reason to believe that having a public health coordinator in a big share of position will be endowed with a positive attitude because county municipalities need to have an address for the initiatives the 2011 act on health promotions mandate them to take. These initiatives will add to the discursive shaping of local government health promotion and what is considered as appropriate for municipalities' health promotion over time can be transformed.

CONCLUSION

Living conditions are part of the health promotion agenda in Norway. However, this is first and foremost at a rhetoric or discursive level. It is the large municipalities that also have the greatest socio-economic challenges that respond to this and thus acknowledge living conditions as challenges to health. Municipalities governed by left wing parties acknowledge income and inclusion as a challenge to health. Nevertheless there are no visible differences between the political blocks according to local government health promotion. This also implies that there are no political barriers for the development of policies and interventions to reduce social health inequalities at the local level. This indicates a potential for stronger institutionalization in the future. However, the focus on health behaviour has a strong position. Implications that can be drawn from this for future research is that the variegated capacity of municipalities to implement public health policies and interventions comprising both individual health behaviour and the social determinants needs to be tended to. Research as well needs to be conducted on how municipalities are able to use the customized knowledge they are receiving on health determinants.

REFERENCES

Barstad, A. S. (2011). Ressurser, behov og subjektiv livskvalitet. En analyse av Levekårsundersøkelsen 2008. *Tidsskrift for velferdsforskning*, *14*(3), 163–180.

Bore, R. R. (2010). På liv og død. Helsestatistikk i 150 år. Statistics Norway, Oslo-Kongssvinger.

Braubach, M., & Fairburn, J. (2010). Social inequities in environmental risk associated with housing and residential location – A review of evidence. *European Journal of Public Health*, *20*(1), 36–42.

Christensen, T., Fimreite, A. L., & Lægreid, P. (2007). Reform and the employment and welfare administrations – The challenges of coordinating diverse public organizations. *International Review of Administrative Sciences*, *73*, 389.

Dahl, E. (2002). Health inequalities and health policy: The Norwegian case. *Norsk Epidemiologi*, *12*(1), 69–75.

Dahlgren, G., & Whitehead, M. (1991/2007). *Policies and strategies to promote social equity in health*. Background document to WHO – Strategy paper for Europe. Working Paper No. 2007:14. Institute for Future Studies, Stockholm.

Directorate of Health. (2005). *Gradientutfordringen - Sosial- og helsedirektoratets handlingsplan mot sosiale ulikheter i helse. [The gradient challenge – Action plan to combat social inequalities in health.]* Report IS-1229. Oslo: Directorate of Health.

Directorate of Health. (2009). *Aktivitetshåndboken - fysisk aktivitet i forebygging og behandling. [Physical activity a handbook – Physical activity in prevention and treatment.]* Report IS-1592. Oslo: Directorate of Health.

Directorate of Health. (2013). Retrieved from http://helsedirektoratet.no/folkehelse/tobakk/tobakkskampanjer/Sider/kampanje-royker-royker-ikke.aspx. Accessed on February 6, 2013.

Directorate of Health. (2010a). *Public health – The road to good health for everybody*. Oslo: Directorate of Health.

Directorate of Health. (2010b). *Physical activity – A handbook. Physical activity in prevention and treatment*. Oslo: Directorate of Health.

Directorate of Health. (2011). *Dietary advice to promote health and prevent chronic disease. Methodologies and scientific knowledgebase*. Oslo: Directorate of Health.

Directorate of Health. (2012). *Policy report on public health*. Oslo: Directorate of Health.

Dyb, E., Solheim, L. J., & Ytrehus, S. (2004). *Sosialt perspektiv på bolig*. Oslo: Abstrakt forlag.

Elstad, J. I. (2005). *Socio-economic inequalities in health, theories and explanations*. Oslo: Directorate of Health.

Esping-Andersen, G. (1990). *The three worlds of welfare capitalism*. Cambridge: Polity Press.

Fosse, E. (2009). Norwegian public health policy: Revitalization of the social democratic welfare state? *International Journal of Health Services*, *39*(2), 287–300.

Fosse, E. (2012). Norwegian experiences. In D. Raphael (Ed.), *Tackling health inequalities. Lessons from international experiences.* Toronto: Canadian Scholar's Press Inc.

Fosse, E., & Strand, M. (2010). Politikk for å redusere sosiale ulikheter i helse i Norge: Fornyet politisering av folkehelsespørsmål. *Tidsskrift for velferdsforskning*, *13*(1), 14–25.

Gains, F., John, P. C., & Stoker, G. (2005). Path dependency and the reform of English local government. *Public Administration*, *83*(1), 25–45.

Graham, H. (2002). Building an inter-disciplinary science of health inequalities: The example of life course research. *Social Science and Medicine*, *55*, 2005–2016.

Graham, H. (2004). Social determinants and their unequal distribution: Clarifying policy understandings. *The Milbank Quarterly*, *82*, 101–124.

Grimm, M., Helgesen, M., & Fosse, E. (submitted). Health Policy. http://dx.doi.org/10.1016/j.healthpol.2013.09.019. The Norwegian public health act: A milestone towards reducing social inequities in health at local levels?

Grøholt, E. K., Dahl, E., & Elstad, J. I. (2007). Health inequalities and the welfare state. *Norsk Epidemiologi*, *17*(1), 3–8.

Helgesen, M. K. (2012). Styring av folkehelsepolitikk i relasjonen mellom stat, fylkeskommuner og kommuner [Steering of public health policies in the state-county-municipal relation]. In G. Sandkjær Hanssen, J. E. Klausen, & O. Langeland (Eds.), *Det regionale Norge 1950 til 2050*. Oslo: Abstrakt forlag.

Helgesen, M. K., & Hofstad, H. (2012). *Regionalt og lokalt folkehelsearbeid. Ressurser, organisering og koordinering. En baselineundersøkelse.* Norwegian Institute for Urban and Regional Research (NIBR). Retrieved from http://www.nibr.no/pub1584

Heløe, L. A. (2010). *Velferd på avveie? Utviklingslinjer og dilemmaer i helse- og omsorgspolitikken.* Oslo: Abstrakt forlag.

Hofstad, H. (2011). Healthy urban planning: Ambitions, practices and prospects in a Norwegian context. *Planning Theory & Practice*, *12*(3), 387–406.

Hofstad, H., & Vestby, G. M. (2009). *Lokalt folkehelsearbeid- Underveisevaluering av Helse i Plan og Partnerskap for folkehelse.* NIBR Working Paper 2009:102. Norwegian Institute for Urban and Regional Research, Oslo.

Immergut, E. M. (1998). The theoretical core of the new institutionalism. *Politics & Society*, *26*(1), 5–34.

Kartez, J. D., & Casto, M. P. (2008). Information into action: Biodiversity data outreach and municipal land conservation. *Journal of the American Planning Association*, *74*(4), 467–480.

Katznelson, I. & Milner, H. (Eds.). (2002). Historical institutionalism in contemporary political science. In *Political science: State of the discipline*. New York, NY: Norton & Co.

Kelly, M. P. (2006). Mapping the life-world: A future research priority for public health. In A. Killoran, C. Swann, & M. P. Kelly (Eds.), *Public health evidence: Tackling health inequalities*. Oxford: Oxford University Press.

Mackenbach, J. P. (2012). The persistence of health inequalities in modern welfare states: The explanation of a paradox. *Social Science and Medicine*, *75*, 761–769.

March, J. G., & Olsen, J. P. (2009). *The logic of appropriateness*. ARENA Working Paper No. 04/09. University of Oslo, Oslo.

March, J., & Olsen, J. P. (1989). *Rediscovering institutions: The organizational basis of politics*. New York, NY: The Free Press.

Marmot, M. (2007). Achieving health equity: From root causes to fair outcomes. *Lancet, 370*, 1153–1163.

Navarro, V. (2009). What we mean by social determinants of health. *Global Health Promotion, 16*(1), 5–16.

Navarro, V., Muntaner, C., Borell, C., Benach, J., Quiroga, Á., Rodriguez-Sanz, M., ... Pasarin, M. I. (2006). Politics and health outcomes. *Lancet, 368*, 1033–1037.

North, D. C. (1993). Economic performance through time. The Nobel Foundation. *Revista Universidad Eafit, 93*, 9–18.

Norwegian Ministries. (2005). *Sammen for fysisk aktivitet, handlingsplan for fysisk aktivitet 2005–2009. [Action plan for physical activity.]*

Ouff, S. M., Bergem, R., Hanche-Dahlseth, M., Vestby, G. M., Hofstad, H., & Helgesen, M. (2010). Partnerskap for folkehelse og Helse i Plan. Sluttrapport. *Møreforskning*, rapport nr. 7.

Prop 90L. (2010–2011). *Lov om folkehelsearbeid (folkehelseloven)*, Helse- og omsorgsdepartementet [Proposition to the Parliament, Public Health Law].

Raphael, D. (2011). A discourse analysis of the social determinants of health. *Critical Public Health, 21*(2), 221–236.

Raphael, D. (2012). The political economy of health promotion: Part 1, national commitments to provision of the prerequisites of health. *Health Promotion International, 28*(1), 95–111.

Report No. 16. (2002–2003). *Prescriptions for a healthier Norway*. Oslo: Ministry of Health and Care.

Report No. 20. (2006–2007). *National strategy to reduce social inequalities in health*. Oslo: Ministry of Health and Care.

Report No. 34. (2012–2013). *The report on public health: Good health – A common responsibility*. Oslo: Ministry of Health and Care.

Robertson, A., & Minkler, M. (1994). New health promotion movement: A critical examination. *Health Education & Behavior, 21*, 295.

Samdal, O., & Wold, B. (2012). Introduction to health promotion. In B. Wold & O. Samdal (Eds.), *An ecological perspective on health promotion: Systems, settings and social processes*. Norway: University of Bergen, Bentham eBooks.

Schmidt, V. (2008). Discursive institutionalism: The explanatory power of ideas and discourse. *Annual Review of Political Science, 11*, 303–326.

Schmidt, V. (2010). Taking ideas and discourse seriously: Explaining change through discursive institutionalism as the fourth new institutionalism. *European Political Science Review, 2*(1), 1–25.

Scott, W. R. (1995). *Institutions and organizations*. Thousand Oaks, CA: Sage.

Siegrist, J., & Marmont, M. (2006). Introduction. In J. Siegrist & M. Marmont (Eds.), *Social inequalities in health. New evidence and policy implications*. Oxford: Oxford University Press.

Stenvoll, D., Elvbakken, K. T., & Malterud, K. (2005). Blir norsk forebyggingspolitikk mer individorientert? *Tidsskrift for Den Norske Lægeforening, 125*(5), 603–605.

Strand, B. H., & Næss, Ø. (2010). Forskning på sosial ulikhet i helse. In R. R. Bore (Ed.), *På liv og død. Helsestatistikk i 150 år*. Oslo-Kongssvinger: Statistisk sentralbyrå.

Strand, M., Brown, C., Torgersen, T. P., & Giæver, Ø. (2010). Setting the political agenda to tackle health inequities in Norway. *Studies on social and economic determinants of population health* (No. 4). Copenhagen: WHO Regional Office for Europe.

Sund, E. R. (2010). *Geographical and social inequalities in health and health behaviour in the Nord-Trøndelag health study (HUNT)*. Thesis for the degree of Philosophiae Doctor, Norwegian University of Science and Technology, NTNU Trondheim.

Sund, E. R., & Jørgensen, S. H. (2009). Folkehelsens geografiske fordeling. In J. G. Mæland (Ed.), *Sosial epidemiologi: Sosiale årsaker til sykdom og helsesvikt*. Oslo: Gyldendal akademisk.

Thelen, K., & Steinmo, S. (1992). Historical institutionalism in comparative politics. In S. Steinmo, K. Thelen, & F. Longstreth (Eds.), *Structuring politics. Historical institutionalism in comparative analysis*. Cambridge: Cambridge University Press.

Torfing, J. (2001). Path-dependent Danish welfare reforms: The contributions of institutionalisms in understanding evolutionary change. *Scandinavian Political Studies, 24*(4), 277–309.

Torfing, J. (2004). *Det stille sporskiftet i velferdsstaten. En diskursteoretisk beslutningsprosessanalyse*. Aarhus: Aarhus universitetsforlag.

Vallgårda, S. (2011). Addressing individual behaviours and living conditions: Four Nordic public health policies. *Scandinavian Journal of Public Health, 39*(6), 6–10.

WHO. (2009). *Milestones in health promotion statements from global conferences*. Geneva: World Health Organization.

Wilkinson, R., & Pickett, K. (2010). *The spirit level. Why equality is better for everyone*. London: Penguin Books Ltd.

SOCIAL IMPLICATIONS OF LONG TERM CARE INSURANCE IN JAPAN: A REVIEW ☆

Atsuko Kawakami

ABSTRACT

Purpose — *This chapter will review the evaluations of the newly developed elderly care system in Japan, Long Term Care Insurance, and its social implications with the focus on demographic change.*

Methodology/approach — *By reviewing literature, this chapter will examine how demographic and social change over the years has impacted the features of caregivers. Then, how this policy change has demedicalized the aging process will be described. Finally, this chapter will evaluate whether this insurance has shifted the responsibility for elderly care from the family to society as the governmental slogan advertised.*

☆Atsuko Kawakami is currently affiliated to Department of Social Sciences, Tarleton State University, Box T-0660, Stephenville, TX 76402, akawakami@tarleton.edu

Technology, Communication, Disparities and Government Options in Health and Health Care Services
Research in the Sociology of Health Care, Volume 32, 181–198
Copyright © 2014 by Emerald Group Publishing Limited
All rights of reproduction in any form reserved
ISSN: 0275-4959/doi:10.1108/S0275-495920140000032020

Findings — *The new insurance has offered more options in different services and established a new norm of self-reliance and determination for one's own aging however it is doubtful if this new insurance has shifted the responsibility from family to society.*

Research limitations/implications — *Applying the implications of policy reforms for elderly care in Japan to the United States, one can assume the traditional U.S. norms and values can facilitate effective utilization of the elderly care system. However, since each nation faces different problems with its specific condition, continuous studies and observations on the relationship between elderly care, immigration issues, and demographic changes will be necessary in order to offer more specific suggestions for each aging nation.*

Originality/value of chapter — *As Japan's new insurance scheme for the elderly has been studied by many aging nations, recommendations for more comprehensive plans are suggested including building a community-based support system into the Long Term Care Insurance scheme to prevent social isolation and respond to emergency situations for the elderly.*

Keywords: Long Term Care Insurance; Japan; aging; elderly care

Traditionally, daughters-in-law have been the caregivers for the elderly in Japan as well as many other Asian countries (Asai & Kameoka, 2005; Ikels, 1997; Ishida, 1971; Lan, 2002; Ogawa & Retherford, 1993). Elderly care has been considered as the domain of the family in Japan; therefore, the government did not actively provide many options for elderly care (Asai & Kameoka, 2005; Ogawa & Retherford, 1993). When the average age of the caregivers was still relatively young and the number of the elderly was relatively small, the government did not develop an initiative for elder care. Due to the cultural practice of home-based care and the lack of governmental involvement in elderly care until the end of the last century, the options and availability of elderly care services were seriously limited in Japan.

Elderly care was the responsibility of the wife of the first son (Asai & Kameoka, 2005; Ishida, 1971; Kondo, 1990, pp. 124–127). This custom is based on the Meiji Civil Code of 1898 which officially outlined Japan's culture of primogeniture. Guided by the samurai family tradition, Meiji Civil Code indicated the first son ought to inherit all property from his parents but his wife ought to provide care and services for the husband's aging parents for the return of inheritance. This family-based caregiving system was a well-established means of social security and elderly people's preference of care-receiving for the elderly until the recent Japanese people's attitudinal change in this custom (Ogawa & Retherford, 1993).

However, one can easily understand how stressful it has been for a daughter-in-law to care for her spouse's parents at home by herself. The seniors also feel uneasy spending most of their daytime being cared for by the daughter-in-law in the same household while their son and grandchildren are at work and school. Uneasiness of both parties often turns into overly critical views toward each other. Chronic conflict between the seniors and daughters-in-law is actually expected and has been very common in Japanese families for many generations. The strife between them and its resolution have been popular topics on television shows, essays, and magazines (Lock, 1996; Long, 1996; Painter, 1996).

A caregiver's burden from providing elderly care at home started to get more attention, along with the financial deficit for medical expenditures, as one of the most serious social problems in Japan. Since the population of the elderly, their longevity, and the number of separated households from children's family have increased, the more elders themselves have become the caregiver for other seniors in the same household (Yoshida, 2002). Pressure is on the government to alleviate this situation and tackle the problem of the financial deficit. After implementing several policy reforms in 1980s and 1990s, Japan finally launched a new insurance system, Long Term Care Insurance, in 2000. This insurance aimed to shift the responsibility of elderly care from the family to society to release the pressure and burden of family-based care.

More than a decade after the implementation of the Long Term Care Insurance scheme, it is still debatable whether this new insurance system has shifted the responsibility of elderly care from the family to the society. This new insurance scheme is also aiming to remove the medicalized aspects from the aging processes. Medicalization is a process in which previously non-medical aspects of life or moral issues are defined and treated as medical conditions such as gambling becoming a compulsive disorder (Conrad, 2007). Schmidt (2011, p. 59) argues that the medicalization of aging is problematic because it sees "growing old as a form of social deviance: 'the elderly are punished by isolation and stigmatization for this "deviant" act.'" The handicapped and the elderly are disvalued but told "they are normal and encouraged to act like they are normal while social organization precludes normalcy and acceptance" (Schmidt, 2011, p. 59). Schmidt (2011) sees medicalization of aging takes senior individual's personhood away and makes them less of a person. Indeed, Schmidt (2011, p. 88) argues

The "arc, end, and prolongation of life" with medicalization err on the side of medical diagnosis, treatment, and life extension seemingly regardless of cost, and with significant challenges to individual autonomy and individual and social preference to not medicalize life, to not needlessly prolong life, and ultimately to end life in a demedicalized manner.

In fact, demedicalization of aging is the key element of the discourse on whether the new insurance in Japan has shifted elderly care from the family to society, or put the responsibility back to the family. It can be argued that demedicalization and the new insurance system may even have established a new norm of self-reliance and determination of elderly care in Japan.

This chapter will review the evaluations of the Long Term Insurance scheme and its social implication with the focus on the demographic change in Japan and what needs to be accomplished for better total care for the elderly. First, this chapter will describe how various insurances were developed in Japan, followed by a brief description of the newly developed Long Term Care Insurance system. Next, it will explain how traditional family-based care has been affected by the new Long Term Care Insurance as well as the demographic and social changes. Then, how the new insurance scheme has demedicalized elderly care and the consequences of demedicalization will be described. As this newly created insurance scheme has been getting attention from other aging nations, conclusions will be drawn by reviewing various scholars' recommendations for a better elderly care system and further research possibilities, including how Japan's experiences of the policy reform can be translated into the United States.

HISTORY OF HEALTH INSURANCE FOR THE ELDERLY

Fukawa (2002) briefly reviews the history of national insurance schemes in Japan; it started for the purpose of strengthening the nation's labor force, rather than concern for the elderly. Five years after passing the first Health Insurance Law in Japan, the Health Insurance Law was enacted in 1927 to protect from illness and injury for private sector employees. Even though the law and the benefits were not comprehensive at first, the health insurance system was gradually ameliorated. In 1938, the Ministry of Health and Welfare and region-based National Health Insurance were established. Labor Standard Law and Workers' Accident Compensation Law in 1947 excluded work-related illnesses and injuries from health insurance coverage. In 1948, the National Public Service Mutual Aid Association Law was established to institutionalize various insurance schemes for employed people.

In 1954, for the first time, the government subsidized government-managed health insurance. In 1961, universal public health insurance coverage was finally accomplished. Employer-based health insurance benefits covered 100 percent of costs for insured persons and 50 percent for their dependents, while National Health Insurance covered 50 percent for both heads of households and household members. The coverage of National Health Insurance was raised to 70 percent for subscribers and their dependents by 1973. By 1980, the coverage level of inpatient care for dependents of employer-based health insurance became 80 percent. The Revision of the Health Insurance Law of 1973 set a ceiling on patient's cost; when patient's monthly copayment was higher than the ceiling, insurance funds would pay the excess amount back to the patient. The revision of 1973 also implemented free health service system for the elderly by paying the 30 percent of patient's cost from the public funds. With the extended accessibility and increasing aging population, the health expenditures grew double-digit percentage points every year while Japan's rapid economic growth became stable growth by the mid-1970s.

To deal with the budget deficit and contain health expenditures, the public health insurance system was reformed several times in the 1980s. One of the significant changes was the creation of the health insurance for seniors in 1982 to spread the costs for the elderly among various sickness funds. Another insurance policy change regarding the elderly health care in 1984 is transferring money from the employer-based funds to the National Health Insurance fund to help cover the costs of retired employees. The senior patient's copayment was increased and the method of calculating contributions from sickness funds was also amended in 1987. Reviewing the history of health insurance in Japan, Fukawa (2002) explains that the focus of reforming health insurance for the elderly and effective health services to the nation have always been concentrated on four points: (1) well-coordinated health services and welfare services for the elderly; (2) elimination of unnecessary long term hospitalization; (3) separation of medical training costs at university hospitals from insurance-covered health services; and (4) providing better services for patients. With this in mind, in 1989 the government implemented a new reform called the Golden Plan or the Ten-Year Strategy for the Promotion of Health and Welfare for the Elderly in order to improve home-based and facility-based welfare as well as other services for seniors by 2000.

Finally, as planned, Japan launched a new insurance scheme, Long Term Care Insurance, for the elderly in April 2000. Fifty percent of the budget of the Long Term Care Insurance is from the general tax and another 50 percent is from the premium of the insured individuals age 40 and above. For the individuals who are between 40 and 64 years old, their premium is withheld from the medial insurance premium. Individuals who are age 65 and above pay a premium with deduction from pension or direct payment for insurer according to the individual's pension status. The benefit of Long Term Care Insurance includes home help, bathing service, day care, short stay in nursing home, visiting nurses as well as institutional care in long term care hospitals. For individuals age 65 and above, there is no limitation for the causes of dependency but for individuals between 40 and 64, the eligibility is limited to the age related disabilities such as Alzheimer's disease and stroke.

Tsutsumi and Muramatsu (2005) summarize the two-step assessment process of Long Term Care Insurance which determines the limit of benefits the insured seniors can receive after the application is submitted by the applicants. The insurer is the municipal government. First, on-site assessment is conducted with a standardized 85 item questionnaire. An official computer analyzes each item to classify the applicant into one of six levels of dependency or to reject eligibility. The second step is the assessment conference by health care professionals including a report from the applicant's home doctor. Decision of eligibility is delivered within 30 days. If dissatisfied with the eligibility decision, the applicant may appeal. Each eligibility level entitles the applicant to utilize an explicitly defined monetary amount of services such as home help services, visiting nurse services, visiting bathing service, visiting rehabilitation services, day care services, medial day care services, short stay services, and nursing home. However, no cash or actual monetary assistance is given as the benefit.

Institutional care in the health service facility for the elderly and geriatric ward is now only under the Long Term Care Insurance. The reason for this specific change is that those services used to be covered by the health insurance scheme and many hospitals were actually functioning as nursing homes for elderly patients who require little care. Ikegami and Campbell's report in 2004 explains that "one-fifth of all hospital beds are already paid by a flat per diem rate. This flat rate has acted as a disincentive to admit heavy-care or sub acute patients. One of the objectives of the new Long

Term Care Insurance system was to deal with this problem by transferring long term care hospital beds from the health insurance to Long Term Care Insurance where fees vary by level of disability" (Ikegami & Campbell, 2004, p. 30; see also Campbell & Ikegami, 2003). However, during the initial transition period, relatively few beds had actually been transferred to the Long Term Care Insurance scheme. Therefore, the decline of health insurance expenditure was marginal due to the fact that the municipalities, the Long Term Care insurers, did not want such costly patients to be enrolled in their system; however, the increase in various copayment rates and fee schedule actually led to a reduction of medical expenditure for the first time in history (Ikegami & Campbell, 2004). In that sense, this was the first step and the sign of hope for the successful transformation of insurance scheme in terms of pecuniary point of view.

TRANSITION OF FAMILY-BASED ELDERLY CARE

Asai and Kameoka (2005) argue that many Japanese families feel embarrassed to utilize formal services such as day care and government or commercial based nursing homes because it reflects badly on them; Japanese families fear that their neighbors might perceive them abandoning the family obligation for their elderly members when they are cared for by formal institutions and service providers (see also Momose & Asahara, 1996). Others see that today's Japanese women in their 50s and 60s are open and flexible enough to accept new ideas to fulfill such duty by utilizing outside services or providing care for their own parents instead of in-laws (Long, Campbell, & Nishimura, 2009).

Long et al. (2009) explains that Japanese women in their 50s and 60s are the cohort of people who are expected to care for their in-laws, especially if their husband is the eldest son; however, those women see the practice of biological daughter caregiving positively. The researchers also found that parental satisfaction is higher when they are cared for by their own daughters than cared for by daughters-in-laws; caregivers also receive the higher amount of sibling supports when they are providing care for their own parents while daughters-in-law receive less support when providing care for parent-in-laws (Long et al., 2009). Long et al. (2009) analyze that Long Term Care Insurance is a new option which has created greater uncertainty about who will provide care for the elderly in any given family; however, this flexibility also has allowed for continuity of the family-based care system in Japan, despite the tremendous increased length of the caregiving period due to the prolonged longevity (Long et al., 2009). In other words, the new insurance scheme created more options to support the extended family-based caregiving time rather than releasing the family members from caregiving duty at home.

Meanwhile, a new group of caregivers emerged since the 1990s. They are called "social security parasites" that grow in number with the economic depression and unemployment that prevailed in Japan (Suzuki, 2007). Unlike the stereotypical image of caregivers – married women in 50s and 60s – they are the middle aged non-employed single, mostly male, child who remains in the parental household and controls the parent's social security income in the name of caregiving; however, those "parasites" actually provide minimum care, resulting in physical abuse, neglect, or even homicide (Suzuki, 2007). The increased number of such abuse cases matched the timing of various policy changes, including implementation of the Long Term Care Insurance system. Suzuki (2007) analyzes such a matched timing of the increased number of abuse cases and implementations of various policies indicates the system settings for the Long Term Care Insurance may not be suitable for male caregivers.

In fact, Tamiya, Yamaoka, and Yano (2002) found that characteristics of caregivers significantly affect the use of the services. One of the most popular services, such as day care, was utilized mostly by a wife who is providing care for her husband. Interestingly, when the level of care needed for the insured senior increases, the utilization of such services decreases. Home help is another popular service used mostly by a wife who is taking care of her husband or by elderly individuals without a resident caregiver. It seems that the decision of caregivers is more important than the level of care the insured needs. Therefore, Tamiya et al. (2002) suggest the caregiver situation should be considered for policy making as well as eligibility of various services under Long Term Care Insurance.

DEMOGRAPHICAL CHANGE OF CAREGIVERS

MacAdam (2004) lists three main reasons why Japan mandated and implemented the Long Term Care Insurance program in spite of its scarce financial resources for social welfare as follows: First, Japan is the most rapidly aging nation in the world and, by 2020, the percentage of the elderly age 65 and above will reach 27 percent of the entire population in

Japan. Second, because more women are employed outside the home and the family size has become much smaller, traditional filial care within the family can no longer be sufficient. Lastly, the elders had been cared for in hospitals for a prolonged period of time without any long term care programs and various individualized services due to the shortage of such facilities and providers.

Family-based care is more bearable when caregivers are relatively young and healthy compared to the case when elderly individuals with some functional disability provide care for the oldest old seniors. However, with the current demographic and economic characteristics, the prediction of elderly care gets gloomier as the cohorts move forward to the higher age categories. Muramatsu and Akiyama (2011) describe the demographic characteristics regarding labor participation and support for seniors as follows: When current oldest old individuals (age 85 and above) were young, they moved into metropolitan areas from rural areas, married, and had children. These individuals are the core of the oldest old in today's urban communities. Current oldest old individuals have experienced sheer poverty and know the value of frugality, but baby boomers, who have just started retiring, grew up in the midst of rapid economic growth. Unlike the current oldest old women, the majority of female baby boomers have worked outside the home and have borne fewer children. In 2030, the baby boomers will be the core of the oldest old. They are less likely than the current oldest old to save money for future generations and more likely to depend on their grown up children. On the other hand, their children grew up and started to work when Japan was in the midst of prolonged economic depression. These young adults are more likely to remain single and have even fewer children than their parents. From those observations, Muramatsu and Akiyama (2011, p. 429) maintain that "Japan simply cannot afford having older adults not working. In 2030, they will constitute one third of the total population and can expect limited support from the working-age population. Labor participation among older adults is essential for sustaining the Japanese society."

The Japanese government has encouraged employers to provide more opportunities for the elderly (Martin, 1989) to cover the shortage of labor as well as to raise the eligibility age to receive public pensions. However, the fundamental problems still remain the same. With the increasing number of the elderly with prolonged longevity, not only the middle aged individuals but also elders are now taking care of frail oldest old seniors or an elderly individual providing care for his/her spouse. The stress for the elderly caregivers can be enormous; sometimes the hopelessness leads to homicides or double suicides among caregivers and care receivers to end their misery and burden (Kato, 2005; Oota, 1987; Shimizu, 1980a, 1980b; Yamaguchi, 2001; Yoshida, 2002).

The care providing institutions are also facing the problems of decline of the young population, such as an insufficient number of young laborers in nursing homes and medical facilities. Relatively low wage for the demanding physical work in the long term care facilities (Kibayashi & Amano, 2008) has attributed to the high turnover rate, resulting in the shortage of young laborers in the industry. With the necessity of keeping the service fees affordable, the care providing institutions are struggling to retain young employees. The possibility of accepting foreign workers in the long term care industry has been discussed, but issues of immigration remain controversial. Some of the popular rhetoric for dismissing the possibility of active recruitment of foreign workers is Japanese people's xenophobia, based on the higher crime rate committed by foreigners, and their linguistic barriers. Noro (2002, p. 21) describes "when receiving services, the resistance is strong to let a foreigner enter into the house. Also human-touch services such as nursing, caregiving, housework, and nanny-jobs tend to require high Japanese language skills." Some argue that there is a need to provide linguistic training programs for foreign workers, but some do not see the meaningfulness to spend public funds to educate foreigners to speak fluent Japanese when they tend to go back to their countries in a short time. Although a small number of foreign workers already exist in Japan, it is unlikely to see any drastic change in immigration issues any time soon.

IMPLICATIONS OF LONG TERM CARE INSURANCE: DEMEDICALIZATION AND SHIFT OF RESPONSIBILITY

Many researchers agree that the Long Term Care Insurance is considered an epoch because it means that Japan has moved toward socialization of care for the elderly from the tradition of family-based care (Matsuda & Yamamoto, 2001). Muramatsu and Akiyama (2011, p. 429) call the Long Term Care Insurance an "historic policy" because it "has made a variety of home, community-based, and institutional services, a universal entitlement for every Japanese person aged 65 + years based strictly on physical and mental status, regardless of family availability and economic status." The initial and primary motivation for reforming the public health insurance system in 1980s was to balance the nation's ever increasing budget deficit for health expenditures and pensions for the elderly. However, the new policies also encouraged an increase in the number of home-helper services, short stay services, and nursing homes (Campbell, 1984) which may have encouraged shifting the basic ideology of elderly care itself.

Universal entitlement of Long Term Care Insurance covers all elderly citizens including never-married citizens, childless couples, or those who do not live close to their spouse or children for various reasons. Indeed, this insurance was created based on the governmental slogan, "from care by family to care by society" (Campbell & Ikegami, 2000; Muramatsu & Akiyama, 2011; Tsutsumi & Muramatsu, 2005). This policy also changed how aging processes are understood. Long Term Care Insurance "was to 'de-medicalize' and rationalize the care of elderly persons with disabilities that were characteristic of the process of aging" (Matsuda & Yamamoto, 2001, p. 1). With this new insurance, seniors should be at home rather than staying in the hospital for a long period of time and to be seen as "sick" persons as Schmidt (2011, p. 88) describes "[a] medicalized sick role in aging makes the person a patient, a disease, illness, sickness, disorder, or syndrome, with less personhood and less of a person."

Ogawa and Retherford (1997) agree that under this insurance policy, the government's effort to establish both short term stay services and day care services throughout the country would contribute significantly to improving levels of elderly care since hospitals do not offer such individualized programs, detailed care, and various services for the elderly. However, contrary to the governmental slogan of Long Term Care Insurance, "From Care by Family to Care by Society," Ogawa and Retherford (1997) see this policy as the shift of the responsibility from the social security system back to the families when analyzing it from a financial perspective. Hospitals have played the role of a nursing home by providing long term care for the able-elderly at the expenses of the government; therefore families paid either nothing or very little fees to hospitals before the various insurance policy reforms (Ogawa & Retherford, 1997). In other words, this policy mandates the insured people to pay premium and service fees to receive care mainly at *home* with or without family members.

For seniors who have family members to depend on in the same household, the new insurance may work well because it supplements family-based care with various services. For seniors who have financial resources to purchase the high quality private residential nursing home care or visiting nurse services, implementation of Long Term Care Insurance is not as relevant as the middle class seniors who can benefit the most from the public assistance. For the seniors with limited financial resources and no family members and affordable housing, this policy change definitely took away the option of hospitalization; therefore, it shifted the responsibility and the place of elderly care back to home.

Matsuda and Yamamoto (2001) see that some of the key concepts of Long Term Care Insurance are self-determination and self-reliance since this new insurance system is no longer based on a flat per diem rate at the cost of government. The insured seniors or their family members have to work with a care manger that "is entrusted with the entire responsibility of planning all care and services for individual clients" (Matsuda & Yamamoto, 2001, p. 7). The emergence of care managers in the medical care field also "changed the balance of authority from the physician to the care manager," however, different care providers do not always agree with the authority of care managers; in fact a significant number of care mangers did not come up with any care plans for the insured due to the lack of knowledge and skills (Matsuda & Yamamoto, 2001, p. 7). Hopefully all care managers will gain their authority based on the consensus from other medical professionals by receiving extensive and comprehensive trainings to provide specific and appropriate plans for the insured seniors and their families; however, it is still crucial for any individuals to study the availability of various services and plan ahead for him/herself. This is a significant change as a care receiver compared to the passive nature of care-receiving and planning in the past.

FUTURE CONSIDERATIONS FOR A BETTER ELDERLY CARE

More than a decade after the successful implementation of the historic Long Term Care Insurance scheme, researchers have been identifying shortcomings and the necessity of further measurements and considerations. For example, Tsutsumi and Muramatsu (2005) write that Long Term Care Insurance has been widely accepted in Japanese society within a short period of time; however, several important measurements must be considered for the improvement of the system. It is crucial to build the right incentives into the system for all involved parties such as seniors, family members, service providers, and insurers to promote seniors' functional independence; this will in turn reduce excessive dependency on institutions and the government by promoting preventative services and rewarding providers who contribute to senior's improvement in function and health (Tsutsumi & Muramatsu 2005; Tsutusmi & Muramatsu 2007).

When a caregiver, often a senior person who is providing care for his/ her spouse or very old parents, becomes unable to provide care due to illness caused by the heavy burden of caregiving, "*tomodaore*" may happen. The literal meaning of "*tomodaore*" is the caregiver and care receiver are "falling together." Focusing on caregivers' emotional and psychological health and prevention of "*tomodaore*," Arai et al. (2004) study reveals that caregivers who found utilizing the services "inconvenient" tended to feel a heavier caregiving burden than those who did not. Although those family members and their insured seniors regularly use visiting nurse services, the caregivers feel it was "inconvenient" to use the services because they are not available when they are really needed (Arai et al., 2004). For instance, caregivers have to apply several months in advance to utilize services, therefore, when the caregivers suddenly became ill, neither short stay services nor home help services are available because of the need for long-standing reservations. By recognizing the effectiveness and benefit of the total release from caregiving time for the family members, the researchers suggest that emergency access of the services as needed may alleviate the feelings of burden. In order to achieve such a condition, a certain number of beds for the short stay facilities must be set aside to accommodate the emergency needs on a reservation free basis (Arai et al., 2004). This measurement seems especially important when considering the fact that many caregivers today are also in the category of the "old" population.

Extending with the possibility of total care for the elderly, Muramatsu and Akiyama (2011) point out the Great East Japan Earthquake of 2011 brought attention to the necessity of community-based support systems and emergency readiness for the elderly in addition to the various services under Long Term Care Insurance to support the elderly comprehensively. The hardest hit area of the tsunami in 2011 was the Tohoku district where mostly rural farming lands are located. One in three people in the area was age 65 and above and many of them struggled during the initial period of the tsunami aftermath due to the lack of access, not financial access but physical access, to medications and treatments which may have caused premature death (Muramatsu & Akiyama, 2011).

Although the rural Tohoku district was characterized as a closely knit rural community, it was still difficult for the elderly people to escape quickly due to their functional disabilities even with the neighbor's help. Comparing to the Tohoku area, social isolation is more salient for the oldest old people in urban communities. Universal availability of Long Term Care Insurance would not be enough if their isolation and disabilities are too severe to obtain necessary help when they need it the most. Muramatsu and Akiyama (2011) cited a study of international comparison to warn that Japan ranked last in the frequency of contacts with children who are living in a separate household and the second from the bottom for contacts with their neighbors in a five-country survey with France, Germany, Korea, and the United States. Indeed, Mainichi Shinbun (Mainichi Newspapers) (2012, April 10) listed several cases that received some media attention for the discovery of skeletonized or decomposed bodies in one's household within a few month period, but too many other individuals died alone of natural causes in his/her household or died after the death of their caregiver to be reported by mass media.

Combined with the Long Term Care Insurance system, Muramatsu and Akiyama (2011) suggest that building community-based support systems can be an effective new system if it is based on existing societal structures and systems such as re-building traditional Japanese housing and neighborhood styles. Muramatsu and Akiyama (2011) give the examples of the effort of community building among the tsunami evacuees. For instance, building temporary housing with the traditional Japanese *engawa* (a long veranda on the first floor with sliding doors to protect from outside elements, but open up the doors to make a room for gathering and communicating with neighbors who just stop by) to prevent isolation of the elderly Tsunami evacuees. The effect of the community building efforts such as this example should be studied and incorporated with policy implementation in the future.

Muramatsu and Akiyama (2011) also suggest reinstituting the traditional custom of *kairanban* (periodical circulated bound copies of information on community events and emergency contingency plans) is another effort to build a sense of neighborhood. Members of the neighborhood sign the signature boxes to ensure all members view the information. Those efforts can create social integration for the elderly in an urban community. Muramatsu and Akiyama (2011, p. 431) conclude "[a]lthough tragic, this earthquake provides an opportunity to understand how such a large-scale historic natural disaster can impact people's life course and, in turn, how individual and collective lives can affect societal responses to natural disasters and population aging." Although Long Term Care Insurance may not be a perfect system for everyone, it has transformed how Japanese people perceive elderly care and expanded options in a relatively short time. There is no reason why insurers and municipal governments cannot incorporate the traditional societal structures and systems into the new insurance programs to build a community-based support system which can improve the societal responses to emergency situations for the aging population.

CONCLUSION

Overall, it seems that evaluations of the Long Term Care Insurance scheme are mixed with positives and negatives; increased use of formal care at lower cost to households, reducing medical expenditures, and the necessity to improve caregivers' dissatisfaction toward the system (Tamiya et al., 2011). It is still debatable to whether this policy change has shifted "From Care by Family to Care by Society" as the governmental slogan promotes especially considering the fact that demedicalization of aging process may have shifted a heavy financial burden and the prolonged home care time back to the family. Schmidt (2011, p. 88) sees medicalization of aging leading into the condition in which "choice, planning, implementation, and responsibility are diminished. Normal social responsibilities are excused. Medicalizing social problems in aging reduces law and rule by law and substitutes rule by medicine." As one can see, medicalization has implications for personal liberty. Inversely, demedicalization put responsibility back to individuals, however, this returned responsibility is actually placed on the able-bodied family members when the current senior individuals do not share the values such as individual choice and liberty since interdependency of family members have been the traditional norm in Japan. Therefore, this new policy, for sure, created more options and various services for those families who prefer giving home-based care for their senior members and have been planning to utilize such options. This insurance also forces current younger generations to ponder about their personal responsibility and planning for their own aging; how to take care of oneself without counting on family members regardless of their marital status and/or existence of offspring.

As the planning and effective utilization of services becomes the key for the successful elderly care and aging process with this new insurance, it seems too early to evaluate this system as a successful shift to "self-reliance and self-determination" of elderly care because mandatory Long Term Care Insurance enrollment also created the concern for low income seniors (Hashizume, 2006). It can be translated as a heavy taxation on low-income seniors to offer more options for seniors from the middle class. High-income seniors can purchase the private high quality residential nursing homes but low income without family do not have a cheaper alternative to "live in a hospital" anymore. When "self-reliance and determination" is used to justify the limited access to the services among the low income seniors and families, the Long Term Care Insurance would lose its initial benevolent intention.

The imminent increase in the number of frail elderly people and decrease in the number of young tax payers continue to be a serious concern in Japan. Although a small number of foreign workers already do exist in Japan, the country has not actively recruited immigrants to cover the shortage of health and long term care industry as well as other industries (Muramatsu & Akiyama, 2011; Tsukada, 2010). Noro (2002) sees there is a lack of social support and cultural structures to encourage highly skilled foreign professionals to stay long or permanently in Japan. This lack of support seems to be caused by the ideological reason to keep the nation as homogeneous as possible.

Aging, lack of young labor, and immigration issues are common themes among many industrialized nations; therefore, implementation of this new scheme has been studied by many aging nations. As the United States is finally moving forward to the implementation of universal health care, the United States might have some advantages in terms of supply of young laborers in the elderly care and health care industry as the country is not as resistant to the idea of immigration as Japan.

Self-reliance, self-determination, utilization of formal care such as visiting nurse and short stay services may have been difficult to accept at first for Japanese people because those concepts contradict to some aspects of Japanese traditional norms, values, and life styles. As Muramatsu and Akiyama (2011) suggest, building elder care systems can be effectively accomplished if it is based on existing societal structures. Since self-reliance, self-determination, and utilization of formal care services are not a new idea to people in the United States, it is less likely for American individuals to have the difficulty of psychological adjustment in terms of planning and utilizing formal services for themselves. In that sense, the traditional U.S. norms and values can be the existing societal structure to build a comprehensive elderly care system. However, since each nation faces different problems with its specific condition, continuous studies and observations on the relationship between elderly care, immigration issues, and demographic changes will be necessary in order to offer more specific suggestions for each aging nation.

REFERENCES

Arai, Y., Kumamoto, K., Washio, M., Ueda, T., Miura, H., & Kudo, K. (2004). Factors related to feelings of burden among caregivers looking after impaired elderly in Japan under the long-term care insurance system. *Psychiatry and Clinical Neurosciences, 58,* 396–402.

Asai, M. O., & Kameoka, V. A. (2005). The influence of sekentei on family care giving and underutilization of social services among Japanese caregivers. *Social Work, 50,* 111–118.

Campbell, J. C., & Ikegami, N. (2000). Long-term care insurance comes to Japan. *Health Affairs (Millwood), 19*(3), 26–39.

Campbell, J. C., & Ikegami, N. (2003). Japan's radical reform of long-term care. *Social Policy and Administration, 37*(1), 21–34.

Campbell, R. (1984). Nursing homes and long-term care in Japan. *Pacific Affairs, 57*(1), 78–89.

Conrad, P. (2007). *The medicalization of society: On the transformation of human conditions into treatable disorders.* Baltimore, MD: Johns Hopkins University Press.

Fukawa, T. (2002). *Public health insurance in Japan.* Washington, DC: World Bank Institute. Retrieved from http://siteresources.worldbank.org/WBI/Resources/wbi37201. pdf. Accessed on November 19, 2012.

Hashizume, T. (2006). Kaigohokenseidonominaoshidetowaretakoto: "Teishotokushataisaku" wo chuushinnishite [Questioned issues on the review of long term care insurance system: Focusing on "counter measurement for the low income individuals"]. In Social Policy Studies Editorial Committee (Eds.), *Shakaiseisakukenkyuu* (Vol. 6, pp. 97–114). Tokyo, Japan: Toshindo.

Ikegami, N., & Campbell, J. C. (2004). Japan's health care system: Containing costs and attempting reform. *Health Affairs, 23*(3), 26–36.

Ikels, C. (1997). Long term care and the disabled elderly in urban China. In J. Sokolovsky (Ed.), *The cultural context of aging* (3rd ed.). Westport, CT: Bergin and Garvey.

Ishida, T. (1971). *Japanese society.* New York, NY: Random House.

Kato, E. (2005). Kaigosatsujin: Shihoufukushinoshitenkara *[The caregiving murder: From the view of laws on welfare].* Tokyo, Japan: Kuresu Shppan.

Kibayashi, M., & Amano, Y. (2008). A study of job satisfaction of care workers in a nursing home. *Annual Report of University of Shizuoka Junior College, 22,* 57–66.

Kondo, D. K. (1990). *Crafting selves: Power, gender, and discourses of identity in a Japanese workplace.* Chicago, IL: University of Chicago Press.

Lan, P. C. (2002). Subcontracting filial piety. *Journal of Family Issues, 23,* 812–835.

Lock, M. (1996). Centering the household: The remaking of female maturity in Japan. In A. Imamura (Ed.), *Re-imaging Japanese women* (pp. 73–103). Berkeley, CA: University of California Press.

Long, S. O. (1996). Nurturing and femininity: The ideal of caregiving in postwar Japan. In A. Imamura (Ed.), *Re-imaging Japanese women* (pp. 156–176). Berkeley, CA: University of California Press.

Long, S. O., Campbell, R., & Nishimura, C. (2009). Does it matter who cares? A comparison of daughters versus daughters-in-law in Japanese elder care. *Social Science Japan Journal, 12*(1), 1–21.

MacAdam, M. (2004). Home health care management practice examining home care in other countries. *The Policy Issues, 16,* 393–404.

Mainichi Shinbun (Mainichi Newspapers). (2012, April 10). *Kurozuappu 2012: Kodokushi, seidonohazama teigi toukei nashi fusegushikumi mikakutei (Close Up 2012: Dying alone, between the institutions, no definition, no statistics, not established mechanism for prevention).* Retrieved from http://mainichi.jp/opinion/news/20120408ddm003040063000c4. html. Accessed on January 15, 2013.

Matsuda, S., & Yamamoto, M. (2001). Long-term care insurance and integrated care for the aged in Japan. *International Journal of Integrated Care, September,* 1–11.

Martin, L. G. (1989). The graying of Japan. *Population Bulletin, 44*(2), 1–42.

Momose, Y., & Asahara, K. (1996). Relationship of "sekentei" to utilization of health, social and nursing services by the elderly. *Nihou Koshu Eisei Zasshi, 43*, 209–219.

Muramatsu, N., & Akiyama, H. (2011). Japan: Super-aging society preparing for the future. *The Gerontologist, 51*(4), 425–432.

Noro, N. (2002). *Foreign workers and the reception of immigrants* (pp. 4–25). Dai-ichi Life Research Institute monthly report [Online]. Retrieved from http://group.dai-ichi-life.co. jp/dlri/ldi/report/rp0202.pdf. Accessed on December 9, 2012.

Ogawa, N., & Retherford, R. D. (1993). Care of the elderly in Japan: Changing norms and expectations. *Journal of Marriage and the Family, 55*, 585–597.

Ogawa, N., & Retherford, R. D. (1997). Shifting costs of caring for the elderly back to families in Japan: Will it work? *Population and Development Review, 23*, 59–94.

Oota, T. (1987). Study on problems of home care for the elderly: Through analysis of the 29 criminal cases concerning care of the elderly. *Japanese Society for the Study of Social Welfare, 28*(2), 54–75.

Painter, A. (1996). The telerepresentation of gender in Japan. In A. Imamura (Ed.), *Re-imaging Japanese women* (pp. 46–72). Berkeley, CA: University of California Press.

Schmidt, W. C. (2011). Medicalization of aging: The upside and the downside. *Marquette Elder's Advisor, 13*(1), 55–88.

Shimizu, T. (1980a). Roubyousinjyu (1): Aru takushoku satujinjiken no kousatu [Age related diseases double suicide (1): Thoughts on a contract murder]. *Kangogakuzasshi, 44*, 492–499.

Shimizu, T. (1980b). Roubyoushinjyu (2): 53 rei no bunseki to kousatsu [Age related diseases double suicide (2): Analysis and thoughts on 53 examples]. *Kangogakuzasshi, 44*, 835–841.

Suzuki, T. (2007). Kazokukaigo no motodeno koreishanosatsujin, sinjyujiken [Murder or double suicide of seniors under family-based elderly care]. *The Hiroshima Law Journal, 31*(2), 101–118.

Tamiya, N., Noguchi, H., Nishi, A., Reich, M. R., Ikegami, N., Hashimoto, H., ... Campbell, J. C. (2011). Population ageing and wellbeing: Lessons from Japan's long-term care insurance policy. *The Lancet, 378*(9797), 1183–1192.

Tamiya, N., Yamaoka, K., & Yano, E. (2002). Use of home health services covered by new public long term care insurance in Japan: Impact of the presence and kinship of family caregivers. *International Journal for Quality in Health, 14*(4), 295–303.

Tsukada, N. (2010). Kaigogenbanogaikokujinrodosha: Nihonnokeagenbawadoukawarunoka *[Foreign workers in long-term care: How is long-term care changing in Japan?]*. Tokyo, Japan: Akashishoten.

Tsutsumi, T., & Muramatsu, N. (2005). Care-needs certification in the long-term care insurance system of Japan. *American Geriatrics Society, 53*, 522–527.

Tsutsumi, T., & Muramatsu, N. (2007). Japan's universal long-term care system reform of 2005: Containing costs and realizing a vision. *Journal of the American Geriatrics Society, 55*, 1458–1463.

Yamaguchi, M. (2001). Zaitakukaigotoshinjyuujiken: Naganoshidehasseishitajikenno bunseki-kara [Home care and double suicide: Analysis on the case happened in Nagano city]. *Shakaifukushishi, 8*, 141–148.

Yoshida, T. (2002). Fuufugashitomukaiautoki *[When husband and wife face death]*. Tokyo, Japan: Bungeishunjyu.

HARM TO THE HEALTH OF THE PUBLIC ARISING FROM AGGRESSIVE MARKETING AND SALES OF HEALTH-RELATED PRODUCTS AND SERVICES: ANOTHER ASPECT OF MEDICALIZATION WHICH IS A CAUSE FOR CONCERN?

Kai-Lit Phua

ABSTRACT

Purpose − *To present the view that harm arising from aggressive marketing and sales of health-related products and services (including dangerous and defective ones) in order to maximize profits should be a cause of concern for public health academics and practitioners.*

Technology, Communication, Disparities and Government Options in Health and
Health Care Services
Research in the Sociology of Health Care, Volume 32, 199−212
Copyright © 2014 by Emerald Group Publishing Limited
ISSN: 0275-4959/doi:10.1108/S0275-495920140000032025

Methodology/approach – *The discussion is conducted using biomedical ethics principles and supported using various real-world examples.*

Findings – *Harm arising from aggressive marketing and sales of health-related products and services (including dangerous and defective ones) in order to maximize profits should be a cause of concern for public health academics and practitioners. In the area of products, the most obvious would be tobacco products. In the case of pharmaceutical drugs, it would include overuse or inappropriate use because of aggressive marketing. It would also include harm caused by the continued promotion and sale of a drug in the face of evidence that it has significant negative side effects. Brody and Light's "Inverse Benefit Law," that is, the benefit-to-harm ratio of drugs tends to vary inversely with how aggressively drugs are marketed is discussed. Harm is also evident in health-related services, for example, misuse of ultrasonography for sex-selective abortion. This chapter will discuss how the risk of harm is increased because of questionable marketing strategies used by drug companies.*

Research limitations/implications – *One limitation is that no attempt to quantify the harm done (e.g., through economic evaluation techniques) is carried out.*

Originality/value of chapter – *This chapter presents the view that much more attention should be paid to this aspect of medicalization as a public health threat.*

Keywords: Biomedical ethics; medicalization; marketing; pharmaceutical drugs

INTRODUCTION

Health-related products (such as pharmaceutical drugs) and services play a vital role in the battle against disease and disability. However, the use of pharmaceutical products and medical services are not always beneficial or risk-free. They can give rise to negative effects on a person's health too (Avorn, 2004). The risks increase with one aspect of medicalization (Conrad, 2007), that is, aggressive marketing of such products and services in the quest for maximization of sales or profits resulting in overuse or inappropriate use. Harm has also been caused by the continued marketing and sale of particular pharmaceutical drugs in the face of evidence from post-marketing surveillance that the drugs can cause significant side effects in users. Examples include the pain-killer for arthritis called Rofecoxib (brand name Vioxx) (Ross et al., 2009) and the diabetic drug scandal in France (brand name Mediator) (Schofield, 2011). There has also been harm resulting from aggressive and sometimes unethical marketing or supply of other products (e.g., tobacco, infant formula, fast foods, soft drinks) and services (e.g., plastic surgery).

The "Inverse Benefit Law" proposed by Brody and Light posits that the benefit-to-harm ratio of drugs tends to vary inversely with how aggressively drugs are marketed through the use of six strategies, that is, reducing thresholds for diagnosis of disease, relying on surrogate endpoints, exaggerating safety claims for drugs, exaggerating efficacy claims for drugs, invention of new diseases, and encouraging unapproved (off-label) uses for existing drugs (Brody & Light, 2011).

It should be noted that harm can also arise from aggressive marketing of health-related services. An example is the misuse of ultrasonography for the purpose of sex-selective abortion in countries where there is a culturally derived preference for male babies as compared to female babies (Hesketh & Xing, 2006). This chapter will focus on harm associated with health-related products (especially pharmaceutical drugs).

HARM ARISING FROM AGGRESSIVE MARKETING OF HEALTH-RELATED PRODUCTS: PHARMACEUTICAL DRUGS

Illich, in his provocative book Medical Nemesis (1974), classified ill health resulting directly from medical intervention under the label "clinical iatrogenesis." However, he did not relate this in any way to the pressures generated on healthcare providers who are operating in a market economy and who are also subjected to the impulse to maximize sales or profits.

In the case of pharmaceutical drugs, it is necessary to keep in mind that even if genuine drugs have been correctly prescribed and are being taken properly by the patient, the patient can still be affected negatively, for example, short term side effects such as impaired driving skills, drowsiness, nausea, dry mouth, loss of appetite, or loss of libido; long term side effects that affect the quality of life; elevated risk of developing other conditions; adverse drug reactions; negative drug interactions resulting from polypharmacy; addiction to prescription drugs; increased financial costs and opportunity costs. Overuse and inappropriate use of genuine drugs because of aggressive marketing and sales efforts would contribute to the above.

Examples of long term side effects from taking pharmaceutical drugs and elevated risk of developing other conditions include rhabdomyolysis (muscle wasting) and liver damage from taking statins to lower cholesterol levels (Moynihan & Cassels, 2005). There is even the possibility that drugs prescribed to treat epilepsy (anticonvulsants) or psychiatric conditions such as depression (antidepressants such as the Selective Serotonin Reuptake Inhibitors or SSRIs) may actually increase the risk of suicidal behavior, suicide ideation, or even violent behavior toward other people (Kassirer, 2005; Pringle, 2009).

Adverse drug reactions can be significant or even life-threatening. A notorious example from Singapore concerns the taking of an appetite suppressant drug by an actress named Andrea de Cruz that caused severe damage to her liver. She was saved from dying only because her husband (then fiancé) Pierre Png donated half of his liver for a liver transplant for her. The drug was manufactured in China, contained fenfluramine (banned in the USA for causing damage to valves in the heart) and was marketed under the name "Slim 10." Diet pills such as these are often registered as traditional Asian herbal medicines or health foods and thus, do not have to undergo rigorous drug trials for safety and efficacy (Cullen, 2002). In the United Kingdom, 5% of all hospital admissions are due to adverse drug reactions (House of Commons Health Committee, 2005).

The taking of prescription drugs can result in addiction and strong withdrawal symptoms when patients stop taking the drugs. There is the example of the addiction of the late singer Michael Jackson to prescription drugs. Apparently, it is not difficult to obtain a prescription for addictive pharmaceutical drugs legally from doctors by feigning mental disorders. If this does not work, pharmaceutical drugs can be bought over the Internet (Spicer, 2010).

Unnecessary drug-taking induced by the marketing efforts of pharmaceutical companies (especially the taking of expensive proprietary drugs) will result in higher financial costs − financial harm − to patients, and to third-party payers such as insurance companies and governments. From an economist's point of view, opportunity costs will also be incurred as limited healthcare resources are diverted and used up, with resulting negative effects on allocative efficiency. Higher costs can also be incurred in the treatment of iatrogenic illnesses due to the taking of drugs such as Vioxx and Celebrex (House of Commons Health Committee, 2005).

It has been pointed out that pharmaceutical drugs approved for the market by regulatory agencies such as the Food and Drug Administration of the USA (FDA) are not necessarily completely safe (see, e.g., the list of FDA-approved drugs that were later withdrawn on the "Worst Pills" website http://www.worstpills.org/public/page.cfm?op_id=68 set up by Public Citizen's health group). Phua and Achike (2007) have described problems associated with the process of getting a new pharmaceutical drug onto the market and how these can affect drug safety. The problems begin with drug research and development, clinical trials, presentation and publication of research findings, all the way to approval by public regulators, the writing of clinical practice guidelines, drug marketing by pharmaceutical companies, and post-marketing surveillance.

PROBLEMATIC MARKETING STRATEGIES USED BY PHARMACEUTICAL COMPANIES

As mentioned earlier, Brody and Light (2011) pointed out the aggressive marketing of drugs through the use of six strategies, that is, reducing thresholds for diagnosis of disease, relying on surrogate endpoints, exaggerating safety claims for drugs, exaggerating efficacy claims for drugs, invention of new diseases, and encouraging unapproved (off-label) uses for existing drugs.

Beginning in the 1990s, critics of marketing strategies used by pharmaceutical companies to increase drug sales came up with the term "disease mongers" to denote those who attempt to widen the boundaries of disease – and thus the need for treatment – for financial gain. According to Payer (1992), the disease mongers include pharmaceutical companies and doctors. The primary motivation is to sell more health-related products and services. Moynihan and his co-authors (Moynihan & Cassels, 2005; Moynihan, Heath, & Henry, 2002; Moynihan & Henry, 2006) identified different forms of "disease mongering":

- Medicalization of normal life events and conditions such as menopause and male pattern baldness;
- Portraying mild problems as serious illnesses or particular rare personality traits as more prevalent conditions that need to be treated aggressively with drugs, for example, irritable bowel syndrome and social anxiety disorder;

- Framing risk factors as diseases in themselves, for example, high cholesterol level, high blood pressure, and osteoporosis. A recent example is the decision by the American Medical Association at its 2013 meeting to classify obesity as a disease (Wilson, 2013). Seriousness of risks can also be exaggerated in order to induce those affected to seek treatment;
- Inventing new diagnostic categories, for example, female sexual dysfunction and premenstrual dysphoric disorder (PMDD).

In 2002, the journal *BMJ* initiated a series of articles and discussions on "non-disease" (Smith, 2002). Readers were also asked to suggest non-diseases and to select those that best fit the definition of non-disease as "a human process or problem that some have defined as a medical condition but where people may have better outcomes if the problem or process was not defined that way." Readers responded and some of the top choices included ageing, baldness, unhappiness, pregnancy, road rage, and loneliness.

Psychiatric conditions are very susceptible to medicalization (Conrad, 2007) because the boundary between what is normal and what is a "mental disorder" is often unclear. There was controversy when the previous version of the Diagnostic and Statistical Manual of Mental Disorders (DSM-IV) was undergoing revision as part of the preparation of the current version (DSM-5). Some psychiatrists were worried about the consequences of creation of new diagnostic categories and especially the lowering of thresholds of existing categories, for example, "binge eating disorder" whereby a person would be diagnosed as suffering from the condition by binge eating only *once a week* for three months (PBS Newshour, 2010).The latest version, called DSM-5, has been heavily criticized and the National Institute of Mental Health has even decided not to fund research based on DSM symptom clusters (McKay, 2013).

One marketing strategy used by pharmaceutical companies is the "disease-awareness campaign." Moynihan and Henry (2006) note that disease awareness campaigns are "more often designed to sell drugs than to illuminate or to inform or educate about the prevention of illness or the maintenance of health." Disease awareness campaigns (Koerner, 2002) typically begin with the recruitment of prominent doctors or biomedical scientists – called Key Opinion Leaders in the parlance of the public relations and marketing industry – to proclaim to the public about the high prevalence of a hitherto relatively unknown or unrecognized medical condition such as generalized anxiety disorder. Statistics and findings from corporate-sponsored studies are used to reinforce this message and to inform the public as well as healthcare providers that there is an effective treatment at hand for the medical condition: typically a drug manufactured by the pharmaceutical company sponsoring the studies. Lastly, patient groups (heavily subsidized by the drug company or even operating directly out of the offices of public relations firms hired by the drug company) are established to "... serve as the 'public face' for the condition, supplying quotes and compelling human stories for the media ..." (*ibid.*). The stories are sometimes told via blogs, drug internet chat groups, and websites set up by individuals who may not disclose their financial links to the disease awareness campaign of the pharmaceutical company selling the drug used to treat the particular disease (Consumers International, 2006).

Sometimes, disease awareness campaigns attempt to increase the numbers of the "afflicted" by encouraging self-diagnosis through online quizzes, for example, the drug company-sponsored patient support group website for restless legs syndrome was also designed to encourage self-diagnosis. The "afflicted person" is then encouraged to "see your doctor" and ask for the drug recommended to treat the syndrome (Dear & Webb, 2007). The "see your doctor" strategy to increase drug prescribing by doctors actually works: Kravitz et al. (2005) showed that doctors are more likely to prescribe an antidepressant drug even for mild, temporary distress if the patient directly requests for it.

Marketing of drugs on the part of pharmaceutical companies can include ethically questionable strategies. These include attempts to influence the prescribing patterns of doctors using dubious means (the supply side) and promoting patient awareness of and requests for new drugs from the doctors they consult in misleading ways (demand side) (Phua & Achike, 2007).

Drug advertisements in medical journals read by doctors can contain incomplete or inaccurate information such as leaving out descriptions of side effects or making claims that are not supported by the references they cite (Villanueva, Peiro, Librero, & Pereiro, 2003). Drug companies commonly sponsor doctors on trips to resorts to listen to presentations on the merits of their drugs. "Key Opinion Leaders" such as prominent doctors and biomedical scientists and "product champions" such as sports stars, entertainers, and other celebrities are recruited to help in the promotion of new drugs. There is also direct-to-consumer advertising of new drugs in the USA which have been shown to increase sales (Lyles, 2002). In the European Union countries, direct-to-consumer advertising is not permitted but the pharmaceutical companies use various strategies to get around this, for example, setting up internet chat groups, and launching websites dealing with particular drugs or diseases (Consumers International, 2006).

Drug companies may also attempt to increase usage (and therefore sales) of their drugs by "product stretching." Thus, FDA approval can be obtained to treat new conditions using existing drugs, for example, the antidepressant Prozac − under pressure from generic versions after its patent expired − was repackaged as Sarafem to treat PMDD (Greenslit, 2002). This is because marketing existing drugs for new uses is much cheaper than developing a new drug from scratch. However, Koerner (2002) notes that "to show that a drug works in treating a new disease, the FDA often accepts in-house corporate studies, even when companies refuse to disclose their data or methodologies to other researchers, as is scientific custom."

More questionably, pharmaceutical companies may also attempt to encourage off-label use of their drugs, that is, using a drug for medical conditions other than those for which it has obtained approval to deal with (Kassirer, 2005). An example of off-label use associated with increased risk of harm would be using Hormone Replacement Therapy (HRT) to "prevent osteoporosis." Here, the principle of justice is violated: while drug companies reap the financial benefits from encouraging off-label use of their drugs, the patients are the ones who will bear the cost of bodily harm should any harmful effects occur.

Critics allege that drug companies are not above establishing front groups like the Social Anxiety Disorder Coalition and the Post-Traumatic Stress Disorder Alliance (Koerner, 2002). Drug companies have also sponsored disease or patient support groups such as Mental Health America (Pringle, 2009). Critics fear that some of these patient support groups may become co-opted because of financial sponsorship by drug companies.

In short, drug companies, their marketing staff and the public relations companies they hire have turned diseases and drugs into commodities for mass marketing. Other parties are also complicit in the commodification of pharmaceutical drugs and increased risk of harm, for example, mass media that periodically publicize new drugs as if they are "magic bullets" against particular diseases. As for third-party payers, in order to reduce costs, Koerner (2002) says that primary care doctors in the USA are pressured by health insurance companies to prescribe drugs rather than refer mental health patients for psychotherapy because the latter mode of treatment is more expensive. Furthermore, in the USA, some critics have decried the attempts of drug companies to influence politicians and public policy with respect to pharmaceutical drugs and other medical products through lobbying and financial contributions (Angell, 2004; Relman & Angell, 2002).

Invention of new diseases is likely in the identification of conditions such as restless legs syndrome (Woloshin & Schwartz, 2006), andropause (supposedly the male equivalent of menopause), and prehypertension. There has also been loosening of the criteria for diagnosis of bipolar disorder, determination of high cholesterol level and high blood pressure in order to increase the prevalence rate. In the case of bipolar disorder, people as young as two years of age have been diagnosed as suffering from the condition! (Business Week, 2006; Healy, 2008). "Prehypertension" has been defined as blood pressure range of 120–139 mm Hg systolic or 80–89 mm Hg diastolic and the condition is supposedly present in 70 million Americans (Schunkert, 2006). From a statistical point of view, this definition is clearly highly debatable since the blood pressure for a healthy young adult is about 120 mm Hg systolic and 80 mm Hg diastolic and blood pressure when measured for an entire population is in the shape of a bell curve or "normal distribution." If one accepts this definition of "prehypertension," this would mean that one is saying that the entire right side of the normal distribution – up to the customary cut off point for "borderline hypertension" (140 mm Hg systolic and 90 mm Hg diastolic) – constitutes the condition!

Whatever the merits of re-defining an important risk factor for ill health – obesity – as a "disease" on the part of the American Medical Association, this only promotes the further medicalization of U.S. society. It also results in the strange phenomenon of a significant percentage of the American population being labeled as being "diseased" simply because their Body Mass Index (BMI) is high.

In order to combat breast cancer in women, regular mammograms are recommended for older women so as to detect the disease in its early stages.

There has been some controversy over at what age and how frequently women should go for mammograms. The U.S. Preventive Task Force recommended in late 2009 that women aged between 50 and 74 should get mammograms but only every other year. In contrast, the American Cancer Society stuck to the recommendation of annual mammograms for women beginning at age 40 (Hobson, 2009). It should be remembered that in addition to anxiety (mental health cost) and the additional financial cost of further testing as a result of false positive results, mammograms also cause physical discomfort and increased exposure to radiation to the women undergoing the procedure.

PROBLEMATIC PHARMACEUTICAL MARKETING STRATEGIES AND THE CHALLENGES THEY PRESENT TO BIOMEDICAL ETHICS

Biomedical ethicists commonly look at four things when discussing ethical issues with respect to clinical medicine, that is, autonomy, beneficence, non-maleficence, and justice. From a public health perspective, these can be broadened to include issues such as individual freedom/rights of corporate entities versus social control (by the state via compulsory, restrictive public health laws), and social justice with respect to public expenditure patterns and the outcomes of these patterns.

Supporters of disease awareness campaigns often use the same arguments as those who favor relatively unrestricted advertising of non-medical goods and services (i.e., subject only to truthfulness of claims made in advertisements). They commonly argue that patient autonomy is enhanced because patients get to learn more about their particular medical condition and the drugs that are available to treat it. The principle of beneficence is also supported because disease awareness campaigns can help patients with undiagnosed conditions (and even doctors) to finally understand what the problem is so that the patients will get proper care. Thus, according to these supporters of disease awareness campaigns, why should there be any controversy over direct-to-consumer advertising? (Lyles, 2002).

In more individualistic societies such as the USA, the issue of the rights of individuals and corporate entities − it should be remembered that the corporation is a legal entity in the eyes of the law − versus control by the state via mandatory, restrictive public health laws can be highly contentious.

In fact, some have even argued that restrictions on a corporation's advertising activities are an infringement on the U.S. Constitution's First Amendment rights to freedom of speech (Ringold, 1995). Also, in the USA, there are virtually no restrictions on the pricing of drugs by pharmaceutical companies.

Critics of disease mongering such as Consumers International (2006) have documented numerous cases of dubious strategies and techniques used by pharmaceutical companies and argue that more stringent regulations are needed. Instead of promoting patient autonomy (through informed choice) and beneficence, misleading drug advertising and the fabrication of new but dubious disease categories such as restless legs syndrome only increase the ingestion of drugs and thus increase the risk of harm arising from inappropriate use of drugs. This violates the principle of non-maleficence. Disease mongering can create medically unnecessary consumer demand for health-related goods and services and further worsen the problem of rising person's healthcare costs. It will also add to further strain on the public finances of countries where government spending on healthcare is significant, thus affecting distributive justice or social justice.

Finally, pharmaceutical companies often exaggerate the benefits of treatment and minimize the risks in their disease awareness campaigns (Consumers International, 2006).

CONCLUSIONS

In this chapter, I have discussed some of the threats to public health, using specific examples, arising from the aggressive marketing and provision of health-related products and services (including dangerous and defective ones) in order to maximize sales and profits. This is one aspect of medicalization which should be of concern for public health practitioners.

Following the "Inverse Benefit Law" of Brody and Light, the risk of harm can be increased by the questionable marketing strategies used by some pharmaceutical companies, for example, the deliberate widening of boundaries of disease in order to sell more health-related products and services. These also significant challenges to biomedical ethics.

It is probable that such harm is more likely in the more market-oriented economies or more market-oriented healthcare systems such as that of the USA. Indeed, Moynihan and Henry (2006) declared that:

> ... the broad shift away from government-run programs and towards the marketplace ... and the consequent commercialisation and commodification of health services, may be a useful framework for a more profound explanation of ... (disease mongering). In a climate where governments are encouraging corporations to vigorously pursue for-profit activities within the health-care sector, it is hardly surprising that pharmaceutical companies will use a range of promotional activities to widen the definitions of disease .... (Moynihan & Henry, 2006)

However, looking at the demand side of the equation, the possibility of harm is heightened if there is demand by people for medically unnecessary services and goods, for example, plastic surgery for purely cosmetic purposes and medical consultations and drugs to deal with the stresses and strains of daily life. Moynihan and Henry (2006) regard disease mongering as exploitation of anxiety about human frailty and of faith in scientific progress and believe that allowing panels of specialists "riddled with profes-sional and commercial conflicts of interest" to define disease "is no longer viable."

Heath (2006) further expands this by seeing disease mongering as being due to powerful economic, political, and professional interests that exploit fear of suffering and death to make money, or place emphasis on treatment to minimize "… political responsibility for those fundamental causes of dis-ease that are located within the structure of society …" According to her, disease mongering and encouragement of drug-taking is another example of the individualistic approach (and not a population-based approach) to health problems. Heath makes the plea for more biomedical scientists and healthcare practitioners (and presumably the public as well) to recognize and acknowledge the limits of medical knowledge, extrapolate less beyond research findings and also to use statistics much more responsibly. Finally, it is my view that the public health community can respond to the challenge in the case of drugs by encouraging the authorities to strengthen regulation pertaining to marketing of pharmaceutical drugs and also by supporting consumer advocacy groups such as Worst Pills (to reduce information asymmetry between drug companies on the one hand and drug users on the other hand).

REFERENCES

Angell, M. (2004). *The truth about the drug companies: How they deceive us and what to do about it.* New York, NY: Random House.

Avorn, J. (2004). *Powerful medicines: The benefits, risks, and costs of prescription drugs.* New York, NY: Random House.

Brody, H., & Light, D. W. (2011). The inverse benefit law: How drug marketing undermines patient safety and public health. *American Journal of Public Health, 101*(3), 399–404.

Business Week. (2006). Hey, you don't look so good. *Business Week*, May 8.

Conrad, P. (2007). *The medicalization of society: On the transformation of human conditions into treatable diseases.* Baltimore, MD: Johns Hopkins University Press.

Consumers International. (2006). *Branding the cure.* London: Consumers International.

Cullen, L. T. (2002). Asia's killer diet pills. *Time*, August 5. Retrieved from http://www.time.com/time/magazine/article/0,9171,333902,00.html

Dear, J. W., & Webb, D. J. (2007). Disease mongering – A challenge for everyone involved in healthcare. *British Journal of Clinical Pharmacology, 64*(2), 122–124.

Greenslit, N. (2002). Pharmaceutical branding: Identity, individuality, and illness. *Molecular Interventions, 2*(6), 342–345.

Healy, D. (2008). *Mania: A short history of bipolar disorder.* Baltimore, MD: Johns Hopkins University Press.

Heath, I. (2006). Combating disease mongering: Daunting but nonetheless essential. *PLoS Medicine, 3*(4), e146. doi:10.1371/journal.pmed.0030146

Hesketh, T., & Xing, Z. W. (2006). Abnormal sex ratios in human populations: Causes and consequences. *Proceedings of the National Academy of Sciences of the United States of America, 103*(36), 13271–13275.

Hobson, K. (2009, November 16). *Routine mammograms before 50: Not much point.* U.S. news and world report. Retrieved from http://health.usnews.com/health-news/managing-your-healthcare/cancer/articles/2009/11/16/routine-mammograms-before-50-not-much-point.html

House of Commons Health Committee. (2005). *The influence of the pharmaceutical industry.* London: The Stationery Office Limited.

Illich, I. (1974). *Medical nemesis.* London: Calder and Boyars.

Kassirer, J. (2005). *On the take: How medicine's complicity with big business can endanger your health.* Oxford: Oxford University Press.

Koerner, B. I. (2002). Disorders made to order. *Mother Jones*, July/August. Retrieved from http://motherjones.com/politics/2002/07/disorders-made-order

Kravitz, R. L., Epstein, R. M., Feldman, M. D., Franz, C. E., Azari, R., Azari, M. S., ... Franks, P. (2005). Influence of patients' requests for direct-to-consumer advertised antidepressants: A randomized controlled trial. *Journal of the American Medical Association, 293*, 1995–2002.

Lyles, A. (2002). Direct marketing of pharmaceuticals to consumers. *Annual Review of Public Health, 23*, 73–91.

McKay, M. (2013). Goodbye to the DSM-V. *Huffington Post Science*, May 22. Retrieved from http://www.huffngtonpost.com/new-harbinger-publications-inc/goodbye-to-the-dsmv-b-3307510.html

Moynihan, R., & Cassels, A. (2005). *Selling sickness: How the world's biggest pharmaceutical companies are turning us all into patients.* New York, NY: Nation Books.

Moynihan, R., Heath, I., & Henry, D. (2002). Selling sickness: The pharmaceutical industry and disease mongering. *British Medical Journal, 324*(7342), 886–891.

Moynihan, R., & Henry, D. (2006). The fight against disease mongering: Generating knowledge for action. *PLoS Medicine, 3*(4), e191. doi:10.1371/journal.pmed.0030191

Payer, L. (1992). *Disease mongers: How doctors, drug companies, and insurers are making you feel sick.* New York, NY: Wiley.

PBS Newshour. (2010). *Psychiatrists propose revisions to diagnosis manual.* Retrieved from http://www.pbs.org/newshour/bb/health/jan-june10/mentalillness_02-10.html

Phua, K. L., & Achike, F. I. (2007). Vioxx and other pharmaceutical product withdrawals: Ethical issues in ensuring the integrity of drug and medical device research, development and commercialization. *Clinical Ethics, 2*, 155–162.

Pringle, E. (2009). *4 Part Series Mothers Act disease mongering campaign.* Retrieved from http://evelynpringle.blogspot.com/search/label/Mothers%20Act

Relman, A. S., & Angell, M. (2002). America's other drug problem: How the drug industry distorts medicine and politics. *New Republic, 16*, 27–41.

Ringold, D. J. (1995). Social criticisms of target marketing: Process or product? *American Behavioral Scientist, 38*, 578–592.

Ross, J. S., Madigan, D., Hill, K. P., Egilman, D. S., Wang, Y., & Krumholz, H. M. (2009). Pooled analysis of Rofecoxib placebo-controlled clinical trial data: Lessons for post-market pharmaceutical safety surveillance. *Archives of Internal Medicine, 169*(21), 1976–1985.

Schofield, H. (2011). *France braces for diabetic drug scandal report.* Retrieved from http://www.bbc.co.uk/news/world-europe-12155639

Schunkert, H. (2006). Pharmacotherapy for prehypertension – Mission accomplished? *The New England Journal of Medicine, 354*(16), 1742–1744.

Smith, R. (2002). In search of "non-disease". *British Medical Journal, 2002*(324), 883–885.

Spicer, K. (2010). Brittany Murphy, Michael Jackson, Heath Legder ... America's fatal addiction to prescription drugs. *Sunday Times*, May 2. Retrieved from http://www.cchrint.org/2010/05/03/the-london-times-brittany-murphy-michael-jackson-heath-legder-americas-fatal-addiction-to-prescription-drugs/

Villanueva, P., Peiro, S., Librero, J., & Pereiro, I. (2003). Accuracy of pharmaceutical advertisements in medical journals. *Lancet, 361*, 27–32.

Wilson, J. (2013). Physicians group labels obesity as a disease. *CNN*, June 19. Retrieved from http://edition.cnn.com/2013/06/19/health/ama-obesity-disease-change

Woloshin, S., & Schwartz, L. M. (2006). Giving legs to restless legs: A case study of how the media helps to make people sick. *PLoS Medicine, 3*(4), e170. doi:10.1371/journal.pmed.0030170.

Worst Pills Website. (2010). Retrieved from http://www.worstpills.org

IMPROVING RESIDENT OUTCOMES IN STATE MEDICAID NURSING FACILITY LONG-TERM CARE PROGRAMS: AUGMENTING CMS SURVEYS WITH MODEST CHANGES TO A FEW STATE PROGRAM FEATURES

Charles Lockhart, Kristin Klopfenstein, Jean Giles-Sims and Cathan Coghlan

ABSTRACT

Purpose — *Federal and state governments collaborate on state Medicaid nursing facility long-term care (SMNF-LTC) programs. These programs are increasingly expensive as the baby-boomers retire. Yet serious resident outcome problems continue in spite of the Centers for Medicare and Medicaid Services' (CMS) extensive process-focused regulatory*

Technology, Communication, Disparities and Government Options in Health and Health Care Services
Research in the Sociology of Health Care, Volume 32, 213–234
Copyright © 2014 by Emerald Group Publishing Limited
ISSN: 0275-4959/doi:10.1108/S0275-495920140000032021

efforts. This study identifies a promising and simpler auxiliary path for improving resident outcomes.

Methodology/approach − *Drawing on a longitudinal (1997−2005), 48-state data set and panel-corrected, time-series regression, we compare the effects on resident outcomes of CMS process-focused surveys and four minimally regulated program structural features on which the states vary considerably.*

Findings − *We find that each of these four structural features exerts a greater effect on resident outcomes than process quality.*

Research limitations/implications − *We suggest augmenting current process-focused regulation with a less arduous approach of more extensive regulation of these program features.*

Originality/values of chapter − *To date SMNF-LTC program regulation has focused largely on member facility processes. While regulating processes is appropriate, we show that regulating program structural features directly, an arguably easier task, might well produce considerable improvement in the quality of resident outcomes.*

Keywords: Long-term care; Medicaid; nursing facilities; nursing facility long-term care; nursing facility resident outcomes

Nursing facility long-term care for elders is one of the coverages specified by the Medicaid law of 1965, itself an amendment of the Social Security Act, and the federal and state governments collaborate in its provision through the Medicaid programs of the various states. The two levels of government share the substantial financial expenditures that the provision of this care consumes with the states paying somewhat less than half of the total. Data arising from inspections or "surveys" of nursing facilities which are members of state Medicaid nursing facility long-term care (SMNF-LTC) programs − the vast majority of extant facilities − are collected by state-level survey teams. These survey data are compiled at the state level and sent on to the national Centers for Medicare and Medicaid Services (CMS) which manages the Online Survey, Certification and Reporting (OSCAR) System. States also develop MNF-LTC programs with distinctive structural characteristics.

Federal survey teams periodically survey a sample of facilities for comparative purposes, and CMS provides special teams representing its Quality Improvement Organizations (QIOs) as warranted. The federal government regulates resident care primarily through setting standards for the services that facilities associated with SMNF-LTC programs provide and authorizing "deficiencies" (Ftags) for inadequacies. It also has a relatively infrequently applied and languidly proceeding capacity (shared in part by the states) for sanctioning unacceptable standards through fines (Civil Monetary Penalties − CMPs), withholding Medicaid payment for new program residents or even closing facilities (Harrington, Mullan, & Carrillo, 2004; Li, Harrington, Spector, & Mukamel, 2010).

State MNF-LTC programs are the major payors of the care expenses for two-thirds of their roughly 1.4 million residents (Harrington, Carrillo, Dowdell, Tang, & Woleslagle Blank, 2011), providing an expensive public benefit for a large portion of older citizens and their families. But resident outcomes in these programs are persistently discouraging (USDH&HS, 2009) (U.S. Government Accounting Office [USGAO], 2009), and it is difficult to argue that these public SMNF-LTC funds are optimally spent. Additionally, the United States is an aging society; Americans 65 or older constitute a progressively larger portion of the overall population as the leading edge of the post-World War II baby-boomers retires (He, Sengupta, Velkoff, & DeBarros, 2005). In 2005, the midpoint of this study, Medicaid programs claimed 23 percent of all state budgets, $315 billion nationwide. Medicaid was already the largest single, and a growing, category of state expenditure, and nursing facility long-term care was responsible for about $60 billion (19 percent of total Medicaid expenditures) across the states (Eiken, Burwell, Gold, & Sredl, 2010; Eiken, Burwell, & Schaefter, 2004; National Association of State Budget Officers [NASBO], 2005). These program expenditures are apt to increase as the baby-boomers continue to age. Improving the way these programs are regulated is surely warranted in light of their expense and the persistent deficiencies of resident outcomes. This study suggests a possibility for achieving improvement.

The current study arises from Donabedian's (2003) well-known contention that the structure of medical care institutions (e.g., a SMNF-LTC program's registered nurse hours per resident day) largely determines the quality of their processes (e.g., the proportion of SMNF-LTC program's facilities which is not deficient in preventing resident pressure sores). Further, the quality of these processes heavily influences the quality of patient outcomes (e.g., the proportion of a SMNF-LTC program's residents which avoids pressure sores). We previously examined various aspects of the degree to which this contention characterizes state nursing facility long-term care programs (Lockhart, Giles-Sims, & Klopfenstein, 2008, 2009). In this study, we examine a modest revision of Donabedian's thesis: that certain program structural features and program processes each make independent contributions to program residents' quality of life outcomes. More precisely, we ask how specific program structural characteristics and program process quality compare in their influence on program residents' quality of life outcomes. While we thought that aspects of program structure would have some independent influence on these outcomes, we imagined that the effects of program process quality would be more extensive. But, our results here suggest that particular structural features exhibit stronger influence on residents' outcomes than process quality. Using state program as the unit of analysis for this study illuminates an avenue for improving quality of care not as clearly visible from the facility or resident levels: namely, states regulating certain program structural features directly with an eye toward improving resident outcomes. The balance of this chapter is organized into the following sections: (1) a brief review of relevant theory, (2) our research design and data, (3) our results, and (4) the implications of our results and conclusion.

REVIEW OF RELEVANT THEORY

Relations among Resources, Processes, and Outcomes

With respect to publicly financed medical care generally, Donabedian (2003) maintains that recipient outcomes reflect the various human and material resources a program applies to their situations as well as the proficiency of this application. That is, richness of resources and the appropriateness of their organization (structure) facilitate high-quality delivery processes which in turn translate into positive patient outcomes. From this perspective the Centers for Medicare and Medicaid Services' (CMS) approach of surveying, certifying, and reporting SMNF-LTC processes and – to a somewhat lesser degree – outcomes is an, if not the, obvious way to facilitate improved quality of life outcomes for residents.

But, while among SMNF-LTC programs structural breadth and depth appears to largely determine process quality as measured by CMS, process quality may not be associated with outcome quality as closely as Donabedian (2003) contends (Lockhart & Giles-Sims, 2007). In acute medicine, for instance, Fisher et al. (2003a, 2003b) find no link between structure and processes on one hand and outcomes on the other in the care delivered to older citizens through Medicare. What appears to be a refined organization of resources among diverse specialists may foster excessive and wasteful resource utilization (Baicker & Chandra, 2004; Barnato et al., 2007; Cooper, 2009; Fisher et al., 2003a, 2003b). Fisher et al. find that patients frequently have better therapeutic outcomes when their care is directed by a primary care physician who, while lacking the expertise of a cast of specialists, synthesizes information, and focuses on the overall picture. As a result of what Fisher et al. argue is disproportionate reliance on specialists, who frequently focus only on that aspect of a patient's situation relevant to their expertise, Medicare spends twice as much on patients in Miami as on patients with similar maladies in Minneapolis, where specialist involvement is less pronounced, without any evidence of improved quality, accessibility of care, and better patient outcomes.

Fisher et al. (2003a, 2003b) foster recognition that related situations may arise in SMNF-LTC programs. The association of poor quality of care with for-profit nursing facilities in the literature (e.g., Harrington, Wollhandler, Mullan, Carrillo, & Himmelstein, 2001) offers, for instance, the suggestion of poor utilization of resources. Strong incentives exist to divert for-profit facility revenues from resident care to other goals such as investor profits or luxurious public areas designed to entice the families of potential residents. But our point here is not that evaluating SMNF-LTC program processes in order to assure service recipients' adequate outcomes is misguided. Rather, it is that evaluating these processes is a complicated, difficult, and expensive activity, and it has remained insufficient for assuring adequate resident outcomes across a quarter century (USGAO, 2009). If it were possible to augment it with another − in some respects less demanding − regulatory approach, the pace of improvement might increase.

Four SMNF-LTC Program Structural Features

Four program structural features appear prominently and repeatedly in the literature seeking to explain SMNF-LTC program residents' quality of life outcomes. One of these is occupancy rate. Nursing facilities and SMNF-LTC programs generally have better resident outcomes as occupancy rates rise, presumably because the programs' facilities experience decreasing marginal costs while revenues rise (e.g., Elliott, 2010; Harrington et al., 2004).

Also, the relative presence of registered nurses (i.e., improved staffing) in nursing facilities and SMNF-LTC programs is, as we discuss below, repeatedly associated with improved resident outcomes (e.g., Anderson, Hsieh, & Su, 1998; Bowblis, 2011; Castle, 2008; Harrington, Zimmerman, Karon, Robinson, & Beutel, 2000; Horn, Buerhaus, Bergstrom, & Smout, 2005; Konetzka, Stearns, & Park, 2008; Schnelle et al., 2004).

In contrast, nursing facilities and SMNF-LTC programs with high proportions of residents for whom Medicaid is the primary payor routinely exhibit poorer resident outcomes. High proportions of Medicaid-funded residents may reduce revenues because Medicaid's reimbursement rates are generally lower than private pay rates (e.g., USGAO, 2009; Wagner et al., 2008). Additionally, for-profit nursing facilities and SMNF-LTC programs with a high proportion of proprietary facilities share this tendency of poor resident outcomes. For-profit operation likely raises incentives for using revenues for purposes other than resident care such as advertising (e.g., Aaronson, Zinn, & Rosko, 1994; Comondore et al., 2009; Harrington et al., 2001; Hillmer, Wodchis, Gill, Anderson, & Rochon, 2005; Horn et al., 2005).

As Table 1 shows, states differ sharply on the structures of their MNF-LTC programs with respect to these four specific characteristics. Across the period of this study (1997–2005), SMNF-LTC program occupancy rates varied from 64.7 to 98.4 percent, registered nurse hours per resident day ran from 0.2 to 1, the proportions of program residents with Medicaid as

Table 1. Descriptive Statistics and Predicted Effects of the Independent Variables.

Variables	Mean	Standard Deviation	Minimum	Maximum	Predicted Effect
Dependent variable					
Resident outcomes	0	3.42	−9.09	5.24	N.A.
Independent variables					
Process quality	0	2.81	−7.29	6.41	+
Occupancy rate	85.37	6.99	64.7	98.4	+
Registered nurses	0.58	0.15	0.2	1	+
Medicaid payor	65.41	6.79	49.2	82.9	−
For-profit	62.78	15.56	6.4	86.1	−
Control variables					
Case-mix	99.31	11.61	69.8	127.3	−
HCBS$	0.13	0.18	0	1.38	near 0

Note: N = 192.

their primary payor ranged from 49.2 to 82.9 percent, and the percentage of for-profit facilities in state programs stretched from 6.4 to 86.1.

Drawing on this literature about the varying structural features of SMNF-LTC programs we decided to examine whether there might be any payoff in terms of residents' quality of life outcomes from augmenting existing regulation of processes through additional legal requirements with respect to specific program structural characteristics. This question lies at the root of this study.

RESEARCH DESIGN AND DATA

Our central research question then is how SMNF-LTC program process quality and various features of program structure compare in contributing to program recipients' quality of life outcomes. Our data consist of 192 cases, one for each of the contiguous 48 states for the odd-numbered years 1997 through 2005. Our independent variables are lagged two years (one legislative session in most states). So the dependent variable data cover the odd years 1999−2005; the independent variable data cover the odd years 1997−2003. We analyze these data with panel-corrected, time-series regression. Because of well-known instability and lack of representativeness of many individual state program measures, we follow Mor et al. (2003) in using multi-items scales to measure SMNF-LTC processes and outcomes. Our scales provide incomplete operationalization of SMNF-LTC process quality and outcome quality, but they are more adequate than any of their individual scale elements. Our diagnostic tests (item-scale correlations; multi-method, multi-trait convergent-discriminant analysis; principle component analysis; comparison of full-scale with individual element regression models, and Cronbach's alpha) support relying on these multi-item scales rather than on individual variables. Each of these scales transcends its various elements sufficiently to be considered a generic measure of the concept it represents.

We stress that all of our variables are aspects of SMNF-LTC *programs*. We do not move from one level of analysis to another or commit an ecological fallacy by linking certain program structural features or processes to outcomes in terms of the *proportions* of program residents avoiding several undesirable circumstances. For instance, our *dependent* variable represents the varying *proportions* of SMNF-LTC programs' residents avoiding certain undesirable outcomes. One *independent* variable is couched in terms of the different *proportions* of SMNF-LTC programs' facilities avoiding certain deficiencies. These variables are central to addressing our research question: in comparison to the effects of certain SMNF-LTC programs' structural features on reducing undesirable outcomes for the programs' residents, how strong is the effect of the degree to which the processes of SMNF- LTC programs' facilities are judged sufficient?

Dependent Variable

SMNF-LTC Program Residents' Quality of Life Outcomes (hereafter, *resident outcomes*): To assure that *resident outcomes* retains some separation from one of the independent variables used in conjunction with it and, especially, that it avoids some of the reliability and validity problems of the Online Survey, Certification and Reporting (OSCAR) System deficiency data, we eschew using OSCAR *deficiency* data for measuring *resident outcomes*. Since CMS remains the best, if sometimes problematic, source for data on these programs, we use instead CMS data on what Harrington et al. (2011) call "resident characteristics." Our scale, formed from adding the z-scores of its four elements, is constructed from the proportions of a state's nursing facility residents who *avoid*: being bed-ridden, being restrained, having pressure sores and being nourished through a feeding tube (Harrington et al., 2011; Harrington, Carrillo, & LaCava, 2006, tables 14, 15, 18, and 21, respectively). The alpha for this scale is 0.84.

While Harrington et al. (2011) refer to these as "characteristics," they are obviously "outcomes" as well. Further, Harrington et al. contend that good nursing facility care can sharply reduce the incidence of, even eliminate, these four distressing outcomes. Other recent research concurs and suggests that the appearance of these outcomes frequently serves program and facility convenience more than resident wellbeing (McCullough, 2008; Teno et al., 2010). So, we draw on the incidence of largely preventable outcomes which are either inherently dangerous (e.g., pressure sores) and/or involve the withdrawal of a previous freedom or pleasure (e.g., being restrained or nourishing via a feeding tube). These outcomes reflect official CMS assessments of the proportions of a SMNF-LTC program's residents experiencing undesirable conditions. Our choices, as described above, were also influenced by the necessity of acquiring a coherent scale. See Table 1 for summary data on all variables and the predicted effects of independent variables on the dependent variable.

Independent Variables

In addition to the variables described below, we control for specific time effects.

Quality of SMNF-LTC program processes (hereafter *process quality*): There are 185 CMS OSCAR evaluation measures, largely for nursing facility processes. OSCAR evaluation measures suffer from well-documented reliability and validity limitations (Angelelli, Mor, Intrator, Feng, & Zinn, 2003; Grabowski, Angelelli, & Mor, 2004; Klopfenstein, Lockhart, & Giles-Sims, 2011). Instability of individual measures (limited reliability) and cross-item disparities (validity challenges) occur even among the 40 measures that Mullan and Harrington (2001) sanction on the basis of several sensible criteria. But they are the best data currently available. Despite the fact that there is currently no single "best" summary measure for *process quality*, the index we describe below transcends its individual elements sufficiently to be considered a generic measure of program process quality. We are reassured in this regard by the fact that our scale correlates predictably with Harrington et al. (2004) related index which draws entirely on different elements (Lockhart, Klopfenstein, & Giles-Sims, 2009). Our scale for the quality of SMNF-LTC program processes is calculated by adding the z-scores of its four elements: proportions of a SMNF-LTC program's facilities *without* deficiencies with respect to: preserving resident dignity, maintaining good housekeeping, fostering an accident-free environment and sustaining food sanitation (Harrington et al., 2011, 2006, tables 38, 40, 45, and 48, respectively). This scale produces an alpha of 0.79.

Our logic for generating the quality of SMNF-LTC program processes scale in this way is as follows. While nursing facility long-term care has some essential medical components, the recipients are referred to as residents rather than patients for a reason. They reside in the facility, often until their death. For many of them, how they are treated and food quality are as, if not more, important than the more technical aspects of their care. To generate this scale, we start with a concern for salience in the sense of problem frequency by focusing on the 10 OSCAR elements which receive the highest incidence of deficiencies (Harrington et al., 2011, 2006). Working from this list, we follow three guides in forming *process quality*. First, all our elements come from the 40 that Mullan and Harrington (2001) have vetted. Following the order in our text above these are F241, F253, F323, and F371, respectively. Second, we represent the domains (i.e., administration, nursing, residents' rights, food service, and environment) which Mukamel and Spector (2003) distinguish, save for administration. Third, we narrow as necessary to attain credible scale coherence which we assess with a variety of criteria (see text above). We anticipate that *process quality* will exert a positive effect on *resident outcomes,* but we were initially uncertain as to how the strength of this effect would compare with the effects of the four program structural characteristics which follow below.

Comments on previous versions of this chapter have sometimes suggested that we should use process scale elements as substantively similar as possible to our outcome scale elements (e.g., the percentage of a SMNF-LTC program's facilities without deficiencies for having avoidable pressure sores in conjunction with the percentage of the program's residents avoiding pressure sores as an outcome) so as not to understate the effect of program processes. We had initially thought that this approach would represent too easy a test of generic quality, but we examined the possibilities of this suggestion. Two of our outcome items, pressure sores and physical restraints, have close substantive correspondence with two process deficiency measures not included in our process index (F314 and F221). Through analyses in which with these two process items replaced our originals we found that relying on such substantively similar process-outcome pairs did not lead to quality indicators' fostering better resident outcomes in comparison to the four program structural feature measures employed in this study.

SMNF-LTC program occupancy rate (hereafter, *occupancy rate*): This is the proportion of a SMNF-LTC program's beds occupied by residents (Harrington et al., 2011, 2006, table 4). We anticipate that *occupancy rate* will produce a positive effect on *resident outcomes.*

SMNF-LTC program registered nurse hours per resident day (hereafter, *registered nurses*): This is a SMNF-LTC program's registered nurse hours per resident day (Harrington et al., 2011, 2006, table 25). We expect that this variable will exert a positive effect on *resident outcomes.*

Medicaid primary payor (hereafter, *Medicaid payor*): This is the proportion of a SMNF-LTC program's residents who have Medicaid as their primary payor (Harrington et al., 2011, 2006, table 6). We anticipate that this variable will have a negative effect on *resident outcomes.*

SMNF-LTC program facilities for-profit (hereafter, *for-profit*): This is the proportion of a SMNF-LTC program's facilities which are operated on a proprietary or for-profit basis (Harrington et al., 2011, 2006, table 7). We expect that *for-profit* will exert a negative effect on *resident outcomes.*

Control Variables

SMNF-LTC Program Case-Mix (hereafter, *case-mix*): This is the average degree of care required by a SMNF-LTC program's residents (i.e., the state program's nursing facility residents' average summary acuity index; Harrington et al., 2011, 2006, table 13). This variable allows us to control for cross-state differences in the depth or difficulty of care required by SMNF-LTC programs' residents. States influence case-mix through their disability requirements for Medicaid access to long-term care. The stiffer these requirements, the more difficult the care required per resident in a state's MNF-LTC program. So, we expect that *case-mix* will exert a negative effect on *resident outcomes*. Yet to a greater extent than for the four preceding variables, this measure is also contingent on the health of a state's population, particularly elders, and other factors largely beyond the control of public officials. Thus, we consider it a control variable rather than a program structural characteristic.

State HCBS aged/disabled waiver expenditures/SMNF-LTC program expenditures (hereafter, *HCBS$*): Another concern is how thoroughly a state's overall Medicaid long-term care program relies on (and its MNF-LTC program is perhaps displaced by) Home and Community Based Services (HCBS) alternatives to nursing facility care (Eiken et al., 2010, table 3; Eiken et al., 2004, table 1; USDH&HS, 1999, 2001, 2003, table 110; USDH&HS, 2005, table 13.26). We utilize as a control variable states' HCBS aged/disabled waiver Medicaid expenditures as a percentage of their SMNF-LTC expenditures. These HCBS aged/disabled waiver expenditures represent the Medicaid funds used to maintain elders needing help with various ADLs in a variety of community, rather than institutional (i.e., nursing facility), settings. This study includes state (Medicaid) HCBS long-term care programs only through this control variable due to the absence of any comparably rigorous state-level process and outcome quality indicators for HCBS care (Lockhart, Giles-Sims, et al., 2009; Mollica & Johnson-Lamarche, 2005).

Older citizens needing professional assistance with activities of daily living (ADLs), such as toileting or bathing, routinely prefer either to remain in their own homes or live in community-based congregate settings such as assisted-living complexes rather than to enter institutions such as nursing facilities (Kane & Kane, 2001). Since the U.S. Supreme Court's *Olmstead v. L.C.* ruling in 1999, states have made greater efforts to employ these alternatives to nursing facility care. This ruling encouraged states to offer these options, and alternatives to nursing facility care are usually less expensive per person served. As the use of HCBS long-term care within a state increases, the state's MNF-LTC program is generally burdened with a more demanding case-mix. However, to the extent that nursing facilities improve their services to compete with HCBS alternatives, program-wide performance may not decline. Due to these cross-pressures, we anticipate that *HCBS$* will not produce strong positive or negative effects on *resident outcomes*.

RESULTS

Table 2 presents the results of a panel-corrected, time-series regression model with *resident outcomes* as the dependent variable. All of the independent variables exert effects consistent with our expectations expressed above and in Table 1. All four of the specific program structural characteristics that we introduced above (*occupancy rate, registered nurses, Medicaid payor*, and *for-profit*) produce statistically significant effects in the direction that we predicted. *Process quality* produces a positive effect on *resident outcomes*, but its effect is not strong or statistically significant. Overall this model explains (statistically) about 80 percent of the cross-state variation in *resident outcomes*. A two-stage least squares (2SLS) analysis, using global SMNR-LTC program resources (overall depth and breadth of program beds and finances) as an instrument for process quality, produces similar

Table 2. Panel-Corrected, Time-Series Regression.

Independent and Control Variables	Dependent Variable: Resident Outcomes
Process quality	0.056 (0.064)
Occupancy rate	0.120*** (0.031)
Registered nurses	3.203* (1.554)
Medicaid payor	−0.110** (0.036)
For-profit	−0.037* (0.014)
Case-mix	−0.162*** (0.021)
HCBS$	1.437 (0.935)
Adjusted R^2	0.806

Notes: Significant at $< 0.05 = *$; at $< 0.01 = **$; at $< 0.001 = ***$. N for all variables is 192. Robust standard errors (i.e., corrected for clustering on states) are in parentheses. Dummy variables controlling for time-specific effects are included in the model. The dependent variable data cover odd-numbered years 1999–2005. The independent variable data cover odd-numbered years 1997–2003.

results, suggesting no significant endogeneity between *process quality* and *resident outcomes* at least at this level of aggregation. This global resource measure correlates well with *process quality*, but poorly with *resident outcomes*.

DISCUSSION

This study covers a modest amount of time. It also includes a limited number of control variables. Since it focuses on relations internal to SMNF-LTC programs (i.e., structural features, processes, and outcomes) rather than on how a state's broader political context affects, for instance, global program resources (e.g., Grogan, 1994, 1999; Kane, Kane, Ladd, & Veazle, 1998; Lockhart, Giles-Sims, et al., 2009), it includes only two prominent controls relating to this external context. Thus, the results are vulnerable to omitted variable bias as are, in varying degree, results of virtually all social science studies. But, there is no obvious reason why most external contextual factors (i.e., factors beyond the structure, processes, outcomes path) would influence *process quality's* effect on *resident outcomes* so differently from the effects of certain structural features as to reveal a stronger effect for process quality were these contextual variables to be explicitly controlled.

In essence, our results show that, while the quality of a SMNF-LTC program's processes exerts a positive effect on the program residents' quality of life outcome, this effect is modest in comparison to the positive and negative effects of specific program structural characteristics. It is difficult to avoid the conclusion that augmenting existing CMS efforts to assess the quality of SMNF-LTC programs' processes with regulatory measures focused directly on these program structural characteristics might well produce benefits for program residents' quality of life. These additional measures would entail constraining program occupancy rates within certain parameters, upgrading program registered nurse hours, assuring that program residents relying on Medicare were not concentrated in a small minority of program facilities, and nudging (Thaler & Sunstein, 2008) state programs toward lower levels of for-profit facilities.

We propose neither curtailing CMS's current surveying, certifying, and reporting regime nor adding additional measures of the same type. CMS's procedures are arguably essential (Mukamel, Weimer, Harrington, Spector, & Ladd, 2012), but they are complex, difficult, and expensive, and to date they have been insufficient (USGAO, 2009). Therefore, we seek to augment them with different, more straightforward measures in a new venue, the program level. Adding any regulation to SMNF-LTC programs will be difficult. At the national level creating the momentum to initiate new regulatory measures will have an extremely tough time acquiring attention from other important matters and overcoming the resistance of conservatives and likely major proprietary nursing facility care providers. Many state governments have political cultures adverse to public regulation, difficult fiscal circumstances, and/or strong provider interest groups opposed to further regulation (Edelman, 1998; Freeman, 1998; Harrington et al., 2004; Sparer, 1993). So adopting the changes we identified in the previous paragraph would likely initially fall to a few sympathetic state governments.

But, if the new regulations we introduced above were initiated, they might have some advantages over the current CMS regulatory regime. First, while some aspects (e.g., increased registered nurse hours) would mean greater provider costs, additional public sector costs would likely be marginal (Mukamel et al., 2011). In comparison to funding multiple survey teams which roam the state and engage in a continuing process of examining a myriad SMNF-LTC program facility practices, having central state officials keep track of four program-level CMS survey statistics and negotiate adjustments in them would likely be less expensive. Second, in comparison to poring through multiple resident cases to ascertain whether a facility is, for example, preserving the dignity of its residents, using state-level CMS survey data for determining whether a SMNF-LTC program meets the criterion for registered nurse hours per resident day or the currently acceptable proportion of facilities run on a for-profit basis would be less ambiguous and difficult.

We should address why we think that regulating these four structural features would improve resident outcomes as well as the general nature of these regulations. As a SMNF-LTC program's occupancy rates fall, a growing number of its facilities may suffer increasing marginal costs as revenues decline. Several potential responses are available to program administrators to relieve this problem: refusing to issue new Certificates of Need (CONs) which authorize additional program beds, facilitating the consolidation of neighboring struggling facilities, and shifting existing residents with no community ties from heavily populated facilities to (or minimally placing similarly unconnected new residents in) under-occupied facilities. Raising program registered nurse hours per resident day could be addressed by setting state-level mandates at levels requiring facilities with the lowest existing levels to add additional registered nurses to their staffs. We explain below why we think this step is apt to improve resident outcomes.

Further, even if SMNF-LTC programs have limited control over the proportion of program residents with Medicaid as their primary payor, they can influence the consequences of high proportions of residents paying low reimbursement rates by shifting existing Medicaid primary-payor residents with no community ties to (or minimally placing similarly unconnected new residents in) facilities with relatively low proportions of such residents. This approach leaves the program proportion unchanged, but may nonetheless improve program resident outcomes by avoiding the concentration of these residents in a few facilities. Such concentrations tend to reduce the quality of life for all residents in these facilities and thus likely have stronger negative effects on program-wide resident outcomes than having residents with low payment rates spread out across a state program. Nudging (Thaler & Sunstein, 2008) SMNF-LTC programs toward lower proportions of proprietary facilities is presumably associated with better resident outcomes because it increases the proportion of program facilities which have less need to use program resources for investor profits, fancy public areas designed to appeal to the families of prospective residents, or advertising. Raising this proportion might be achieved by encouraging non-profit entities with start-up grants – loosely modeled on the tax abatements employed to attract business – to create new facilities. It could also be furthered by using state experience to justify greater caution in issuing CON's to proprietary providers.

We were surprised by the relative strength, vis-à-vis the effect of program process quality, of the effects on program residents' outcomes of the four program structural characteristics on which we have focused. While we can at this point only speculate about the bases of this disparity, we draw on the nursing facility quality literature to offer some possible explanations. We raise three considerations.

First, SMNF-LTC programs differ from acute medical care in several ways, one of which is particularly relevant here. Nursing facilities deal primarily with chronic problems from which persons are not expected to recover. Licensed staff in these facilities can address and perhaps mitigate these problems through careful monitoring of medication, sponsoring organized exercise groups, or fostering social interaction. But most of the tasks of nursing facilities are custodial rather than medical. Staffers help residents with various ADLs. They prepare and serve meals, make beds and clean, and try to keep residents safe from accidents. The majority of "front-line" staff in nursing facilities at any given time is not composed of medical or related professionals (e.g., social workers); they are relatively unskilled nurses' aides and similarly skilled other workers, earning barely above the minimum wage with few if any benefits (Harrington et al., 2011). Assessing the adequacy of these (technically) low-skill tasks, which may rest on subtle feelings about interpersonal relations between care givers and residents may be more difficult than measuring the success of acute medical treatments which are more easily observable.

Fostering positive feelings between staff and residents may be one underlying basis for the relative presence of registered nurses being associated with improved nursing facility care. These nurses may be particularly useful in fostering something analogous to what has been referred to as "bedside manner" with respect to physicians in acute care that contributes to resident quality of life outcomes: a willingness to listen, a predisposition toward comforting verbal responses and particularly an informed inclination to help in practical ways (e.g., proactive with respect to pressure sores and hesitancy with regard to restraints). Positive orientations toward caring for others through mundane tasks and training that develops the capacity to do so in a SMNF-LTC program context may be crucial to how well these activities are conducted from the perspective of the residents.

Registered nurses (RNs) are more apt to exhibit this orientation than are most other front-line staff. They have generally chosen *careers* as registered nurses. They have much more training for their jobs than their nursing facility licensed nurse (Licensed Practical Nurses (LPNs) and Licensed Vocational Nurses (LVNs)), and nurses' aide (NAs) coworkers. Registered nurses are also routinely in demand and can generally choose to work in a variety of settings other than nursing facilities. In comparison to most other nursing facility staff, they are well paid for their work, and their position near the apex of the front-line staff hierarchy facilitates their ability to influence the work of others. Nursing facility front-line work, however essential, is often trying, dirty, and uninspiring. So infusing SMNF-LTC program front-line staff with larger doses of the likely salutary influence of registered nurses is, understandably, a promising way to improve SMNF-LTC program residents' quality of life outcomes. The federal government requires that SMNF-LTC facilities must have one registered nurse for at least eight hours straight per day, seven days a week — Centers for Medicare and Medicaid Services (CMS), 2010, chapter 7, section 7014.1). A state with the mean average facility size (105.1 residents — Harrington et al., 2011, 2006) and the mean occupancy rate (85.37, see Table 1) that adhered to this minimum standard would have only 0.089 registered nurse hours (a bit over five minutes) per resident day. Across the period of this study all states exceeded this federal minimum requirement, but we think further upgrading actual register nurse hours per resident day would likely contribute importantly to improved resident quality of life outcomes.

Second, the current focus of SMNF-LTC regulation, while certainly appropriate, gives both public sector policy makers as well as regulators (both federal and state-level) and various categories of providers (for-profit, private but non-profit, public sector) incentives for doing well on CMS surveys at the expense of focusing on other relevant matters (Edelman, 1998; Miller, 2007). Similarly to some public school students with short-term incentives to essentially memorize answers to questions on standardized tests rather than acquire basic skills and substantive material, the member facilities of SMNF-LTC programs arguably have greater incentives to focus on having their processes pass muster on CMS surveys than on assuring important resident outcomes. Across time CMS has sought to augment the facility-process focus of its surveying, certifying, and reporting system to include resident outcomes, but the majority of its current 185 deficiency items either focus on processes or are at least difficult to distinguish from processes. Consider, for instance, F314 (see text above) on the presence of unwarranted pressure sores. While a resident having pressure sores represents an outcome, the outcome is presumably unwarranted because the processes of caring for the resident have been inadequate in some manner or manners.

Accordingly, SMNF-LTC programs and their member facilities share interests in avoiding process deficiencies. They relieve themselves thereby of bad publicity (e.g., on CMS' "Nursing Home Compare" website); time-consuming hassles with state survey teams; possible further legal problems with CMS; and even − though rarely − CMPs, withdrawal of Medicaid support for new residents, or facility closure (Li et al., 2010). All these problems are more apt to arise from evaluation of *process quality* rather than from *resident outcomes*. Generally, unless someone can demonstrate that a facility has violated a procedure, it is difficult to extract penalties for the fact that a resident has needlessly been placed on a feeding tube or experienced another undesirable outcome (Edelman, 1998).

Thus while a program may well have, for instance, a relatively low rate of process deficiencies, it may not do a good job of producing positive resident outcomes to which CMS directs less regulatory attention. As Sparer states about California: "(t)he industry, which is dominated by proprietary facilities, has adjusted" (to low reimbursement rates − explanation added) "by keeping employee wages low and by spending relatively little on efforts to improve patient care" (1993, p. 15). But Table 2 shows that program

residents' outcomes are importantly affected by program structural characteristics which often arise in separate, state-level venues largely unregulated
by CMS or frequently the states. Expanding the scope of state and/or federal regulation of SMNF-LTC programs thus offers hope of improving
program residents' quality of life outcomes (Bowblis & Lucas, 2012; Kelly,
Liebig, & Edwards, 2008).

Third, the decisions responsible for the four structural features on which
we have focused often arise in generally low-profile interactions among
loose policy networks involving state legislators and public administrators,
who are frequently divided across lines of public health versus payment
agencies (Miller, 2007; Sparer, 1993), as well as the representatives of distinct proprietary and non-profit provider interests. As Freeman (1998)
reports, while the often poorly organized, inexperienced and financially
strapped groups representing resident interests may succeed in attracting
considerable public attention to their concerns in the aftermath of serious
disasters – often attributable to provider shortcomings – appearing in the
mass media, this attention tends to atrophy rapidly while the concerns of
various generally better organized, more experienced, and frequently weal-
thier provider interests have greater staying power (see also Edelman,
1998). So state decisions on these program structural characteristics, similarly to those on "tax expenditures" (Howard, 1997), tend to fly largely
"under the radar" of public scrutiny, leaving them largely to the discression
of relevant public officials and private providers who may be torn between
looking good on CMS surveys and being good to program residents. As
Freeman notes with respect to Minnesota: "Hardly anyone noticed when
the annual public health inspections of nursing homes were downgraded to
biennial to reduce costs over the objection of consumer advocates" (1998,
p. 45). Low public scrutiny may be facilitated by changes in public perceptions of elders from generally positive (Cook & Barrett, 1992; Schneider &
Ingram, 1993) to more skeptical, particularly in terms of their disproportionate consumption of public social program funds (Binstock, 2005;
Freeman, 1998).

In conclusion, CMS's efforts to assess the adequacy of SMNF-LTC programs' care, while complex, difficult – and thus criticized – as well as
expensive, surely represent an appropriate endeavor. However, across the
last several decades a host of program shortcomings have remained alar-
mingly high. Augmenting CMS's current regulatory regime with efforts to
nudge (Thaler & Sunstein, 2008) certain structural characteristics of
SMNF-LTC programs in directions suggesting that improved resident outcomes will follow seems warranted. While this augmentation will be

politically challenging to initiate, it is likely to be less complex, demanding, and intrusive for providers to maintain and for regulators to monitor.

REFERENCES

Aaronson, W. D., Zinn, J. S., & Rosko, M. D. (1994). Do for-profit and not-for-profit nursing homes behave differently? *The Gerontologist, 38*(6), 775–786.

Anderson, R. A., Hsieh, P.-C., & Su, H.-F. (1998). Resource allocation and resident outcomes in nursing homes: Comparisons between the best and worst. *Research in Nursing and Health, 21*(4), 297–313.

Angelelli, J., Mor, V., Intrator, O., Feng, Z., & Zinn, J. (2003). Oversight of nursing homes: Pruning the tree or just spotting bad apples? *Gerontologist, 43*(Special Issue II), 67–75.

Baicker, K., & Chandra, A. (2004, April 7). Medicare spending, the physician workforce and beneficiaries' quality of care. *Health Affairs (online version),* W4–184.

Barnato, A. E., Herndon, M. B., Anthony, D. L., Gallagher, P. M., Skinner, J. S., Bynum, J. P. W., & Fisher, E. S. (2007). Are regional variations in end-of-life care intensity explained by patient preferences? *Medical Care, 45*(5), 386–393.

Binstock, R. H. (2005). Old-age policies, politics and aging. *Generations, 29*(3), 73–78.

Bowblis, J. R. (2011). Staffing ratios and quality: An analysis of minimum direct care staffing requirements for nursing homes. *Health Services Research, 46*(5), 1495–1516.

Bowblis, J. R., & Lucas, J. A. (2012). The impact of state regulations on nursing home care practices. *Journal of Regulatory Economics, 42*(1), 52–72.

Castle, N. G. (2008). Nursing home caregiver staffing levels and quality of care. *Journal of Applied Gerontology, 27*(4), 375–405.

Centers for Medicare and Medicaid Services. (2010). *State operations manual.* Retrieved from http://www.cms.gov/manuals.downloads/som107c7/pdf

Comondore, V. R., Devereaux, P. J., Zhou, Q., Stone, S. B., Busse, J. W., Ravindran, N. C., Guyatt, G. H (2009). Quality of care in for-profit and not-for profit nursing homes: Systematic review and meta-analysis. *British Medical Journal, 339,* 2732–2747.

Cook, F. L., & Barrett, E. J. (1992). *Support for the American welfare state: The views of congress and the public.* New York, NY: Columbia University Press.

Cooper, R. A. (2009). States with more health care spending have better-quality health care: Lessons about Medicare. *Health Affairs, 28*(1), w103– w117.

Donabedian, A. (2003). *An introduction to quality assurance in health care.* New York, NY: Oxford University Press.

Edelman, T. S. (1998). The politics of long-term care at the federal level and its implications for quality. *Generations, 21*(4), 37–41.

Eiken, S., Burwell, B., Gold, L., & Sredl, K. (2010). *Medicaid HCBS waiver expenditures, FY 2004 through FY 2009.* Retrieved from http://hcbs.org

Eiken, S., Burwell, B., & Schaefter, M. (2004). *Medicaid HCBS waiver expenditures, FY 1998–2003.* Retrieved from http//hcbs.org

Elliott, A. E. (2010). Occupancy and revenue gains from culture change in nursing homes: A win-win innovation for a new age of long-term care. *Seniors House & Care Journal, 18*(1), 61–76.

Fisher, E. S., Wennberg, D. E., Stukel, T. A., Gottlieb, D. J., Lucas, F. L., & Pinder, É. L. (2003a). The implications of regional variations in Medicare spending. Part 1: The content, quality and accessibility of care. *Annals of Internal Medicine, 138*(4), 273–287.

Fisher, E. S., Wennberg, D. E., Stukel, T. A., Gottlieb, D. J., Lucas, F. L., & Pinder, É. L. (2003b). The implications of regional variations in Medicare spending. Part 2: Health outcomes and satisfaction with care. *Annals of Internal Medicine, 138*(4), 288–299.

Freeman, I. C. (1998). Nursing home politics at the state level and implications for quality: The Minnesota example. *Generations, 21*(4), 44–48.

Grabowski, D. C., Angelelli, J. J., & Mor, V. (2004). Medicaid payment and risk-adjusted nursing home quality measures. *Health Affairs, 23*(5), 243–252.

Grogan, C. M. (1994). Political-economic factors influencing state Medicaid policy. *Political Research Quarterly, 47*(5), 589–622.

Grogan, C. M. (1999). The influence of federal mandates on state Medicaid and AFDC decision-making. *Publius: The Journal of Federalism, 29*(3), 1999.

Harrington, C., Carrillo, H., Dowdell, M., Tang, P. P., & Woleslagle Blank, B. (2011). *Nursing facilities, staffing, residents and facility deficiencies: 2005–2010.* San Francisco, CA: Department of Social and Behavioral Science, University of California.

Harrington, C., Carrillo, H., & LaCava, C. (2006). *Nursing facilities, staffing, residents, and facility deficiencies, 1999 through 2005.* San Francisco, CA: Department of Social and Behavioral Sciences, University of California.

Harrington, C., Mullan, J. T., & Carrillo, H. (2004). State nursing home enforcement systems. *Journal of Health Politics, Policy and Law, 29*(1), 43–73.

Harrington, C., Woolhandler, S., Mullan, J. T., Carrillo, H., & Himmelstein, D. U. (2001). Does investor ownership of nursing homes compromise the quality of care? *American Journal of Public Health, 91*(9), 1452–1455.

Harrington, C., Zimmerman, D., Karon, S. L., Robinson, J., & Beutel, P. (2000). Nursing home staffing and its relationship to deficiencies. *Journal of Gerontology: Social Sciences, 55B*(5), S278–S287.

He, W., Sengupta, M., Velkoff, V. A., & DeBarros, K. A. (2005). *65 + in the United States: 2005.* Washington, DC: Census Bureau, U.S. Department of Commerce and National Institutes of Health, U.S. Department of Health and Human Services.

Hillmer, M. P., Wodchis, W. P., Gill, S. S., Anderson, G. M., & Rochon, P. A. (2005). Nursing home profit status and quality of care: Is there any evidence of an association? *Medical Care Research and Review, 62*(2), 139–166.

Horn, S. D., Buerhaus, P., Bergstrom, N., & Smout, R. J. (2005). RN staffing time and outcomes of long-stay nursing home residents. *American Journal of Nursing, 105*(11), 58–70.

Howard, C. (1997). *The hidden welfare state: Tax expenditures and social policy in the United States.* Princeton, NJ: Princeton University Press.

Kane, R. A., & Kane, R. L. (2001). What older people want from long-term care, and how they can get it. *Health Affairs, 20*(6), 114–127.

Kane, R. L., Kane, R. A., Ladd, R. C., & Veazle, W. N. (1998). Variation in state spending for long-term care: Factors associated with more balanced systems. *Journal of Health Politics, Policy and Law, 23*(2), 363–390.

Kelly, C. M., Liebig, P. S., & Edwards, L. J. (2008). Nursing home deficiencies: An exploratory study of interstate variations in regulatory activity. *Journal of Aging and Social Policy, 20*(4), 398–414.

Klopfenstein, K., Lockhart, C., & Giles-Sims, J. (2011). Do high rates of OSCAR deficiencies prompt improved nursing facility processes and outcomes? *Journal of Aging and Social Policy, 23*(1), 384–407.

Konetzka, R. T., Stearns, S. C., & Park, J. (2008). The staffing-outcomes relationship in nursing homes. *Health Services Research, 43*(3), 1025–1042.

Li, Y., Harrington, C., Spector, W. D., & Mukamel, D. B. (2010). State regulatory enforcement and nursing home termination from the Medicare and Medicaid programs. *Health Services Research, 45*(6, Pt. 1), 1796–1814.

Lockhart, C., & Giles-Sims, J. (2007). Cross-state variation in conceptions of quality of nursing facility long-term care for the elderly. *Journal of Aging and Social Policy, 19*(4), 1–19.

Lockhart, C., Giles-Sims, J., & Klopfenstein, K. (2008). Cross-state variation in Medicaid support for older citizens in long-term care nursing facilities. *State and Local Government Review, 40*(3), 173–185.

Lockhart, C., Giles-Sims, J., & Klopfenstein, K. (2009). Comparing states' Medicaid nursing facilities and HCBS long-term care programs: Quality and fit with inclination, capacity and need. *Journal of Aging and Social Policy, 21*(1), 52–74.

Lockhart, C., Klopfenstein, K., & Giles-Sims, J. (2009). Distinguishing quality of nursing facility care from stringency of enforcement. In J. J. Kronenfeld (Ed.), *Social sources of disparities in health and health care and linkages to policy, population concerns and providers of care* (Vol. 27, pp. 213–234). Research in the sociology of health care. Bingley, UK: Emerald Publishing Group.

McCullough, D. (2008). *My mother, your mother: Embracing "slow medicine," the compassionate approach to care for your aging loved ones.* New York, NY: Harper-Collins.

Miller, E. A. (2007). Federal administrative and judicial oversight of Medicaid: Policy legacies and tandem institutions under the Boren amendment. *Publius, 38*(2), 315–342.

Mollica, R., & Johnson-Lamarche, H. (2005). *State residential and assisted living: 2004.* Washington, DC: Department of Health and Human Services.

Mor, V., Berg, K., Angelelli, J., Gifford, D., Morris, J., & Moore, T. (2003). The quality of quality measurement in U.S. nursing homes. *Gerontologist, 43*(Special Issue II), 37–46.

Mukamel, D. B., Li, Y., Harrington, C., Spector, W. D., Weimer, D. L., & Bailey, L. (2011). Does state regulation of quality impose costs on nursing homes? *Medical Care, 49*(6), 529–534.

Mukamel, D. B., & Spector, W. D. (2003). Quality report cards and nursing home quality. *Gerontologist, 43*(Special Issue II), 58–66.

Mukamel, D. B., Weimer, D. L., Harrington, C., Spector, W. D., & Ladd, H. (2012). The effect of state regulatory stringency in nursing home quality. *Health Services Review, 47*(5), 1791–1813.

Mullan, J. T., & Harrington, C. (2001). Nursing home deficiencies in the United States: A confirmatory factor analysis. *Research on Aging, 23*(5), 503–531.

National Association of State Budget Officers. (2005). *State expenditure report.* Retrieved from http://www.nasbo.org/sites/default/files/ER_2006.pdf

Schneider, A., & Ingram, H. (1993). Social construction of target populations: Implications for politics and policy. *American Political Science Review, 87*(2), 334–348.

Schnelle, J. E., Simmons, S. F., Harrington, C., Cadogan, M., Garcia, E., & Bates-Jenson, B. M. (2004). Relationship of nursing home staffing to quality of care. *Health Services Research, 39*(2), 225–250.

Sparer, M. S. (1993). States in a reformed health system: Lessons from nursing home policy. *Health Affairs, 12*(1), 7–20.

Teno, J. M., Mitchell, S. L., Gonzalo, P. L., Dosa, D., Hsu, A., Intrator, O., & Mor, V. (2010). Hospital characteristics associated with feeding tube placement in nursing home residents with advanced cognitive impairment. *Journal of the American Medical Association, 303*(6), 544–550.

Thaler, R. H., & Sunstein, C. R. (2008). *Nudge: improving decisions about health, wealth, and happiness.* New Haven, CT: Yale University Press.

U.S. Department of Health and Human Services (USDH&HS). (1999). *Health care financing review: Medicare and medicaid statistical supplement.* Washington, DC: U.S. Department of Health and Human Services.

U.S. Department of Health and Human Services (USDH&HS). (2001). *Health care financing review: Medicare and medicaid statistical supplement.* Washington, DC: U.S. Department of Health and Human Services.

U.S. Department of Health and Human Services (USDH&HS). (2003). *Health care financing review: Medicare and medicaid statistical supplement.* Washington, DC: U.S. Department of Health and Human Services.

U.S. Department of Health and Human Services (USDH&HS). (2005). *Health care financing review: Medicare and medicaid statistical supplement.* Washington, DC: U.S. Department of Health and Human Services.

U.S. Department of Health and Human Services (USDH&HS). (2009). *National clearing house for long-term care information.* Retrieved from http://www.longtermcare.gov/LTC/ Main_Site/Paying_LTC/Costs_Of_Care/Costs_of_Care.aspx

U.S. Government Accounting Office. (2009). *Nursing homes: Federal monitoring surveys demonstrate continued understatement of serious care problems and CMS oversight weakness.* Washington, DC: USGAO. (GAO-08-517).

Wagner, L. M., Capezuti, E., Brush, B. L., Clevenger, C., Boltz, M., & Renz, S. (2008). Contractures in frail nursing home residents. *Geriatric Nursing, 29*(4), 259–266.

PART V
HEALTH DISPARITIES

FUNDAMENTAL CAUSES OF HEALTH DISPARITIES: ASSOCIATIONS BETWEEN ADVERSE SOCIOECONOMIC RESOURCES AND MULTIPLE MEASURES OF HEALTH

Katie Kerstetter and John J. Green

ABSTRACT

Purpose — *This study tests the first two tenets of the fundamental causes theory — that socioeconomic status influences a variety of risk factors for poor health and that it affects multiple health outcomes — by examining the associations between adverse socioeconomic circumstances and five measures of health.*

Methodology/approach — *We employ bivariate and logistic regression analyses of data from the Centers Disease Control and Prevention 2011 Behavioral Risk Factor Surveillance Survey (BRFSS) to test the*

Technology, Communication, Disparities and Government Options in Health and Health Care Services
Research in the Sociology of Health Care, Volume 32, 237–257
Copyright © 2014 by Emerald Group Publishing Limited
ISSN: 0275-4959/doi:10.1108/S0275-495920140000032022

individual and cumulative associations between three measures of socioeconomic position and five measures of health risk factors and outcomes.

Findings – *The analysis demonstrates support for the fundamental causes theory, indicating that measures of adverse socioeconomic conditions have independent and cumulative associations with multiple health outcomes and risk factors among U.S. adults aged 18–64.*

Research limitations/implications – *The findings of this chapter are generalizable to adults aged 18–64 living in the United States and may not apply to individuals living outside the United States, older Americans, and children.*

Originality/value of chapter – *Adverse socioeconomic circumstances are not only associated with self-rated health but are also associated with the two leading causes of death in the United States (cancer and heart disease) and risk factors that contribute to these causes of death (smoking and high blood pressure). Improving access to socioeconomic resources is critical to reducing health disparities in leading causes of death and health risk factors in the United States.*

Keywords: Fundamental causes theory; health disparities; social shaping approach; risk factors; socioeconomic status; self-rated health

INTRODUCTION

Improvements in health-related knowledge and technology have dramatically increased life expectancy for Americans over the past century. From 1900 to 2007, U.S. residents' life expectancy at birth increased from 47 years to 78 years (National Center for Health Statistics, 2009). Infant mortality rates decreased from 47.02 per 1000 live births in 1940 to 6.75 per 1000 live births in 2007 (Xu, Kochanek, Murphy, & Tejada-Vera, 2010). With small exceptions, age-adjusted death rates have decreased steadily for stroke since 1958, for heart disease since 1980, and for cancer since 1993 (Xu et al., 2010). A review of Americans' self-rated health as measured by the General Social Survey found that increasing numbers of individuals across age groups reported good or excellent health from 1972 to 2004 (Warren & Hernandez, 2007).

However, amidst increasing longevity, disparities in mortality and disease have persisted among groups based on race, gender, level of formal education, and household income. Lower-income U.S. residents report experiencing fewer healthy days, on average, than their higher-income counterparts (Centers for Disease Control and Prevention, 2011a). A review of the relationship between education and health (Cutler & Lleras-Muney, 2006) found that better educated individuals tend to have more positive health outcomes, even when controlling for income, occupational characteristics, and family background. An investigation of health disparities by the Centers for Disease Control and Prevention (2011a) reported that men are more likely to die from coronary heart disease than women, and African Americans are more likely to die from heart disease and stroke compared to whites (Centers for Disease Control and Prevention, 2011a). Given the persistence of health disparities in the face of increasing health knowledge and technology, research attention over the past two decades has been directed toward explaining this phenomenon (Adler & Ostrove, 1999).

One major theoretical approach to studying the social determinants of health has been the "fundamental causes" theory, which posits that the uneven distribution of macro-level socioeconomic resources – such as education, occupation, and income – produces health disparities, regardless of the particular mechanism that links health outcomes to these resources. According to this theory, individuals use flexible resources such as "knowledge, power, money, prestige, and beneficial social connections" to maintain or improve their quality of life and health (Link, 2008, p. 73). This chapter tests the validity of two aspects of the fundamental causes theory: that socioeconomic status affects multiple health outcomes and that it also influences a variety of risk factors for poor health and mortality. Our analysis finds support for these hypotheses in that it demonstrates significant associations between individual and cumulative measures of adverse socioeconomic position and self-rated health, smoking, and diagnoses of high blood pressure, heart disease, and cancer.

LITERATURE REVIEW

According to the fundamental causes theory (House, Kessler, & Herzog, 1990; Link & Phelan, 1995), socioeconomic status has a direct effect on health, independent of mechanisms that may connect socioeconomic resources to a particular disease. Factors such as knowledge, power, money, prestige, and beneficial social connections represent flexible resources that individuals use across many settings to maintain and improve their health (Link, 2008). These factors are termed "fundamental causes" because they persist as factors influencing health disparities, even after the mechanisms linking them to health problems have been eliminated. For example, in the mid-twentieth century, sociologists and medical professionals predicted that with improvements in sanitation, increases in the standard of living, and the growing availability of immunizations, health disparities by social class would disappear (Link & Phelan, 1995). However, while these risk factors were mitigated and general health improved, health disparities by socioeconomic status did not improve. Instead, health disparities by socioeconomic position persisted as new risk factors emerged (Link & Phelan, 1995).

The social shaping approach (Link, 2008) helps to explain how health disparities by socioeconomic status have persisted over time. As medical knowledge and technology have improved, this information "has shifted the causes and consequences of disease from fate, accident, and bad luck to factors that are under some human control" (Link, 2008, p. 367). This shift has meant that social factors, such as information about beneficial health practices and access to high quality care, play an increasingly important role in explaining health disparities. Several empirical studies have provided support for this approach. Phelan, Link, Diez-Roux, Kawachi, and Levin (2004) found a stronger relationship between mortality and socioeconomic status for causes of death where knowledge about prevention and treatment is high, compared to those where knowledge is low. Phelan and Link (2005) also found that socioeconomic and racial disparities in health tended to increase historically during periods where the ability to prevent or treat certain health problems has improved. Finally, a study of socioeconomic disparities in lung cancer mortality rates in the United States since 1954 demonstrated a lag in the belief among lower socioeconomic status (SES) respondents that smoking causes cancer (Link, 2008). The study noted that lung cancer mortality began to slow and decline for men living in higher SES counties much earlier than those living in lower-SES counties. Thus, it appears that once new public health knowledge is discovered and disseminated, those with the greatest material and social resources are the most likely to benefit.

In order to test the validity of the fundamental causes theory, empirical research must demonstrate that (1) socioeconomic status influences a variety of risk factors for poor health and mortality, (2) socioeconomic status affects multiple health outcomes, (3) the use of "flexible resources" (e.g., knowledge, income, social connections) is important to explaining disparities in health by socioeconomic status, and (4) the relationship between socioeconomic status and health persists over time through the replacement of mechanisms that link socioeconomic resources and health outcomes (Phelan, Link, & Tehranifar, 2010). This chapter contributes to a developing literature that tests the first two components of this theory – the association of socioeconomic status with multiple risk factors and health outcomes. This analysis also provides information about the cumulative effect of experiencing multiple measures of socioeconomic disadvantage on health – a perspective that is often missing from existing studies.

Many studies examining the relationship between socioeconomic position and health use education, occupation, or income – or a combination of two or more of these measures – to represent socioeconomic status. This practice has a theoretical basis in Weber's (1946) conception of social class (Liberatos, Link, & Kelsey, 1988). Weber (1946) employed a multidimensional approach to describing social stratification, emphasizing the contributions of class (individuals' relationship to the means of production), status (prestige based on group membership), and party (political and social power distributed among associative groups). Weber's theoretical approach is reflected in the diversity of "flexible resources" that are included in the fundamental causes theory. Flexible resources include material resources such as income, status resources such as occupational prestige, and resources that combine elements of class and status such as education (Liberatos et al., 1988).

In practice, empirical studies of health disparities often have used measures of education, income, and occupational status interchangeably to measure socioeconomic status (Adler & Ostrove, 1999). For example, measures of educational attainment have been used alone (Grzywacz, Almeida, Neupert, & Ettner, 2004; Link, 2008; Miech, Pampel, Kim, & Rogers, 2011) or in combination with measures of household income (e.g., House et al., 1990; Lantz et al., 1998; Link, Northridge, Phelan, & Ganz, 1998) to study the impact of socioeconomic status on physical and mental health. Increasingly, scholars have used a multidimensional conceptualization of socioeconomic position that takes into account multiple measures of material deprivation and status disadvantage. For example, Pampel and Rogers (2004) use four measures of socioeconomic status – educational attainment, household income, labor force participation, and occupational prestige – to examine the interactive effects of cigarette smoking and socioeconomic status on health. Similarly, in an examination of historic trends in the relationship of socioeconomic status and self-rated health, Warren and Hernandez (2007) include relative childhood family income, father's occupation, respondents' educational attainment, and respondents' educational income as measures of socioeconomic status. While they were not explicitly designed to test the fundamental causes theory, studies that have used a measure of the cumulative impact of various measurements of socioeconomic position (Lawlor, Ebrahim, & Davey Smith, 2005) or adverse financial circumstances (Bisgaier & Rhodes, 2011) have found that individuals with more exposure to adverse circumstances are significantly more likely to have poorer health than those who have experienced fewer disadvantages.

Considering multiple measures of socioeconomic status when examining the social dimensions of health is important because measures of education, income, and occupation tend to be only moderately correlated with one another (Adler & Ostrove, 1999) and associations between health and socioeconomic position tend to vary based on the measures of socioeconomic status and health that are used (Macintyre, McKay, Der, & Rosemary, 2003). Our study employs a multidimensional measure of socioeconomic resources by examining the independent and cumulative contribution of three measures of socioeconomic disadvantage — lacking a high school diploma, unemployment, and poverty-level income — on health.

We also contribute to the developing literature on fundamental causes theory by including multiple disease-specific health outcomes and risk factors in our analysis. Many studies that have tested aspects of the fundamental causes theory have done so using general measures of health and mortality (e.g., Lantz et al., 1998; Pampel & Rogers, 2004; Warren & Hernandez, 2007), which has led for calls for empirical research that tests the validity of the theory across more specific health outcomes and risk factors (Miech et al., 2011). Some notable exceptions are Link et al. (1998) examination of the structuring of pap tests and mammography screens by socioeconomic status and Link's (2008) assessment of the association between education and smoking behavior. Empirical evidence from the larger social determinants of health literature finds significant associations between socioeconomic resources and heart disease, diabetes, arthritis, and adverse birth outcomes among different populations and using different measures of socioeconomic status (Adler & Ostrove, 1999). Our analysis draws from a nationally representative sample of adults in the United States aged 18−64 and finds a significant association between individual and cumulative measures of socioeconomic status on self-rated health, smoking, and diagnoses of cancer, high blood pressure, and heart disease.

METHODS

This study uses data from the 2011 Behavioral Risk Factor Surveillance Survey (BRFSS) to test the independent and cumulative associations between measures of socioeconomic status and health outcomes and risk factors. The BRFSS is a nationally representative telephone survey administered by the Centers for Disease Control and Prevention in collaboration with state health departments that measures behavioral risk factors among adults aged 18 years or older who live in households. In 2011, the survey's sample of 506,022 households included cell phone users without landlines for the first time and also adjusted its weighting methodology to more accurately represent groups that are underrepresented in the sample (Centers for Disease Control and Prevention, 2012). The results presented here use weighted data.

Five measures of health and health risk factors were included as dependent variables for this analysis: self-rated health, smoking prevalence, and high blood pressure, heart disease, and cancer diagnoses. In addition to serving as a subjective measure of health, self-rated health has been found to be a valid predictor of mortality across a variety of contexts (Idler & Benyamini, 1997). Smoking represents a health risk factor that is associated with numerous negative health outcomes, including heart disease, stroke, and lung cancer (Centers for Disease Control and Prevention, 2011c), and a diagnosis of high blood pressure places individuals at risk of two of the leading causes of death in the United States: a stroke and heart disease (Centers for Disease Control and Prevention, 2011b). Cancer and heart disease diagnoses were included in our analysis because they were the top two causes of death in the United States in 2011 (Hoyert & Xu, 2012). Thus, our dependent variables allow us to test the validity of the fundamental causes theory by examining the relationship of socioeconomic position to multiple measures of health and health risk factors.

In the survey, self-rated health was measured by asking the question, "Would you say that in general your health is excellent, very good, good, fair, or poor?" The self-rated health variable was recoded to a binary variable, with 0 = good, very good, or excellent health and 1 = fair or poor health. Smoking prevalence was measured in the survey by asking respondents "Do you now smoke cigarettes every day, some days, or not at all?" The variable was recoded to a binary variable with 0 = do not smoke cigarettes and 1 = smoke cigarettes.

High blood pressure was measured in the survey by asking respondents "Have you ever been told by a doctor, nurse or other health professional that you have high blood pressure?" The variable was recoded to a binary variable with 0 = never diagnosed with high blood pressure and 1 = has been diagnosed with high blood pressure. Heart disease diagnosis was measured in the survey by asking respondents "Were you ever told you had angina or coronary heart disease?" The variable was recoded to a binary variable with 0 = never diagnosed with angina or coronary heart disease and 1 = has been diagnosed with angina or coronary heart disease. The BRFSS measures cancer diagnosis using two questions, one that asks whether respondents were ever diagnosed with skin cancer and another that asks whether respondents were ever diagnosed with any other type of cancer. These two variables were combined to create a single binary variable with 0 = never diagnosed with any type of cancer and 1 = has been diagnosed with any type of cancer.

Three measures of socioeconomic position – education, employment, and income – were included as independent variables in this analysis. These objective measures of socioeconomic status represent many of the flexible resources that, when unevenly distributed, lead to disparities in health. Lower levels of formal education are associated with higher levels of poor self-rated health, life-threatening illness, and mortality (Link, Phelan, Miech, & Leckman Westin, 2008). In the survey, respondents' highest level of education was measured as an ordinal variable, originally in six categories. For this analysis, education was recoded into a binary variable, with 0 = at least a high school diploma and 1 = less than a high school diploma.

Employment directly and indirectly impacts health outcomes. Employment provides income and often provides access to health insurance benefits. Individuals who work also often receive subjective benefits such as social connections to co-workers and a sense of purpose and self-worth. Research on the social determinants of health has documented the negative impact of poor economic conditions and unemployment on individuals' perceptions of their health (Åhs & Westerling, 2006; Burgard, Brand, & House, 2009; Kondo, Subramanian, Kawachi, Takeda, & Yamagata, 2008) as well as the positive health benefits associated with employment (Ross & Mirowsky, 1995). In the survey, employment was measured using eight categories. This variable was recoded into a binary variable with 0 = employed for wages or self-employed and 1 = out of work for more than a year, unable to work, student, homemaker, or retired.

Income provides the means with which individuals can directly purchase health care services as well as gain access to resources that have been demonstrated to be beneficial to health, such as "medical care resources and good housing; less exposure to a noxious environment; and a good diet, good working conditions, and more social amenities" (Liberatos et al., 1988, p. 89). The BRFSS measures income by asking respondents to indicate which of eight categories best represents their household income from all sources. This variable was recoded into a binary variable with 0 = household income equal to or greater than $25,000 and 1 = household income less than $25,000. This cut point was chosen to roughly approximate the Census Bureau's poverty threshold, which was $18,123 for a family of three with two children and $22,811 for a family of four with two children in 2011 (U.S. Census Bureau, 2012).

The cumulative effect of the three adverse socioeconomic circumstances was measured by creating an index. Each of the three independent variables was summed to create the index, which ranged from zero to three adverse socioeconomic circumstances. The index was then recoded into a polytomous set of variables, with 0 = no adverse socioeconomic circumstances, 1 = one adverse circumstance, 2 = two adverse circumstances, and 3 = three adverse circumstances. When analyzing the polytomous variables, each additional adverse circumstance is compared with experiencing none of the adverse circumstances.

Seven control variables measuring race, gender, age, insurance coverage, and rural/urban status also were incorporated into the analysis. Race was measured in the survey by asking participants "Which one or more of the following would you say is your race?" It was recoded as a series of binary variables with White serving as the reference group. Ethnicity was measured by asking respondents "Are you Hispanic or Latino?" The variable was recoded to a binary variable with 0 = does not identify as Hispanic/Latino and 1 = identifies as Hispanic/Latino. Gender was coded by interviewers and was recoded to a binary variable for this analysis with 0 = Female and 1 = Male. Age was measured by asking respondents to report their age in years and was included as a continuous variable in this analysis. Respondents aged 65 and older were excluded to eliminate the confounding effects associated with retirement and widespread Medicare coverage. A variable measuring age squared was also included in our regression equations to take into account the likely non-linear relationship between age and our dependent variables.

We included a variable to control for health insurance coverage. The BRFSS measures health insurance by asking "Do you have any kind of health care coverage, including health insurance, prepaid plans such as HMOs, or government plans such as Medicare, or Indian Health Service?" This variable was recoded to a binary variable with 0 = no health insurance coverage and 1 = public or private health insurance coverage. A variable measuring whether a respondent lived in a rural or urban area was included in this analysis to account for lower levels of access to health care services that may be present in rural areas (Smith, Humphreys, & Wilson, 2008). Following Bethea, Lopez, Cozier, White, and McClean (2012), we designated a rural area as one that was located outside of a metropolitan statistical area (MSA). We recoded the BRFSS variable for metropolitan statistical code into a binary variable with 0 = living inside an MSA and 1 = living outside an MSA.

Bivariate analysis and logistic regression were used to assess the relationship of socioeconomic circumstances to health. We calculated bivariate analyses (Chi-Square and Cramer's V) to test the significance and strength of the relationships between our five measures of health and the scale for cumulative adverse circumstances. To assess the independent contribution of each measure of socioeconomic status, we constructed logistic regression equations for each measure of health, entering the four measures of socioeconomic resources as independent variables, and controlling for race, ethnicity, gender, age, health insurance coverage, and rural status. We tested for multicollinearity among the independent variables and found that none of the correlations exceeded a Pearson's r of 0.32. To measure the cumulative contribution of adverse socioeconomic status, we performed a second set of logistic regression analyses for each measure of health, entering the index of adverse circumstances as a polytomous variable set and controlling for race, ethnicity, gender, age, health insurance coverage, and rural status.

FINDINGS

In 2011, nearly half (49 percent) of adults aged 18–64 living in the United States experienced at least one adverse socioeconomic circumstance, and 22 percent of all respondents experienced more than one adverse socioeconomic circumstance. Very few respondents (6 percent) experienced all three measures of adverse socioeconomic position. Of the three measures of socioeconomic disadvantage, not working was the most prevalent, with 45 percent of all respondents reporting that they were not currently working for wages or self-employed. About a third of the BRFSS sample reported an annual household income of below $25,000, and 15 percent did not have a high school degree. Examining the demographic variables, we find that respondents aged 35–49 years are significantly less likely to experience socioeconomic disadvantage than younger (aged 18–34) and older (aged 50–64) respondents. Respondents who identify as Black or Hispanic are significantly more likely to experience multiple adverse circumstances than those who do not identify as Black or Hispanic, and women are significantly more likely than men to experience one or more adverse circumstances. Those living in rural areas are significantly more likely to experience multiple adverse socioeconomic circumstances compared to those living outside rural areas.

Through bivariate analysis, we found that self-rated health, smoking prevalence, and diagnoses of high blood pressure, heart disease and cancer are all significantly associated with adverse socioeconomic circumstances (Table 1). As the number of negative socioeconomic circumstances increases, the likelihood that a respondent reports negative health outcomes or risk behaviors increases, with the exception of cancer diagnosis, where the likelihood slightly decreases after experiencing the first adverse socioeconomic circumstance. There is a very strong relationship between cumulative adverse socioeconomic circumstances and self-rated health, a moderate relationship between adverse socioeconomic position and high blood pressure diagnosis, smoking, and heart disease diagnosis, and a weak relationship between cumulative adverse socioeconomic circumstances and cancer.

With the exception of cancer diagnosis, there is a "dose-response" relationship between adverse socioeconomic position and health outcomes and risk factors: for each additional adverse socioeconomic circumstance experienced, an individual is increasingly likely to experience a risk factor or poor health outcome. For example, only 11 percent of individuals experiencing no adverse circumstances rated their health as fair or poor compared to 17 percent experiencing one adverse circumstance, 34 percent experiencing two adverse circumstances, and 49 percent experiencing three adverse circumstances.

To control for the effects of gender, race, ethnicity, age, insurance coverage, and rural status on the relationship between adverse socioeconomic circumstances and health, we developed two logistic regression models. The first examines the independent contributions of each adverse socioeconomic circumstance on health, while the second assesses the cumulative effects of the three measures of socioeconomic position. Table 2 shows the results of the first regression model. Holding gender, race, ethnicity, age, health insurance coverage, and rural status constant, we find that there are

Table 1. Associations between Adverse Socioeconomic Circumstances, Health Problems, and Health Risk Factors.

	Number of Adverse Socioeconomic Circumstances				Measures of Association
	0	1	2	3	
Self-rated health	(n = 122,066,983)	(n = 62,025,918)	(n = 39, 793,782)	(n = 6,357,749)	χ^2 = 19,774,705.255***
Fair/poor	10.5%	16.8%	33.8%	48.8%	V = 0.289***
High B.P.	(n = 32,154,298)	(n = 62,136,655)	(n = 15,622,134)	(n = 13,085,882)	χ^2 = 4,305,708.378***
Yes	26.3%	33.7%	39.1%	47.7%	V = 0.135***
Heart disease	(n = 3,030,887)	(n = 3,147,597)	(n = 39,640,090)	(n = 12,907,100)	χ^2 = 2,612, 223.562***
Yes	2.5%	5.1%	6.9%	9.6%	V = 0.105***
Cancer	(n = 10,322,207)	(n = 8,790,159)	(n = 4,935,901)	(n = 13,142,504)	χ^2 = 1,625,166.250***
Yes	8.4%	14.1%	12.3%	13.6%	V = 0.083***
Smoker	(n = 121,851,749)	(n = 62,011,208)	(n = 39,862,573)	(n = 13,075,863)	χ^2 = 3,295,781.163***
Yes	16.9%	19.1%	27.8%	31.1%	V = 0.118***

Source: Behavioral Risk Factor Surveillance System (2011); analyses use weighted data.
*$p \leq 0.05$, **$p \leq 0.01$, ***$p \leq 0.001$.

Table 2. Logistic Regression – Impact of Adverse Socioeconomic Circumstances on Health for Adults Aged 18–64.

Health Problems and Risk Behaviors		*B*	Exp (*B*)	
Fair/poor self-rated health	No H.S. diploma	0.645***	1.906	*n* = 119,444,067
	Not working	1.039***	2.826	−2 Log likelihood =
	Low income	1.100***	3.005	86,044,474.701
	Uninsured	0.046***	1.047	Model Chi-square =
	Black, non-Hispanic	0.324***	1.383	16,636,003.546***
	Other race, non-Hispanic	0.202***	1.224	
	Multi-racial, non-Hispanic	0.437***	1.549	
	Hispanic	0.479***	1.615	
	Male	0.107***	1.113	
	Age	0.118***	1.126	
	Age squared	−0.001***	0.999	
	Rural	0.199***	1.221	
	Constant	−6.265***	0.002	
High blood pressure diagnosis	No H.S. diploma	0.087***	1.091	*n* = 119,683,698
	Not working	0.310***	1.363	−2 Log likelihood =
	Low income	0.397***	1.487	124,300,000.000
	Uninsured	−0.143***	0.866	Model Chi-square
	Black, non-Hispanic	0.722***	2.059	=16,836,308.601***
	Other race, non-Hispanic	−0.014***	0.987	
	Multi-racial, non-Hispanic	0.093***	1.098	
	Hispanic	−0.041***	0.960	
	Male	0.415***	1.514	
	Age	0.078***	1.081	
	Age squared	0.000***	1.000	
	Rural	0.184***	1.202	
	Constant	−4.787***	0.008	
Heart disease diagnosis	No H.S. diploma	0.128***	1.136	*n* =119,428,805
	Not working	0.830***	2.294	−2 Log likelihood =
	Low income	0.731***	2.078	26,401,579.956
	Uninsured	−0.328***	0.721	Model Chi-square =
	Black, non-Hispanic	0.014***	1.014	4,336,381.821***
	Other race, non-Hispanic	0.221***	1.247	
	Multi-racial, non-Hispanic	0.012**	1.012	
	Hispanic	−0.261***	0.771	
	Male	0.660***	1.935	
	Age	0.159***	1.172	
	Rural	0.105***	1.111	
	Constant	−10.295***	0.000	
Cancer diagnosis	No H.S. diploma	0.039***	1.040	*n* =119,824,897
	Not working	0.298***	1.348	−2 Log likelihood =
	Low income	0.117***	1.124	59,467,361.738
	Uninsured	−0.311***	0.733	

Table 2. (*Continued*)

Health Problems and Risk Behaviors		B	Exp (B)	
	Black, non-Hispanic	−0.977***	0.376	Model Chi-square = 6,791,286.309***
	Other race, non-Hispanic	−0.860***	0.423	
	Multi-racial, non-Hispanic	−0.222***	0.801	
	Hispanic	−0.923***	0.397	
	Male	−0.366***	0.694	
	Age	0.077***	1.080	
	Age squared	0.000***	1.000	
	Rural	0.000	1.000	
	Constant	−5.576***	0.004	
Smoker	No H.S. diploma	0.588***	1.801	n = 119,487,434
	Not working	0.261***	1.298	−2 Log likelihood =
	Low income	0.786***	2.194	112,200,000.000
	Uninsured	0.443***	1.558	Model Chi-square =
	Black, non-Hispanic	−0.226***	0.798	7,360,856.421***
	Other race, non-Hispanic	−0.581***	0.569	
	Multi-racial, non-Hispanic	0.332***	1.393	
	Hispanic	−1.132***	0.322	
	Male	0.245***	1.277	
	Age	0.079***	1.083	
	Age squared	−0.001***	0.999	
	Rural	0.171***	1.187	
	Constant	−3.233***	0.039	

Source: Behavioral Risk Factor Surveillance System (2011); analyses use weighted data.
*$p \leq 0.05$, **$p \leq 0.01$, ***$p \leq 0.001$.

significant associations between the three measures of socioeconomic circumstances and each health outcome or risk factor. Individuals without a high school diploma are significantly more likely to rate their health as fair or poor, to smoke, and to be diagnosed with high blood pressure, heart disease, or cancer than individuals with at least a high school diploma. Unemployed individuals are significantly more likely to experience negative health outcomes and risk factors than employed individuals. Individuals with incomes below $25,000 a year are significantly more likely to rate their health negatively, to smoke, and to be diagnosed with high blood pressure, heart disease, or cancer.

Examining the odds ratios in our regression models, we find some variation in the relationship between individual measures of socioeconomic circumstances and our five measures of health outcomes and risk factors.

Individuals without a high school diploma are about twice as likely to rate their health as fair or poor and to report smoking than individuals with a high school diploma, about 1.09 times more likely to be diagnosed with high blood pressure or heart disease, and 1.04 times as likely to be diagnosed with cancer than individuals with a high school diploma. Respondents who are not currently employed are nearly three times as likely to rate their health as fair or poor, more than twice as likely to be diagnosed with heart disease, and about 1.30 times as likely to smoke or be diagnosed with high blood pressure or cancer than those who are currently employed. Individuals with a household income less than $25,000 per year are three times as likely to rate their health as fair or poor, twice as likely to be diagnosed with heart disease or to report smoking, 1.5 times as likely to be diagnosed with high blood pressure, and 1.1 times as likely to be diagnosed with cancer than individuals with a household income of more than $25,000 per year.

Table 3 presents the results of the second regression model, which examines the cumulative effects of education, employment, and income on health. This analysis also includes race, ethnicity, gender, age, health insurance coverage, and rural status as control variables. Individuals with no adverse socioeconomic circumstances served as the reference group. Our findings demonstrate that cumulative adverse socioeconomic circumstances are significantly related to respondents' self-rated health, smoking prevalence, and diagnosis of high blood pressure, heart disease, and cancer. Each additional negative circumstance (e.g., lacking a high school diploma, not working, having a low income) is significantly associated with each of our dependent variables. As the number of adverse socioeconomic circumstances increases, so does the likelihood that respondents will rate their health as fair or poor, smoke cigarettes, and be diagnosed with high blood pressure, heart disease, or cancer.

Respondents with one adverse socioeconomic circumstance are about twice as likely to rate their health as fair or poor, while those experiencing the three adverse circumstances are nearly nine times as likely to rate their health negatively compared to respondents with no adverse socioeconomic circumstances. For smoking prevalence, individuals with three adverse circumstances are nearly four times as likely to report smoking as those with no adverse socioeconomic circumstances. Individuals experiencing three adverse socioeconomic circumstances are twice as likely to report being diagnosed with high blood pressure, more than four times as likely to be diagnosed with heart disease, and about one and a half times as likely to be diagnosed with cancer as individuals who are not experiencing any adverse circumstances.

Table 3. Logistic Regression – Impact of Cumulative Adverse Socioeconomic Circumstances on Health Problems and Health Risk Behaviors, Holding Race, Gender, Age, and Rural Status Constant for Adults Aged 18–64.

	Number of Adverse Circumstances	B	Exp(B)	
Fair/poor self-rated health	0	–	–	$n = 135,745,100$
	1	0.712***	2.039	−2 Log likelihood =102,400,000
	2	1.729***	5.636	Model Chi-square = 15,395,715.486***
	3	2.164***	8.708	
High blood pressure diagnosis	0	–	–	$n = 135,970,429$
	1	0.165***	1.179	−2 Log likelihood = 139,800,000.000
	2	0.589***	1.802	Model Chi-square = 19,298,722.111***
	3	0.791***	2.206	
Heart disease diagnosis	0	–	–	$n = 135,680,975$
	1	0.562***	1.754	−2 Log likelihood = 29,879,547.082
	2	1.253***	3.500	Model Chi-square = 4,600,973.317***
	3	1.538***	4.657	
Cancer diagnosis	0	–	–	$n = 136,195,098$
	1	0.174***	1.190	−2 Log likelihood = 66,693,050.194
	2	0.360***	1.434	Model Chi-square = 7,750,344.572***
	3	0.464***	1.591	
Smoker	0	–	–	$n = 133,731,627$
	1	0.361***	1.435	−2 Log likelihood = 122,800,000.000
	2	0.948***	2.580	Model Chi-square = 7,336,217.789***
	3	1.379***	3.972	

Source: Behavioral Risk Factor Surveillance System (2011); analyses use weighted data.
*$p \leq 0.05$, **$p \leq 0.01$, ***$p \leq 0.001$.

DISCUSSION

This study examined the validity of two aspects of the fundamental causes theory: that socioeconomic resources are significantly associated with multiple health risk factors and that they are significantly associated with multiple health outcomes (Phelan et al., 2010). In doing so, we assessed the independent and cumulative association between education, employment, and income on self-rated health, smoking, and diagnoses of cancer, heart disease, and high blood pressure. This analysis has demonstrated support for the fundamental causes theory, indicating that measures of socioeconomic status have an independent and a cumulative association with multiple health outcomes and risk factors among U.S. adults aged 18–64. Alone and in combination with each other, low levels of formal education, unemployment, and household income negatively impact individuals' health in critical ways. Self-rated health, a general indicator associated with mortality, and the two leading causes of death in the United States (heart disease and cancer) are significantly associated with socioeconomic status. Smoking and high blood pressure, which are two risk factors associated with leading causes of death, also are significantly related to measures of socioeconomic position.

Both independent and cumulative measures of socioeconomic status are significantly associated with each of our five measures of health. Lacking a high school diploma, unemployment, and low household income are each significantly associated with self-rated health, smoking, and diagnoses of high blood pressure, heart disease, and cancer. When we examined the cumulative effects of education, employment, and income, our logistic regression analyses demonstrated a dose-response relationship between measures of poor health and each additional adverse socioeconomic circumstance for all measures of health. Respondents with three adverse socioeconomic circumstances are nearly nine times as likely to rate their health as fair or poor, more than four times as likely to be diagnosed with heart disease, nearly four times as likely to report smoking, twice as likely to be diagnosed with high blood pressure, and one and a half times as likely to be diagnosed with cancer. These results complement Bisgaier and Rhodes' (2011) analysis, which found significant relationships between cumulative adverse financial circumstances and smoking and self-rated health (among other measures of health) for a sample of urban emergency department patients, and Lawlor et al. (2005) study that found a significant relationship between a cumulative measure of ten aspects of socioeconomic position on coronary heart disease risk among a sample of British women.

Our analysis also uncovered variation in the relationship between our multiple measures of socioeconomic status and the five health outcomes and risk factors included in this analysis. We found the highest odds ratios for associations between adverse socioeconomic circumstances and self-rated health and the lowest odds ratios for associations between adverse socioeconomic position and cancer. The odds ratios for cancer diagnosis may be lower due to the differential relationship between socioeconomic status and certain types of cancer. For example, the incidence of breast cancer and skin cancer has been found to be more prevalent among individuals with a higher socioeconomic position due to delayed childbearing and recreational tanning (Adler & Ostrove, 1999).

We tested this relationship in our model by running our regression models separately for the two cancer variables included in the BRFSS: skin cancer and all other cancers. We found variation in our independent and cumulative models that support previous findings about the relationship between socioeconomic position and skin cancer. In our model that tested the independent contributions of adverse socioeconomic circumstances, we found that education, employment, and income were significantly associated with skin cancer ($p < 0.05$), but the direction of the association changed for education and income, such that individuals with more education and higher incomes were significantly more likely to be diagnosed with skin cancer. Similarly, in our cumulative model, experiencing multiple adverse socioeconomic circumstances is not significantly associated with skin cancer diagnosis ($p > 0.2$). For other types of cancer, we found significant associations between experiencing multiple adverse socioeconomic circumstances and being diagnosed with a type of cancer other than skin cancer ($p < 0.001$). We also found that education is not significantly associated with the diagnosis of other types of cancer ($p > 0.2$), but there is a significant relationship between employment and income ($p < 0.001$) and other cancer diagnosis. These findings underscore the need to test the validity of the fundamental causes theory with multiple disease-specific outcomes. It could be that diagnosis-related complexities result from people in lower socioeconomic groups being less likely to access health care and thereby receive a diagnosis. In all, more research on this issue is needed.

The findings of this study are generalizable to adults aged 18–64 living in the United States and may not apply to individuals living outside the United States, older Americans, and children. Our study also is limited in the measures of socioeconomic status and health outcomes we were able to examine. For example, the BRFSS does not include any data about occupational type or any questions about childhood disadvantage and does not include variables for specific types of cancer other than skin cancer. Our use of cross-sectional data from the BRFSS does not allow us to measure cumulative effects of socioeconomic disadvantage over time for the same individuals. In addition, the new data collection methodology employed by the BRFSS in 2011, which included cell phone users for the first time, does not allow us to easily compare the results of our analysis to previous samples of U.S. residents. Warren and Hernandez's (2007) analysis, which examines the impact of multiple measures of socioeconomic status on self-rated health during the twentieth century using the General Social Survey, suggests that relationships between socioeconomic position and self-rated health have remained relatively consistent over time. However, it is not clear the extent to which this finding also applies to the other health outcomes and risk factors we included in this study.

If education, employment, and income represent "fundamental causes" that will continue to reproduce health disparities over time, mitigating health disparities will require reducing inequalities in individuals' access to these resources (Phelan et al., 2010). In order to know how to target these efforts, it is helpful to have a better understanding about the strength and magnitude of the relationships between particular socioeconomic resources and health outcomes. Our chapter has contributed to this effort by assessing the cumulative and independent contributions of traditional measures of socioeconomic status on multiple health outcomes. This analysis also serves as a reminder that local, state, and federal efforts to improve population health and access to socioeconomic resources should not proceed along separate lines. Increasing the number of students who graduate from high school as well as increasing access to employment, and particularly to well-paying jobs, is critical to reducing health disparities and improving well-being in the United States over the next decade and beyond. In light of the Patient Protection and Affordable Care Act of 2010, and the U.S. Supreme Court ruling that upheld many features of the law (National Federation of Independent Business [NFIB] v. Sebelius, 2012), health insurance coverage is likely to increase dramatically in the coming years. While broader insurance coverage is a major step forward in increasing access to health care, it is important to increase access to other socioeconomic issues of importance to health, as demonstrated in this study.

REFERENCES

Adler, N. E., & Ostrove, J. M. (1999). Socioeconomic status and health: What we know and what we don't. *Annals of the New York Academy of Sciences, 896*(1), 3−15.

Åhs, A., & Westerling, R. (2006). Self-rated health in relation to employment status during periods of high and of low levels of unemployment. *The European Journal of Public Health, 16*(3), 294−304.

Bethea, T. N., Lopez, R. P., Cozier, Y. C., White, L. F., & McClean, M. D. (2012). The relationship between rural status, individual characteristics, and self-rated health in the behavioral risk factor surveillance system. *The Journal of Rural Health, 28*(4), 327−338.

Bisgaier, J., & Rhodes, K. V. (2011). Cumulative adverse financial circumstances: Associations with patient health status and behaviors. *Health & Social Work, 36*(2), 129−137.

Burgard, S. A., Brand, J. E., & House, J. S. (2009). Perceived job insecurity and worker health in the United States. *Social Science & Medicine, 69*(5), 777−785.

Centers for Disease Control and Prevention. (2011a). *CDC health disparities and inequalities report: United States, 2011.* Retrieved from http://www.cdc.gov/mmwr/pdf/other/su6001.pdf

Centers for Disease Control and Prevention. (2011b). *High blood pressure fact sheet.* Retrieved from http://www.cdc.gov/dhdsp/data_statistics/fact_sheets/fs_bloodpressure.htm

Centers for Disease Control and Prevention. (2011c). *Smoking and tobacco use; fact sheets on smoking and tobacco use.* Retrieved from http://www.cdc.gov/tobacco/data_statistics/fact_sheets/health_effects/effects_cig_smoking/

Centers for Disease Control and Prevention. (2012). *Overview: BRFSS 2011.* Atlanta, GA. Retrieved from http://www.cdc.gov/brfss/technical_infodata/surveydata/2011.htm

Cutler, D. M., & Lleras-Muney, A. (2006). *Education and health: Evaluating theories and evidence.* Cambridge, MA: National Bureau of Economic Research. Retrieved from http://www.nber.org/papers/w12352

Grzywacz, J. G., Almeida, D. M., Neupert, S. D., & Ettner, S. L. (2004). Socioeconomic status and health: A micro-level analysis of exposure and vulnerability to daily stressors. *Journal of Health & Social Behavior, 45*(1), 1−16.

House, J. S., Kessler, R. C., & Herzog, A. R. (1990). Age, socioeconomic status, and health. *The Milbank Quarterly, 68*(3), 383−411.

Hoyert, D. L., & Xu, J. (2012). *Deaths: Preliminary data for 2011.* Hyattsville, MD: National Center for Health Statistics.

Idler, E. L., & Benyamini, Y. (1997). Self-rated health and mortality: A review of twenty-seven community studies. *Journal of Health and Social Behavior, 38*(1), 21−37.

Kondo, N., Subramanian, S. V., Kawachi, I., Takeda, Y., & Yamagata, Z. (2008). Economic recession and health inequalities in Japan: Analysis with a national sample, 1986−2001. *Journal of Epidemiology & Community Health, 62*(10), 869−875.

Lantz, P. M., House, J. S., Lepkowski, J. M., Williams, D. R., Mero, R. P., & Chen, J. (1998). Socioeconomic factors, health behaviors, and mortality: Results from a nationally representative prospective study of U.S. adults. *Journal of the American Medical Association, 279*(21), 1703−1708.

Lawlor, D. A., Ebrahim, S., & Davey Smith, G. (2005). Adverse socioeconomic position across the lifecourse increases coronary heart disease risk cumulatively: Findings from the British women's heart and health study. *Journal of Epidemiology and Community Health, 59*(9), 785−793.

Liberatos, P., Link, B., & Kelsey, J. L. (1988). The measurement of social class in epidemiology. *Epidemiologic Reviews, 10*, 87−121.

Link, B. G. (2008). Epidemiological sociology and the social shaping of population health. *Journal of Health and Social Behavior*, *49*(4), 367–384.

Link, B. G., Northridge, M. E., Phelan, J. C., & Ganz, M. L. (1998). Social epidemiology and the fundamental cause concept: On the structuring of effective cancer screens by socioeconomic status. *The Milbank Quarterly*, *76*(3), 375–402.

Link, B. G., & Phelan, J. (1995). Social conditions as fundamental causes of disease. *Journal of Health & Social Behavior*, *36*, 80–94.

Link, B. G., Phelan, J. C., Miech, R., & Leckman Westin, E. (2008). The resources that matter: Fundamental social causes of health disparities and the challenge of intelligence. *Journal of Health and Social Behavior*, *49*(1), 72–91.

Macintyre, S., McKay, L., Der, G., & Rosemary, H. (2003). Socio-economic position and health: What you observe depends on how you measure it. *Journal of Public Health*, *25*(4), 288–294.

Miech, R., Pampel, F., Kim, J., & Rogers, R. G. (2011). The enduring association between education and mortality. *American Sociological Review*, *76*(6), 913–934.

National Center for Health Statistics. (2009). *Life expectancy at birth, at 65 years of age, and at 75 years of age, by race and sex: United States, selected years 1900–2007*. Retrieved from http://www.cdc.gov/nchs/data/hus/hus10.pdf#022

National Federation of Independent Business v. Sebelius. (2012). 132 S. Ct. 2566.

Pampel, F. C., & Rogers, R. G. (2004). Socioeconomic status, smoking, and health: A test of competing theories of cumulative advantage. *Journal of Health and Social Behavior*, *45*(3), 306–321.

Patient Protection and Affordable Care Act. (2010). Pub. L. No. 111–148, §2702, 124 Stat. 119, pp. 318–319.

Phelan, J. C., & Link, B. G. (2005). Controlling disease and creating disparities: A fundamental cause perspective. *The Journals of Gerontology Series B: Psychological Sciences and Social Sciences*, *60*(Special issue 2), S27–S33.

Phelan, J. C., Link, B. G., Diez-Roux, A., Kawachi, I., & Levin, B. (2004). Fundamental causes' of social inequalities in mortality: A test of the theory. *Journal of Health and Social Behavior*, *45*(3), 265–285.

Phelan, J. C., Link, B. G., & Tehranifar, P. (2010). Social conditions as fundamental causes of health inequalities: Theory, evidence, and policy implications. *Journal of Health & Social Behavior*, *51*(1), S28–S40.

Ross, C. E., & Mirowsky, J. (1995). Does employment affect health? *Journal of Health and Social Behavior*, *36*(3), 230–243.

Smith, K. B., Humphreys, J. S., & Wilson, M. G. A. (2008). Addressing the health disadvantage of rural populations: How does epidemiological evidence inform rural health policies and research? *Australian Journal of Rural Health*, *16*(2), 56–66.

U.S. Census Bureau. (2012). *Poverty thresholds by size of family and number of children*. Retrieved from http://www.census.gov/hhes/www/poverty/data/threshld/index.html

Warren, J. R., & Hernandez, E. M. (2007). Did socioeconomic inequalities in morbidity and mortality change in the United States over the course of the twentieth century? *Journal of Health and Social Behavior*, *48*(4), 335–351.

Weber, M. (1946). Class, status, party. In Hans H. Gerth and C. Wright Mills (Eds.), *From Max Weber: Essays in sociology*. New York, NY: Oxford University Press.

Xu, J., Kochanek, K. D., Murphy, S. L., & Tejada-Vera, B. (2010). *Deaths: Final data for 2007*. Hyattsville, MD: National Center for Health Statistics. Retrieved from http://www.cdc.gov/NCHS/data/nvsr/nvsr58/nvsr58_19.pdf

PREDICTORS OF RURAL HEALTH CLINIC MANAGERS' WILLINGNESS TO JOIN ACCOUNTABLE CARE ORGANIZATIONS

Thomas T. H. Wan, Maysoun Dimachkie Masri and Judith Ortiz

ABSTRACT

Purpose – *The implementation of the Patient Protection and Affordable Care Act has facilitated the development of an innovative and integrated delivery care system, Accountable Care Organizations (ACOs). It is timely, to identify how health care managers in rural health clinics (RHCs) are responding to the ACO model. This research examines RHC managers' perceived benefits and barriers for implementing ACOs from an organizational ecology perspective.*

Methodology/approach – *A survey was conducted in spring of 2012 covering the present RHC network working infrastructures –*

Technology, Communication, Disparities and Government Options in Health and Health Care Services
Research in the Sociology of Health Care, Volume 32, 259–273
ISSN: 0275-4959/doi:10.1108/S0275-495920140000032023

(1) Organizational social network; (2) organizational care delivery structure; (3) ACO knowledge, perceived benefits, and perceived barriers; (4) quality and disease management programs; and (5) health information technology (HIT) infrastructure. One thousand one hundred sixty clinics were surveyed in the United States. They cover eight southeastern states (Alabama, Florida, Georgia, Kentucky, Mississippi, North Carolina, South Carolina, and Tennessee) and California. A total of 91 responses were received.

Findings *– RHC managers' personal perceptions on ACO's benefits and knowledge level explained the most variance in their willingness to join ACOs. Individual perceptions appear to be more influential than organizational and context factors in the predictive analysis.*

Research limitations/implications *– The study is primarily focused in the Southeastern region of the United States. The generalizability is limited to this region. The predictors of RHCs' participation in ACOs are germane to guide the development of organizational strategies for enhancing the general knowledge about the innovativeness of delivering coordinated care and containing health care costs inspired by the Affordable Care Act.*

Originality/value of chapter *– RHCs are lagged behind the growth curve of ACO adoption. The diffusion of new knowledge about pros and cons of ACO is essential to reinforce the health care reform in the United States.*

Keywords: Rural health clinics; Accountable Care Organizations (ACOs); Patient Protection and Affordable Care Act (PPACA); information technology

BACKGROUND

The implementation of the Patient Protection and Affordable Care Act (PPACA) has facilitated the development and transformation of health care delivery systems such as Accountable Care Organizations (ACOs). ACOs are provider-run groups (of physicians, hospitals, and/or other health care organizations) that accept responsibility for the cost and quality of care of a defined population. To date, little is known about how managers of Rural Health Clinics (RHCs) will navigate their strategic move and participate in ACOs.

RHCs were developed under the Rural Health Clinics Act (P.L. 95-210). The Act was passed by Congress and signed into law by President Carter in 1977. The main goal of this Act was to (1) promote a collaborative model of health care delivery and encourage the utilization of nurse practitioners, physician assistants, certified nurse midwives, psychologists, and clinical social workers in non-urbanized areas under RHCs; (2) create a cost-based reimbursement mechanism for services provided at clinics located in underserved rural areas (Health Resources and Services Administration [HRSA], 2006). Today, like many health care organizations RHCs are faced by the challenge of providing effective and affordable health services as emphasized under the new Healthcare Reform legislation, the Patient Protection and Affordable Care Act (PPACA).

The PPACA was passed in December 2009 and signed into law in March 2010 by the U.S. Senate. Access to good-quality services in rural underserved areas has been a continuous challenge for the United States (Ortiz, Meemon, Tang, & Wan, 2011; Utz, Nelson, & Dien, 2011). For more than thirty years, RHCs have played an important role in meeting the needs of the rural elderly and other vulnerable populations. Some of the challenges faced by RHCs included difficulties in recruitment and retention of qualified health care professionals, major reimbursement barriers, and information technology and source barriers (Ortiz et al., 2011). Although, according to some policy analysts rural populations will benefit from the PPACA, the effects are still to be studied (Bailey, 2010; Murray, 2011). Furthermore, the ACO model is still evolving in its early stages. Thus, it is timely to identify how health care managers in RHCs are responding to its development.

This research examined RHC health care managers' perceived benefits and barriers to participating in ACOs from an organizational ecology perspective. Organizational ecology was the theoretical framework used to guide the model development and specification for this study (Hannan & Freeman, 1989). Because RHC managers are nested within different states whereby organizational and contextual differences may be observed, it is imperative to determine the net influence of predictor variables on the willingness to participate in ACOs while all other contextual factors are being held constant. A risk adjustment methodology is therefore needed in the analysis of net influences of individual predictors of ACO participation while the effects of organizational and contextual variables are hold constant (Bickel, 2007; Heckman, Ichimura, & Todd, 1998; Heckman, LaLonde, & Smith, 1999; Iezzoni, 1994; King, 1997).

Individuals are seen as possessing different degrees of willingness to adopt innovations (Rogers, 1995). As such, diffusion research was used to analyze the conditions which increase or decrease the likelihood that a new idea (in this case, participating in an ACO), will be adopted by RHC managers. The innovation-diffusion construct was also used to frame the major research question: Do RHC managers' perceptions of ACOs benefits, barriers, and organizational factors, such as social capital and the use of health information technology, influence their willingness to participate in ACOs? It is hypothesized that health care managers' perceived benefits and knowledge level about ACOs have a stronger influence on the willingness to participate in ACOs than organizational factors, holding the contextual factor which is the community propensity score factor (PSF) of high likelihood of ACO's adoption constant.

METHODS

Current secondary sources of RHC data do not include important information on a RHC's organizational structure and culture, implementation of disease and quality management programs, or the use of information technology. The unavailability of this type of data created the need to develop and conduct a survey to capture all this information and identify the organizational and community contexts that may serve as predictor variables for estimating PSF of high likelihood of ACO's adoption. Because certain organizational and community characteristics such as large hospitals and integrated care delivery systems (IDSs) are more likely to form organizational alliances and develop diversification strategies than small RHCs, it was necessary to perform a propensity score analysis to eliminate any potential selection bias factor such as size, volume, payer mix, case mix, referral medical center for remote areas, and presence of ACOs in the community.

A structured mail-survey tool (37 Likert-scale question items), covering the present RHC network working infrastructures – (1) Organizational social network; (2) organizational care delivery structure; (3) ACO participation, benefits, and barriers; (4) quality and disease management programs; and (5) health information technology infrastructure was developed. The survey questionnaire was reviewed and approved by the University IRB Office. No names were obtained from the survey. Thus, the anonymity of respondents was ensured.

In turn, a causal model of predictors of rural health care managers' willingness to participate in ACOs (ACO_join) was formulated, using the PSF as the correction variable of biased selection in a predictive equation. In this analysis, ACO_join was considered the endogenous variable ($Y1$), whereas predictor variables (X_i) included perceived benefits, perceived barriers, knowledge level about ACOs, RHCs organizational factors such as organizational social capital, adoption of electronic medical records (EMRs), and the contextual variable which is the PSF predictor variable identified as high likelihood of expected markets for ACO adoption and development.

The Propensity Score Approach

A propensity score of having a high expectation to be involved with ACOs (a dummy dependent variable; $1 =$ high presence of ACOs in a state with two or more ACOs established and $0 =$ low presence of ACOs in a state with less than two ACOs established in 2012) is estimated from multiple ecological and contextual variables in the propensity score analysis, using R-Project.Org with the subroutine of Matchit (upon request, scores could be obtained from principal investigator). The list of ecological variables include: (1) health information technology adoption rate; (2) disparities index; (3) percentage of elderly population; (4) regional location; (5) urban population size; (6) uninsured population size; (7) physician–population ratio; and (8) volunteerism rate. Logit analysis generated the propensity score for each state.

Measurements and Analysis

The willingness to participate in ACOs, an endogenous variable, is measured by an analog scale, ranging from the lowest (0) to highest (10) score. Predictors included several Likert-scale measures of the theoretical constructs such as perceived benefits, perceived barriers, and organizational social capital were developed and validated using structural equation modeling. Covariance structure analysis was performed to validate a theoretically specified model of predictors of rural health care managers' willingness to participate in ACOs (Wan, 2002). The propensity score for a state with high-expected involvement in ACOs was the control variable in order to adjust the state-level variation in ACO involvement in the analysis.

RESULTS

Survey Results

One thousand one hundred sixty RHC managers from eight southeastern states (Alabama, Florida, Georgia, Kentucky, Mississippi, North Carolina, South Carolina, and Tennessee) and California were surveyed either by regular mail or electronic mail using Qualtrics. A total of 91 responses were received. After eliminating the missing cases, only 89 respondents were included in the analysis. Of the 89 respondents, 37.6 percent belonged to a provider-based practice. About 83 percent of them did not have sufficient knowledge about ACOs. Health care managers from the provider-based rural clinics had a statistically significant higher perception of the ACO benefits than those in the independent practice (Table 1). Only 8 percent of the respondents reported that their clinics were affiliated with an integrated delivery system (IDS). However, 22 percent of provider-based clinics had an affiliation with IDS.

Propensity Score Analysis Results

The propensity score matching and analysis was performed for 50 states plus District of Columbia. The matching analysis eliminated nine states (Idaho, Iowa, Kansas, Maine, Montana, Nebraska, North Dakota, Oklahoma and South Dakota). The score ranged from 0.1930 (the lowest) for Alaska to 0.9231 (the highest) for Florida. The propensity scores for the nine study states were: Alabama (0.8605), California (0.4757), Florida (0.9231), Georgia (0.8957), Kentucky (0.8577), Mississippi (0.8365), North Carolina (0.8809), South Carolina (0.8579), and Tennessee (0.8879). The eight southeastern states experienced a higher likelihood of adoption rate of ACOs than other states in the United States.

Measurement Models for the Predictor (Latent) Variables

Three latent variables were constructed using multiple indicators. Each of these theoretical constructs or latent variables was independently evaluated, using confirmatory factor analysis. The summary statistics for these measurement models are presented in Table 2.

Table 1. Means and Standard Deviations of Selected Study Variables for 89 Respondents by Ownership Status of Rural Health Clinics (RHCs).

Study Variables	Total Mean	Provider-Based RHC Mean	Independent RHC Mean	Provider-Based RHC SD	Independent RHC SD	F-Value
Knowledge about ACOs (ranging from 1 to 4)	1.716	1.839	1.649	0.735	0.790	1.213
No. perceived benefits (ranging from 0 to 6)	2.022	2.656	1.672	2.223	2.180	4.143*
No. perceived barriers (ranging from 0 to 6)	2.267	2.156	2.328	1.668	1.877	0.186
IDS affiliated (1 = affiliated; 0 otherwise)	0.08	0.220	0.000	0.420	0.000	15.879*

*Statistically significant at 0.05 or lower level.

Table 2. Summary Statistics of Measurement Models for Three Exogenous Latent Variables.

Latent Variable and Indicators	Parameter Estimate	SE	Critical Value	Standardized Parameter Estimate
Perceived benefits: Cronbach's alpha =0.883				
Improve population health (ACOhlth)	1.000			**0.750**
Improve quality of care (ACOPtcare)	1.147	0.118	9.682*	**0.817**
Improve patient-focused care (ACOPtfoc)	1.288	0.150	8.605*	**0.926**
Physicians led (ACOPhys)	0.885	0.128	6.895*	**0.728**
Lower costs (ACOcost)	1.029	0.142	7.226*	**0.760**
Share savings (ACOSav)	0.470	0.131	3.581*	**0.393**
Summary of goodness of fit statistics:				
Chi-square value (degrees of freedom)	3.034 (7)			
P value	0.882			
CFI	1			
GFI	0.980			
AGFI	0.967			
RMSEA	0.034			
Perceived barriers: Cronbach's alpha = 0.822				
Legal barrier (ACOLegal)	1.000			**0.495**
Not a mission of RHCs (ACO Msn)	0.913	0.281	3.324*	**0.505**
Lose autonomy (ACOAuto)	0.565	0.223	2.532*	**0.296**
Not large enough population (ACOPop)	0.596	0.265	2.251*	**0.305**
Inadequate capitals (ACOCap)	1.237	0.342	3.623*	**0.629**
Limited payments (ACOpay)	1.586	0.426	3.718*	**0.784**
Summary of goodness of fit statistics:				
Chi-square value (degrees of freedom)	8.918 (8)			
P value	0.349			
CFI	0.988			
GFI	0.966			
AGFI	0.910			
RMSEA	0.036			

Org. Social Capital: Cronbach's alpha = 0.681			
Fully trust each other (Trust)	1.000		0.854
Share a same vision (Vision)	1.131	0.123	9.177*	0.833
Collectively solve problems (ProSolve)	1.045	0.109	9.604*	0.871
Do teamwork (Teamwk)	0.671	0.178	3.777*	0.406
Interact socially outside workplace (Interact)	0.437	0.139	3.140*	0.348
Summary of goodness of fit statistics:			
Chi-square value (degrees of freedom)	5.761 (5)		
P value	0.330		
CFI	0.995		
GFI	0.968		
AGFI	0.904		
RMSEA	0.041		

*Statistically significant at 0.05 or lower level.

The variance in perceived benefits of ACOs is shared in common by six indicators such as (1) improve population health, (2) improve quality of care, (3) improve patient-focused care, (4) improve physicians' leadership, (5) lower costs of care, and (6) share savings. These indicators were found statistically significant at 0.05 or lower level, with the strongest factor loading observed for "improve patient-focused care" as the most dominant or influential indicator and the lowest one observed for "share savings" (Fig. 1). The summary of goodness of fit (GOF) statistics for the "perceived benefits" measurement model showed that the measurement model fits the data very well, with Chi-square value of 3.036 for 7 degrees of freedom, P value of 0.882, CFI of 1, GFI of 0.980, AGFI of 0.967, and RMSEA of 0.034 (Table 2).

The measurement model of perceived barriers was examined with six indicators, namely (1) legal barriers, (2) ACO is not a mission for RHC, (3) lose autonomy, (4) not large enough population to serve, (5) inadequate capital, and (6) limited payments. The results showed that the indicator for a limited ACO payment has the largest factor loading (0.784) with the latent construct of perceived barriers (Fig. 2). All six indicators were statistically significantly related to the common construct although "lose autonomy" has a factor loading of 0.296. The overall GOF statistics showed that

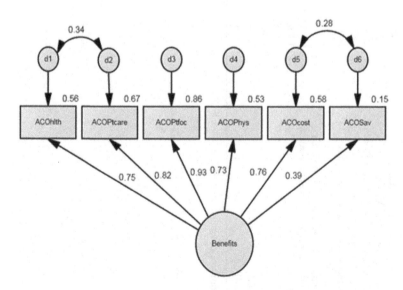

Fig. 1. The Measurement Model of Perceived Benefits of ACOs.

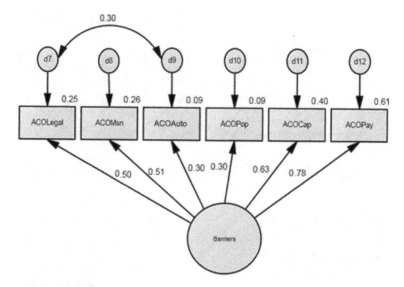

Fig. 2. The Measurement Model of Perceived Barriers of ACOs.

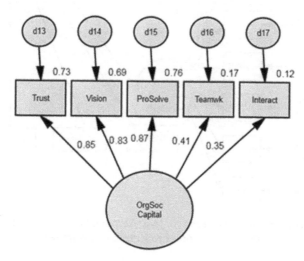

Fig. 3. Measurement Model of Organizational Social Capital.

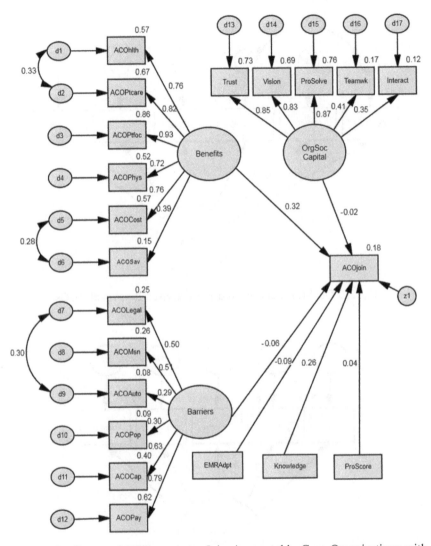

Fig. 4. Predictors of Willingness to Join Accountable Care Organizations with Propensity Score (ProScore) as an Adjuster.

this was an excellent fitted measurement model for perceived barriers, with Chi-square value of 9.918 for 8 degrees of freedom, CFI of 0.988, GFI of 0.966, AGFL of 0.910, and RMSEA of 0.036.

Five indicators in terms of mutual trust, shared vision, collective problem-solving, teamwork, and interactions with colleagues socially outside workplace were reflective of organizational social capital (OSC, see Fig. 3). The first three indicators had relatively large factor loadings associated with the common construct, OSC. The last indicator was considered the weakest one (0.348) although it was statistically significant. The overall GOF statistics showed that this measurement model was also well-fitted with the data, having Chi-square value of 5.761 for 5 degrees of freedom, a *P* value of 0.330, CFI of 0.995, GFI of 0.968, AGFI of 0.904, and RMSEA of 0.041.

Five predictor variables and one control variables were regressed on the willingness to join ACOs (Fig. 4). They accounted for 18.3 percent of the total variance in this endogenous variable. The statistical results are summarized in Table 3. Only two predictor variables were statistically significant at 0.05 level; perceived benefit (standardized regression coefficient = 0.318) and the ACO knowledge level (0.265) were positively associated with the willingness to join ACOs. Other variables exerted a relatively weak or no influence on this endogenous variable. The propensity score, a contextual variable as an adjuster, did not appear to be influential in this analysis.

Table 3. Predictors of the Willingness to Join Accountable Care Organizations.

Predictors	Parameter Estimate	Standard Error	Critical Value	*P* value	Standardized Estimate
Benefits	55.128	23.868	2.310*	0.021	**0.318**
Barriers	−4.183	8.986	−0.466	0.642	**−0.052**
Org. Social Capital	−1.258	6.401	−0.197	0.844	**−0.022**
EMR adoption	−1.149	1.421	−0.829	0.419	**−0.085**
Knowledge about ACO	9.968	4.017	2.481*	0.013	**0.265**
Propensity score	5.989	16.284	0.368	0.713	**0.039**

Notes: Summary of Goodness of Fit Statistics: Chi-square = 215.727 with 184 degrees of freedom; CFI = 0.943; TLI = 0.939; and RMSEA = 0.045.
*Statistically significant at 0.05 or lower level.

IMPLICATIONS AND CONCLUSIONS

The study findings showed that RHC managers' personal perceptions on ACO's benefits and knowledge level explained the most variance in their willingness to join ACOs. Individual perceptions appeared to be more influential than organizational and context factors in this analysis. Should ACOs be the future health care delivery system within the United States, a joined effort should be made to provide evidence of clinical and operational effectiveness in patient care for both rural and urban areas. In addition, it is imperative to improve the general and specific knowledge about ACOs so that RHC managers are well informed about the pros and cons of varying modalities of ACOs.

The study has several limitations. First, the study focused on eight southeastern states and the state of California. The results may not be generalizable to the entire United States. Second, the response rate of the ACO survey was relatively low. More effort should be made to generate the interest of health care managers in responding to the ACO initiative organized and monitored by the Centers for Medicare and Medicaid Services.

RHCs are lagged behind the growth curve of ACO adoption. The diffusion of new knowledge about pros and cons of ACO is essential to reinforce the health care reform in the United States (Kronenfeld, 2012). The use of organizational ecology guiding the development of research questions can help shape the investigation of personal and contextual determinants of adoption of innovative delivery systems. The predictors of RHCs' willingness to participate in ACOs are germane to guide the development of organizational strategies for enhancing the knowledge about the innovativeness of delivering coordinated care and containing health care costs promoted by the Affordable Care Act.

ACKNOWLEDGMENT

This research, in part, is supported by a federal grant U24MD006954 from the National Institute on Minority Health and Health Disparities, NIH. The content is solely the responsibility of the authors and does not necessarily represent the official views of the National Institutes of Health.

REFERENCES

Bailey, J. (2010). *Why healthcare reform can't wait: The benefits of health reform for rural America*. Lyons, NE: Center for Rural Affairs.

Bickel, R. (2007). *Multilevel analysis for applied research*. New York, NY: Guilford Press.

Hannan, M. T., & Freeman, J. (1989). Organizations and social structure. In *Organizational ecology* (pp. 3–27). Cambridge: Harvard University Press.

Health Resources and Services Administration (HRSA). (2006). *Comparison of the rural health clinic and federally qualified health centers program*. Retrieved from http://www.ask. hrsa.gov/downloads/fqhc-rhccomparison.pdf

Heckman, J., Ichimura, H., & Todd, P. (1998). Matching as an econometric evaluation estimator. *Review of Economic Studies, 65*(2), 261–294.

Heckman, J., LaLonde, R., & Smith, J. (1999). The economics and econometrics of active labor market programs. In O. Ashenfelter & D. Card (Eds.), *Handbook of labor economics* (Vol. 3, pp. 1865–2097). Amsterdam: Elsevier.

Iezzoni, L. I. (1994). *Risk adjustment for measuring health care outcomes*. Ann Arbor, MI: Health Administration Press.

King, G. (1997). *A solution to the ecological inference problem: Reconstructing individual behavior from aggregate data*. Princeton, NJ: Princeton University Press.

Kronenfeld, J. J. (2012). Systems of health-care delivery: Sociological issues linked to health reform and roles of patients and providers. In J. J. Kronenfeld (Ed.), *Access to care and factors that impact access, patients as partners in care and changing roles of health providers* (Vol. 29, pp. 3–17). Research in the Sociology of Health Care. Bingley, UK: Emerald Group Publishing Limited.

Murray, L. R. (2011). Health reform to have significant benefits for rural Americans. *The Nation's Health, 41*(4), 3.

Ortiz, J., Meemon, N., Tang, C. Y., & Wan, T. T. H. (2011). Rural health clinic efficiency and effectiveness: Insight from a nationwide survey. *Journal of Medical Systems, 35*, 671–681.

Rogers, E. M. (1995). *Diffusion of innovations* (4th ed.). New York, NY: The Free Press.

Utz, R. L., Nelson, R., & Dien, P. (2011). American health care: Public opinion differences in the confidence, affordability, and need for reform. In J. J. Kronenfeld (Ed.), *Access to care and factors that impact access, patients as partners in care and changing roles of health providers* (Vol. 29, pp. 243–272). Research in the Sociology of Health Care. Bingley, UK: Emerald Group Publishing Limited.

Wan, T. T. H. (2002). *Evidence-based health care management: Multivariate modeling approaches*. Boston, MA: Kluwer Academic Publishers.

AGING PUERTO RICANS' EXPERIENCES OF DEPRESSION TREATMENT: A NEW ETHNOGRAPHIC EXPLORATION

Marta B. Rodríguez-Galán and Luis M. Falcón

ABSTRACT

Purpose – *To examine aging Puerto Ricans' experiences with and perceptions of depression treatment.*

Methodology/approach – *In-depth analysis of eight exemplary cases from ethnographic interviews with a subsample of 16 aging Puerto Ricans in the Boston area who are part of the Boston Puerto Rican Health Study.*

Findings – *The results show that respondents were resistant to accepting pharmacological treatment for their depression, and they often characterized antidepressants as "dope." Moreover, they claimed that in addition to their health problems, social stressors such as financial strain, lack of jobs, housing problems, and social isolation are triggering or contributing to their depression. Because of this, they express reluctance in accepting clinical treatment only, and suggest that broader social*

Technology, Communication, Disparities and Government Options in Health and Health Care Services
Research in the Sociology of Health Care, Volume 32, 275–303
ISSN: 0275-4959/doi:10.1108/S0275-495920140000032024

issues and other health needs ought to be addressed as part of an effective treatment. For many, pharmacological treatment is acceptable only in the more severe forms of depression.

Research limitations/implications — *These results have important implications for improving the quality of depression treatment and reducing health disparities for mainland Puerto Ricans.*

Originality/value of chapter — *Even though recent studies continue to show a high frequency of depression among Puerto Ricans, issues of treatment quality are still understudied and ethnographic accounts are especially lacking. Our study offers an exploratory investigation of this unresolved research issue.*

Keywords: Puerto Ricans; Latinos/Hispanics; depression; mental health disparities; depression treatment

INTRODUCTION

The disproportionate prevalence of depression among aging Hispanics is well documented, particularly among Puerto Ricans who — among all Hispanic subgroups — exhibit the highest rates. Key social and medical factors are associated with the prevalence of depression for this U.S. population and these include: being female, having lower education levels, health problems and problems with access to medical care (Falcón & Tucker, 2000; Kemp, Staples, & Lopez-Aqueres, 1987; Ramos, 2005; Robinson, Gruman, Gaztambide, & Blank, 2002; Rodríguez-Galán & Falcón, 2009). According to a report by the Department of Health and Human Services published a decade ago, Hispanics in general and other older adults are less likely to receive depression treatment that meets the general quality treatment guidelines. In this regard, language barriers may impede access to specialty mental health care, especially because Spanish speaking mental health providers are underrepresented in those professions (DHHS, 1999). These institutional barriers seem to still affect mental health treatment for Hispanics today. Moreover, personal and cultural barriers such as attitudes, social norms, and beliefs regarding treatment for depression may prevent some from seeking help or adhering to treatment (Cooper et al., 2003; Keyes et al., 2012). Although several studies have addressed health disparities for Puerto Ricans, the general question of access to quality depression treatment, and especially the experiences with various types of treatment and their perceived effectiveness from the subject's own point of view, have received little to none scholarly attention. Our study offers an exploratory investigation of this unresolved research issue.

The purpose of this chapter is to investigate Puerto Ricans' experiences with treatment through the use of in-depth, semi-structured ethnographic interviews with a small sample of aging Puerto Ricans (age 50 and above) in the Boston area. In so doing, our aim was to offer a micro-level investigation of reported access to various treatment options and their perceived effectiveness. We hypothesized that a low socioeconomic profile, cultural and language barriers, and the inadequacy of the mental health system and mental health policy in addressing Hispanics and the poor would hinder access to adequate treatment for depression.

Puerto Ricans represent the largest Hispanic group in Massachusetts and share similar characteristics with other Hispanic subgroups, such as language and other cultural similarities. However, they also possess their own sociocultural idiosyncrasies, particularly due to their status as U.S. citizens and the historically uneasy relationship between the island of Puerto Rico and the United States, which has resulted in a peculiar pattern of migratory flux to the mainland, including immigration, outmigration, and circular migration (Baer, 1992; Borjas & Bratsberg, 1996). In this context, Massachusetts has been a secondary site of migration for aging Puerto Ricans, the majority of whom were born in the island. Because of the special legal status of Puerto Ricans and their unique migration experience, it will be necessary to situate our discussion within the larger context of the history of outpatient mental health policy in the United States, especially as it relates to treating both immigrant and minority populations.

As was the case of other minority immigrant populations in the past (see Vander Stoep & Link, 1998, for a discussion of the Irish) psychiatric epidemiological research on Puerto Ricans has been plagued by ethnocentric biases in many instances. Not only have Hispanics in general been challenged in terms of gaining access to mental health services, but they have also had an often traumatic relationship with the mainstream of U.S. psychiatry and psychology, in large measure due to a lack of cultural understanding of this population, which has often led to misdiagnosis and stigmatizing psychiatric labels such as the so called "Puerto Rican Syndrome." This form of mental distress was first observed by U.S. psychiatrists in Puerto Rican soldiers who had been drafted in the island to fight during War World II (Gherovici, 2003).

Both mental illness and physical illness for that matter are now generally understood as a complex phenomenon involving the interplay of biological, environmental, and socioeconomic factors. Although popular misconceptions about the nature of "race" and "ethnicity" persist even among health researchers today (Baer et al., 2013), most social scientists now conceive race as a social construct, rather than a biological structure. Observed health disparities among minority groups, women, and the poor are largely explained by social and economic factors in the research literature (Kuzawa & Sweet, 2009). Because of the social and economic basis for this excess of mental health issues in a community, Alegría and colleagues have further posited that not only mental health but also public policies in general play a crucial role in eliminating mental health disparities, which are driven by housing, education and income factors that affect U.S. minority groups disproportionally (Alegría, Perez, & Williams, 2003).

Recent epidemiological studies on mental health in Puerto Rican populations have used the Center for Epidemiologic Studies Scale (CES-D) and the NIMH Diagnostic Interview Schedule (DIS) to assess symptoms of depression. The former has been proven a more valid measure of depression in Puerto Rican populations (Robinson et al., 2002). Using this scale, the Hispanic Health and Nutrition Examination Survey confirmed the higher prevalence of depression symptoms among Puerto Ricans compared to both Mexican-Americans and Cuban-Americans. Additionally, researchers found support for the social stress hypothesis, in other words, psychological distress among Puerto Ricans was associated with their higher rates of unemployment, lower income, and marital disruption when compared to Mexican-Americans or Cuban-Americans (Angel & Guarnaccia, 1989).

Another recent survey, the Massachusetts Hispanic Elders Study, examined the prevalence and correlates of depression of older Hispanics (Puerto Rican, Dominican, and other Hispanic origin) in the state and a comparison group of Non-Hispanic Whites. This study found higher rates of depression symptoms for Hispanics than ever reported, especially for Puerto Ricans. Depression for this Latino sub-group was associated with being female, living alone, and having a high number of health problems. In fact, chronic health conditions were the factors most consistently associated with depression in this Massachusetts sample (Falcón & Tucker, 2000). Moreover, Hispanics as a whole, and Puerto Ricans in particular, were more likely than Non-Hispanic Whites to experience problems with access to medical care. For Puerto Ricans being female, living alone, possessing low education levels, having high numbers of health problems, disability, and access to medical care problems were all independently associated with depression symptoms (Rodríguez-Galán & Falcón, 2009). Thus, in addition to confirming the social stress hypothesis earlier reported by other researchers (Haberman, 1976; Krause & Carr, 1978; Malzberg, 1956), this Massachusetts study suggests that inequalities in health and health care access help explain most of the disparities in depression among Puerto Ricans.

Not only do Puerto Ricans in Massachusetts exhibit higher rates of mental distress, but — like other minority groups — they also encounter disparities in treatment. However, in comparison to other states, Massachusetts has kept a better record on responding to the mental health needs of minorities. Dickey and colleagues used the state of Massachusetts as an example of a state whose Department of Mental Health had made efforts to address the needs of racial/ethnic minority patients in state hospitals and the community, by using existing data on homicide rate, families in poverty, female-headed households, income level, and adults and children who speak a language different from English to arrive at estimates of need (Dickey et al., 1989). More recent studies continue to show, though, that throughout the nation Hispanics experience disparities in access to mental health treatment in comparison to non-Hispanic whites, particularly poor Hispanics who are less likely to have access to Medicaid specialty services in Latino neighborhoods and also experience language barriers and cultural stigma in seeking help for mental health issues (Alegría et al., 2002).

Under-representation of Latinos in the mental health professions constitutes a major problem; especially given that psychosocial therapy necessitates that the clinician be attuned to the cultural and linguistic background of the client. According to a report by the Department of Health and Human Services, one of the main obstacles for mental health treatment for Latinos is finding Spanish speaking providers (DHHS, 1999). Even though the number of Hispanic staff was relatively high in the CMHC, these workers were concentrated in sub-master's degree types of occupations (Dowell & Ciarlo, 1989; Rochefort, 1989). Furthermore, according to the American Psychological Association, Latinos represent only 1% of all practicing psychologists, whereas 96% of psychologists identify themselves as Whites (DHHS, 1999). Moreover, while the Latino population continues to grow, the numbers of Latinos receiving PhD degrees in psychology have remained stagnant at about 2% of all graduating students (Maton, Kohout, Wicherski, Leary, & Vinokurov, 2006). It is also worth noting that not all self-identified Latinos are fluent in Spanish, a skill that would be necessary in order to offer treatment to the majority of today's older Hispanics seeking psychotherapy. The same report by the Department of Health and Human Services shows evidence from available community studies that point to the insufficient mental health care that Hispanics are receiving. In fact, Latinos were twice as likely to receive treatment for mental health in general health care centers rather than mental health specialized settings (DHHS, 1999). These general health care centers often lack specialized knowledge about the cultural and language differences of minority patients and generally do not reach out or advocate for older Hispanics (Biegel, Farkas, & Song, 1997). Interestingly, one study conducted in Puerto Rico, found that the use of mental health specialists was associated with a higher socioeconomic status, which supports the argument that economic barriers interfere with the use of mental health services in the United States (Vera et al., 1991).

LITERATURE ON TREATMENT OF DEPRESSED ADULT HISPANICS

Older adults are, in general, less likely to receive adequate depression screening and treatment. While this holds true across all racial/ethnic groups, it is particularly prevalent among historically oppressed racial/ethnic groups (Olfson et al., 2002; Young, Klap, Sherbourne, & Wells, 2001). Yet, it has been found that older adults would be inclined to receive psychosocial services, in particular psycho-educational services and psycho-educational programming (Aeran, Alvidrez, Robinson, & Scotia Hicks, 2002). Some scholars have attributed under-treatment among depressed older adults to individual behaviors, such as stigma attached to mental disorders among the elders, as well as to failures in the mental health system. For example, the failure of health care providers to properly identify symptoms of depression in the older population and ageist beliefs among health professionals that impact how aging individuals are treated. General guidelines recommend that, in managing depression care for older adults, it is necessary to assess their health, living conditions and social isolation and require the intervention of other health and social agencies when appropriate (NICE, 2004).

The issue of what constitutes appropriate treatment for depression is in itself the subject of much controversy. In this regard, it is important to note that even though depression is used in this study as a general term, it is certainly a diverse phenomenon. There are different forms of depression, this illness can also be acute or chronic, and there is also a range of degrees of severity. For this reason, the particular kind of treatment/s may vary for each individual case. In general, mental health experts recommend that adequate treatment usually involves both biological therapy (i.e., pharma-cotherapy or ECT) and psychosocial therapy (i.e., cognitive behavioral therapy) (NICE, 2004). However, it is also believed that psychotherapy alone can be as effective as pharmacotherapy in alleviating symptoms in milder forms of depression (Olfson et al., 2002). Still, Hispanic elders are less likely to have received depression treatment that met the general depression guidelines, less likely to use antidepressants and more amenable to prefer psychosocial therapy over medication (Bazargan et al., 2005a; Cooper et al., 2003; Miranda & Cooper, 2004; Miranda, Schoenbaum, Sherbourne, Duan, & Wells, 2004; Olfson et al., 2002; Virnig et al., 2004).

Attitudes, beliefs, and social norms may also play a part in acceptance of treatment (Cooper et al., 2003). Both psychotherapy and antidepressants have proven to be effective in treating depression (Brown & Schulberg, 1998; Schulberg, Pilkonis, & Houck, 1998). However, Hispanics and African Americans are less likely to find antidepressants acceptable for treatment and more likely than Whites to believe that antidepressant medications are addictive and that counseling conjures negative feelings. Nonetheless, even though there are differences in beliefs about treatment modalities, these do not explain the differences in the acceptability of depression treatment (Cooper et al., 2003). Among Hispanics, sociodemographic characteristics such as the ability to speak English and the affordability of treatment have been associated with use of antidepressant medications among subjects diagnosed with depression by health practitioners. On the other hand, the use of alternative medicine has been associated with self-reported depression, financial strain, and problems with accessibility and affordability of conventional medical care (Bazargan et al., 2005b).

Perhaps in large part due to the structural and attitudinal factors mentioned above, Hispanics present disparities in access to outpatient mental health treatment compared to Whites. In fact, Latinos and African Americans are less likely to receive depression care than White patients (Bazargan et al., 2005b; Miranda & Cooper, 2004; et al., 2002; Virnig et al., 2004). They are also less likely to take antidepressant medications or attend specialty mental health care than Whites (Miranda & Cooper, 2004). In addition, Hispanics, African Americans, and Asians receive significantly worse antidepressant management care, such as follow-up rates and antidepressant medication management (Virnig et al., 2004). In this regard, the literature suggests that Latinos and African Americans tend to prefer counseling services rather than medication (Brody, Saxena, Silverman, & Aborzian, 1997; Brody & Hunt, 2006; Cooper et al., 2003; Dwight-Johnson, Sherbourne, Liao, & Wells, 2000). This reported preference for counseling may be at least in part a reflection of the lower availability of mental health professionals who can be ethnically matched with them, since Latinos and African Americans are underrepresented in those professions (Miranda & Cooper, 2004).

Olfson et al. (2002) examined the national trends in outpatient treatment of depression between 1987 and 1997. They found that during this decade there was an increase in the proportion of people who received outpatient depression treatment. This trend was characterized by greater involvement of primary care physicians, greater use of psychotropic medications and increased availability of third party payment, but less psychotherapy and fewer outpatient visits. These changes coincided with the advent of better-tolerated antidepressants, the expansion of managed care, and the development of quick and efficient diagnostic tools for depression in clinical practice. As a result, antidepressant medications became mainstay, physicians assumed a more prominent role and psychotherapy sessions were less common and fewer for those in treatment (Olfson et al., 2002).

In sum, Hispanics in general and aging Puerto Ricans in particular are believed to be vulnerable to under-treatment while simultaneously they are at high risk of experiencing depression. Given the history of outpatient mental health policy and its implications for both minority and immigrant populations, this disadvantageous situation rings especially true with respect to access to quality depression treatment. For this reason, in the present study, we hypothesized that aging Puerto Ricans in Massachusetts would have encountered barriers to obtaining adequate depression treatment and we set out to explore their perceptions and experiences through the use of in-depth ethnographic interviews.

METHODS

This chapter uses data collected for the Boston Puerto Rican Health Study (BPRH) — the main project of the NIH funded Center on Population Health and Health Disparities housed at Tufts and Northeastern Universities. The BPRH is an ongoing longitudinal cohort study (1500 participants at wave 1) that examines how psychosocial stress and the development of allostatic load affect health outcomes for aging Puerto Ricans (Tucker et al., 2010). Extensive data for Puerto Ricans ages 45–75, including dietary intake, genetics, components of allostatic load, anthropometric measures, and health and use and access of health care; it also includes a number of scales including the Perceived Stress Scale (PSS), the Center for Epidemiological Studies (CES-D) depression scale, Life Events Inventory (LEI), the Norbeck Social Support Questionnaire (NSSQ), and an acculturation scale. The cohort data collection is currently in the middle of a third wave of interviews.

One of the sub projects conducted at Northeastern consisted of a qualitative data collection that used semi-structured ethnographic interviews with a randomly selected subsample of subjects ($n = 50$) from the main survey (second author P. I.). A primary goal of this sub project was to better understand stress and social support in the Puerto Rican adult population living in the Boston area. A total of 50 interviews were completed, transcribed, and coded. The main themes of these ethnographic interviews included: general quality of life, social support and social networks, self-rated health/mental health and self-care, sources of stress and ways of coping, religion and spirituality, work and care-giving and aging and retirement. From this subsample, the first author of this chapter conducted 16 interviews, in which issues of depression, copying and treatment, and problems obtaining depression treatment were also explored in depth. In addition, through the interviews we also collected the subject's stories of the reasons for migrating to the United States, major life events that have occurred since first arriving and circumstances that have an effect on their overall mental well-being. The interviews were 1−4 hours long, all conducted in Spanish by the first author and digitally recorded. The interviews were transcribed, then coded and analyzed using the qualitative software MAXQDA. Excerpts discussing the respondent's experiences with depression were extracted and further analyzed. In addition, a set of variables from the cohort study, including age, education, depression score, and acculturation score, were added to the MAXQDA data and matched to the qualitative interviews. The PSS was used to measure level of stress at time of interview. This scale asks individuals to evaluate the extent to which various situations were experienced as stressful and the subject's feelings and thoughts over the previous month on a scale of zero to four ($0 =$ never, $4 =$ very often) in the 14-item scale − the version used in this study. The PSS scores are calculated by reversing the scores in the responses and then adding all the individual scores. It is important to note that the PSS is not a diagnostic tool, and therefore there are no cut-off points that can be used to assess stress clinically. Nonetheless, the mean scores in the population may be used as a possible parameter to evaluate abnormalities. Cohen, Kamarck, and Mermelstein (1983) found that, using the 14-item scale, the mean PSS score for Hispanic populations was 14, with a standard deviation

(SD) of 6.9. In comparison, non-Hispanic whites showed an average PSS of 12.8 and a standard deviation (SD) of 6.2. Thus, Hispanics, as well as African Americans and other minorities, tend to exhibit slightly higher levels of perceived stress in comparison to non-Hispanic whites (Cohen, Karmack, & Mermelstein, 1983).

The CES-D depression scale was used to measure depression symptoms. This instrument is commonly used in epidemiological studies and has been proven a more valid measure for depression in Hispanic and aging Hispanic populations (Mahard, 1989; Robinson et al., 2002). The questions ask subjects to indicate whether or not they have felt various symptoms of depression, and how frequently, during the last two weeks. In this scale, a score of 16 through 40 should be interpreted as an indication of symptoms of clinical depression.

To measure the level of acculturation, a scale was created from a list of seven variables that ask respondents which language they normally utilize for a range of daily activities, such as watching TV, reading newspapers and books, chatting with neighbors, at work, listening to the radio, with their friends and in their families on a scale form 1 (Spanish only) through 5 (English only), with 3 being both languages equally. Thus, the score range in this scale is 7 through 35, in other words, the smaller the number the less acculturated to English the person is, and the higher the number the more Anglo-oriented, or more "assimilated," the person is.

Finally, we selected seven exemplary cases for this chapter in which accounts of depression treatment were more salient in order to present in-depth case studies of the respondents' narratives.

RESULTS

A distinctive health care characteristic of the state of Massachusetts is the near universal health insurance coverage offered to its residents, especially since 2006 when an individual mandate for purchasing health care was enacted. For this reason, lack of insurance is not generally a major barrier to accessing mental health services, as it may be in other states. In this sample, the majority of the Puerto Ricans were insured primarily by MASSHEALTH –the Massachusetts Medicaid program – and Medicare, which included coverage for mental health services. In addition to these, the state also offers a program called FREE CARE, which financially assists those who are uninsured or underinsured in helping to pay for the care needed. Thanks to this state's progressive health policy, financial barriers to minimal or basic health services are not a major issue for the aging Puerto Rican population of Massachusetts, a situation that sets them apart from other Puerto Rican populations across the United States, and more generally has made Massachusetts a model for the Affordable Care Act of 2012 – popularly known as "Obama Care."

The majority of respondents in the study had prior experience with depression and/or they were currently depressed (as measured by the CES-D scale). Moreover, most present a low socioeconomic profile, are not currently working and live in public housing. They also display low acculturation and educational levels and report a series of difficult life events, including health problems. Although most subjects expressed satisfaction with the health services received, when questioned about the treatment they had sought and received for depression the main concern expressed was the use of antidepressants. Prior studies have shown that taking medication for depression is often seen as a difficult step to take for many who suffer from depression not only because of the possible side effects of the medication but also because taking antidepressants signifies entering a stigmatized identity, that of being a mental health patient. Moreover, finding the right medication for each individual patient often presents challenges (Karp, 1996). In this regard, Hispanics are even less likely to find antidepressants acceptable than Whites while they are simultaneously also less likely to have access to psychotherapy. However, the reasons why they are reluctant to follow an antidepressant regimen are still not well understood. Aging Puerto Ricans in this sample gave several reasons for their refusal to take antidepressants.

ACCOUNTS OF TREATMENT OF DEPRESSION THROUGH DRUGS

Taking Antidepressants as Being "on Drugs"

Several subjects reported that they felt "drugged up" after taking antidepressants and/or they feared other secondary effects of the drugs. In addition, subjects lamented that treatment for depression as well as other conditions is primarily focused on pharmaceutical drugs that do not tackle the root causes of their depression. This perceived growing reliance on antidepressants could be explained by the policy changes introduced by managed care organizations and the preponderance of treatment offered at primary care settings in the form of an antidepressant pill, a treatment that may be seen as more cost effective. The perceived predominance of pharmacological treatment for depression may also be result of the relatively low availability of Spanish speaking mental health professionals in relation to the high number of Spanish speaking potential clients. Overall, given their limited options, these respondents rejected pharmacological treatment.

Exemplary Case 1

Mariana is 67 years old and lives in public housing with her divorced son. She has suffered asthma since childhood and reports that because of her condition her parents decided to take her out of school. With only two years of education, she can neither read nor write well in Spanish nor in English, and she confesses that she feels embarrassed to attend seminars or classes regarding health because of her illiteracy. Mariana has been living in Boston for over 30 years but experiences low acculturation to the Anglo culture (acculturation score = 14). A skilled seamstress, she worked first in the textile industry and then ran her own store in the same neighborhood where she resides. She then left the business to work as a foster mother and even adopted and raised two girls. However, because she did not contribute much to social security, now in her retirement Mariana faces problems making ends meet. For example, she recently had to give up her car because it was too expensive to keep. Her financial situation coupled with the difficult divorce case of her son and the fear that he would be put in jail are current sources of stress for Mariana (PSS = 14). She also reports that she went through a depression episode after the death of her father; among other things she felt remorseful because her father told her that she had brought him to the United States to die. Although at the time of the survey Mariana did not present symptoms of depression (CES-D = 5), she recalls her experiences with taking antidepressants during her last depression episode:

> ... Unless something big happens in the family and stuff ... I try to keep my nerves under control [*que eso de los nervios no me ataque mucho*], because when my father died, I got sick [depressed] and I had to be in treatment for over a year, and they had me with ... What was it? Valium? I don't know ... I was almost completely drugged up, I could not even ... I would walk and it seemed as if I was not touching the ground, and since then I said to myself that I would not go back to treatment, for I knew they

would give me drugs for my nerves, and I do not like them. And then they gave me medicine to sleep and I do not like to take them either [...] I do not want so much medicine. (Mariana, age 67)

Mariana explains that her treatment consisted exclusively of antidepressive medications, which produced secondary effects. Because of this, she fears that taking drugs for depression, in addition to the other medicines she takes, may actually worsen her health. Moreover, she complains that, in her experience, talk therapy is not normally offered.

Exemplary Case 2

Jimena is 61 and, like Mariana, she lives in public housing. Jimena has a bachelor's degree in education from a well-known university in the East Coast and was for years a primary school teacher. She is bilingual and highly acculturated to the Anglo culture (Acculturation score = 20). She is also a skilled artist who used to sell her paintings at several New England stores. After living for a while in a suburb in a nearby city, she reports that her children insisted that they wanted to be close to their cousins and grandparents in Puerto Rico and to live next to a palm tree. So she returned to Puerto Rico with her husband (Anglo American) to raise her children and later built a house next to her parents. There she enjoyed gardening with her mother, playing cards with her parents and relatives and taking vacation trips with them. Jimena reports that she lived a comfortable middle class life both in the United States and in Puerto Rico. However, after the death of her parents, especially her father, she started experiencing depression episodes and panic attacks. In addition, Jimena was diagnosed with kidney disease and Crohn's disease; as a consequence, the doctors in Puerto Rico recommended that she return to the United States to obtain better treatment for her kidney condition. According to Jimena, her husband divorced her because of her illnesses; however, he continues to be supportive of her. Additionally, she also reports that both of her children have problems in their marriages and also suffer from depression. Because of her daughter's marital problems and episodes of domestic abuse she often takes care of her infant grandchild, who was in the house during the interview. Besides her own health and financial problems, her children's marital problems cause her a great deal of stress. At the time of the survey, Jimena exhibited extremely high symptoms of depression (CES-D = 48) as well as stress (PSS = 41). Unlike Mariana, Jimena uses antidepressants to calm her nerves, but she is very aware of the physical secondary effects as well as the sociocultural stigma associated with depression drugs:

Interviewer: And how do you cope with the depression?

Jimena: I take the medicines, I try to calm down, I try to keep my mind involved in other things; that is why I want to work.

Interviewer: Yes, aha, and with the medicine, how has your experience with the medicines been like?

Jimena: It has been bad. You do not feel well.

Interviewer: Why has it been bad ... the secondary effects or ...?

Jimena: Secondary effects ... because in our culture it is not accepted ... do you understand? They tell you that you are taking "dope," that this and the other, that it makes you sicker, that you should take teas ... But they do not know what is happening within you. (Jimena, age 61)

Although Jimena relays the discomfort caused by the medication's secondary effects, she states that the major deterrent to using antidepressants is in fact the social and cultural stigma expressed by her network of co-ethnics; for example, the belief that medication will be detrimental to one's health, that antidepressants are "dope," and that self-care using natural folk remedies – such as various teas known to have calming effects – are preferable to medication for "nervios" [nerves]. This finding is consistent with prior studies which showed that the stigma of mental illness may prevent many Hispanics from seeking pharmacological treatment (Cooper et al., 2003; Hansen & Cabassa, 2012). Despite the severity of her depression, Jimena feels conflicted about using antidepressants, possibly because she herself has internalized some of these popular beliefs, but especially because of the fear of criticism by others.

Exemplary Case 3

Luis, age 51, lives with his wife and the youngest of their five children in public housing. He came to the United States at age 19 from a rural central part of *La isla,* as many refer to Puerto Rico's countryside. He still remembers being in awe when he first saw a noisy elevated train that used to run across the city. But that was just one of many things that he had to grow accustomed to; he would also have to work during *Semana Santa* (Holy Week) something that as a devout Catholic he found strange. Luis had heard that in the United States there would be plenty of opportunities to get good jobs and get ahead. However, he soon discovered that due to language barriers and discrimination (acculturation score = 11; 9th grade education), he would have to take the lowest skilled jobs that most Anglos did not want. For example, he once applied for a promotion in a maintenance job he had worked at for years, but the job was assigned to a White American who had been at the company for only one year, even though Luis' job performance was highly rated. After that, hurt by what he thought was an unfair decision, Luis never spoke up or applied for any other promotion but resigned himself to just accept how the "system" worked to keep workers in the lower strata, especially poor Hispanics like himself. Subsequently, Luis suffered a fall at the hospital where he was working and injured his back. As a result, he is unable to work and he suffers permanent disability and recurrent depression, for which he was on treatment for over two years. Luis reports that he is very involved in his Church and volunteers for everything, including doing visits to older Latinos who are sick and homebound. Besides that, and riding his bicycle, he reports lack of activities and boredom. Luis also reports that his priest, who was a good friend and confidant, died recently of a sudden death. At the time of the survey Luis exhibited high symptoms of depression (CES-D = 30) and stress (PSS = 37).

Interviewer: And, how did the treatment work for you?

Luis: More or less, not one hundred per cent effective, no. I ... I have ... I have myself dealt with it [depression] on my own, yes. Because, look, the problem is that here [US] they [doctors] want to solve everything with pills. I do not like this. You go [to the doctor] and they give you a lot of pills, they want to solve everything with little pills and little pills ... and sometimes problems ... I do not know, no, I do not think problems can be solved that way. I am aware that yes, you have to prescribe pills, but they fill you up with so many pills that when you realize it you get worse, sicker, because [the pills] are damaging the other organs in your body. Because, even though the doctors tell you that no, that there are no secondary effects, but [sic] there are always secondary effects, always, yeah. These are chemicals that go into your body.

Interviewer: Yes, everything has some effect. But then, did you take the pills or ...?

Luis: I got to the point I took pills, I got to take pills but no ... I got to take pills, but I tell you, the way they made me feel those pills ... I did not want to be that way. I did not want feel like that, like gone, like I was gone. I do not know, I do not want to be that way, I wanted to be normal, yeah. (Luis, age 51)

Like Jimena, Luis struggled with the decision to take antidepressants but, unlike her, he personally believes that this medication can negatively impact one's health and quality of life, and that its effects are similar to those of other (illegal) drugs whose usage he disapproves. One may argue that the equivalency drawn by respondents between antidepressants and illegal recreational drugs is based upon their perceived effects. Thus, many fear that they will become addicted, that "drugs" will have deleterious effects, and that they could be the object of criticism by others for taking "dope."

Avoiding Antidepressants for Fear of Overmedication

Some scholars have critiqued the overmedication of the older adult population in the United States (Fick et al. 2003). In this sample there is a high prevalence of chronic health problems, for which the respondents take multiple prescription drugs. Because of this, many of the interviewees report that they avoid taking antidepressants, since they consider that depression is a minor illness in comparison to the seriousness of the other illnesses afflicting them, and because they are afraid of the possible pernicious effects of taking a lot of medications or of the interactions among them. Mariana expresses this idea in the following quote:

> ... Because ... imagine! With so many pills that I take! And here all ... I take sometimes twelve pills in the morning, and then in the afternoon sometimes I have to repeat, for example, the one for the pressure, for the calcium now, and all they [the doctors] tell you is: "PILLS, PILLS, PILLS" and that is what is hurting my kidney. Umm, and sometimes I keep to myself the simple things like this [depression] so they [doctors] don't give me so many pills. (Mariana, age 67)

Mariana reports that besides having asthma, anemia, and osteoporosis, she suffers from kidney disease and attributes it to medications taken in the past. For this reason, she is especially fearful of taking too many medications and hides certain ailments from her doctors in order to avoid being prescribed yet another pill.

Underrepresented groups have been found to be less likely to adhere to a prescription drug regimen, but it is still not clear why this is so (Miranda & Cooper, 2004; Virnig et al., 2004). With regard to aging Puerto Ricans and other language minority groups, it is worth pointing out that even though interpreter and translation services have improved at sites that deliver health care services, there is still need for improvement in other aspects of health care services. For example, Balkrishnan (2007) has noted that pharmacies very rarely have translation services available nor do they generally translate the labels placed on prescription drugs. Because of this, limited English speakers might not obtain adequate information or be educated on how to use and adhere to pharmacological treatment (Balkrishnan, 2007).

Taking Antidepressants as a Last Resort in Extreme Cases of Depression

Several interviewees indicated that they would be willing to take antidepressants as a last resort in extreme situations, and only if other measures did not work for them, since they consider these drugs addictive and dangerous. Thus, they stress the fact that their depression arises from difficult and concrete life circumstances and that once their problems are addressed they would feel better. It is generally believed that drugs in most cases are unnecessary and would only cause their condition to worsen. In several cases, subjects report seeking treatment that includes both psychotherapy and drugs, although they only accept, eagerly, the former and refuse to take the antidepressants.

Exemplary Case 4

Carmen, age 66, came to the U.S. mainland from Yabucoa, a rural part of Puerto Rico, over forty years ago. She wanted to leave behind her routine because making a living in Puerto Rico was very hard and jobs there were physically demanding. Carmen had heard from two siblings who lived in Boston that jobs in the United States were better. So she moved to Boston and later met her husband. They subsequently moved to New York and to L.A. with their only child. Carmen reports that her husband worked as a dark room technician developing photographs for large industries and that he, over time, developed work related illnesses, such as migraines and over-sensitivity to sunlight. Moreover, at times he became violent and *desagradecido de la vida* [ungrateful at life]. Carmen thinks that perhaps because he did not want to make her and their child suffer, one unexpected day her husband told her that he wanted a divorce. After the dissolution of her marriage she, and her child, moved back to Boston to be close to relatives who were living in the area. She went back to work in the same factory where she had previously worked — in fact she remained there until recently. During a trip to Puerto Rico, in which she went to spent time with her ailing father, she fell on the ground and broke her left arm. As a consequence, she became disabled and to this day, Carmen cannot close her injured hand. She, currently, receives a social security check and lives in a studio apartment in public housing for seniors and people with disabilities. Three years back, the mother of her grandchild (her son's ex-wife) asked her to assume custody of her autistic grandchild, because she did not feel she could continue doing it herself (she died soon after). Taking full responsibility for this child with special needs has been both a blessing and very stressful, according to Carmen, but she has received the support of several friends in the building where she lives and of her social worker as well as the economic support of her son who lives in Chicago with his new family but provides child support. As someone who does not speak English (acculturation = 14; 4th grade education or less) she often depends on a "friend" to serve as interpreter, whom she has to pay. Another stressor for Carmen is her housing situation. She and her grandchild live in a studio apartment that is too small for them. The doctors tell Carmen that especially because of her grandchild's autistic condition, they need a larger space. Indeed, Carmen has been sleeping on a sofa for two years while her grandchild sleeps in the only bed. She has a long-standing request to the housing authority for a larger apartment but her efforts have been unsuccessful. Because of this, Carmen says that for the first time in her life she has felt discriminated against by the housing authority. This stressful situation (PSS = 34) is reported to have triggered a depression for which Carmen is currently under treatment (CES-D = 30).

Interviewer: And how are you dealing with the depression?

Carmen: Well, I am going to the psychologist, and ... and I did not want to take pills, because ... I have heard a lot of people saying that after you start taking pills, and taking pills, that like they get used to the pills ... and if they do not have the pills that ... and I am not ... I go to her [the counselor] and I talk ... and I try to ... The other day she saw me, she looked for me, because those days I was feeling really bad, and then she said to me "Ay, I think you are going to have to ..." and I said "Ay, no, I still do not want pills, I do not want pills."

While Carmen wants to move to a larger apartment, she does not want to move out of her current building because there she has developed network of supportive relationships and friendships with a group of Spanish speaking elders and she feels that those supportive networks would not so easily be found elsewhere.

Carmen: ... I say: "I do not want to move out of this building, I do not want to move out of here and things ... I say: I am going to stay in this *roto* [dump] until ... [laughter]. But then when I went back to her [the psychologists] and I had already received the letter [a letter from the department of housing] and then, they had already approved the transfer for the handicap, so I was feeling more calmed down, and I told her NO, NO, because she was going to ... she was putting me on a waiting list to see the doctor to prescribe pills for me for the depression. So with respect to that I have not ...."

In the quote above, Carmen suggests that there is an inverse relationship between obtaining a larger apartment and receiving a prescription for depression. In other words, her success in being listed as needing a move because of an existing handicapping condition meant that she would move up on the waiting list at the department of housing. This small victory made Carmen hopeful that what she perceived as the trigger of her depression might be resolved in the near future. Moreover, this new development also allows Carmen to reason with her social worker that she will not need to place her on a waiting list to see a Spanish speaking psychiatrist, and will not need to be prescribed the antidepressants that she so fears.

Taking Antidepressants but Having Inadequate Psychological Treatment

Some of the subjects accepted adhering to a drug regimen for depression but feel that they are not getting adequate psychological treatment.

Exemplary Case 5

María is 62 years old and lives in public housing with her husband in a town adjacent to Boston. She came to the United States from Coamo over 30 years ago and was always a stay-at-home mother. María reported that she and her family were lucky that her husband always worked while she stayed home to care of him and the children, and that they were never on welfare. Occasionally, she worked from home as a babysitter. She seems proud when she says that one of her children is a policeman in Florida and another is a teacher in Massachusetts. María currently baby-sits for some of the grandchildren, although communication with them is not easy at times because they do not speak Spanish and her English is very limited (acculturation = 12; 4th grade education or less). With the last child moving out of the home and a personal diagnosis of facial cancer, as well as other health problems, she reports that these health and family situations triggered a depression that has been ongoing for approximately the past five years. María reports that she often feels lonely and is not involved in out of home social activities besides her therapy group. She does have a friend from the group and maintains telephone contact with her. María became emotional when she confessed that she was very worried about her facial cancer. However, she has not received individual therapy for her depression, only antidepressants and group therapy. At the time of the survey, María exhibited very high symptoms of depression (CES-D = 38) and stress (PSS = 31).

Interviewer: And you told me that you suffer from depression. Are you taking something for the depression?

Maria: Yes, I have ... I have pills for everything.

Interviewer: Pills, aha.

Maria: For sleeping also, for the cholesterol ...

Interviewer: So, you have a collection of pills ...!

Maria: Yes, I have a pharmacy over there (laughter)

Interviewer: (laughter) and do you take all your pills?

Maria: Yes, I put them all in a little box there and that is why it is not difficult at all [to take the pills].

Interviewer: And when did you start with the depression?

Maria: *Ay!* I think that a long time ago, a long time ago, like five years ago.

Interviewer: Around five years, and what kinds of treatment have you received?

Maria: Well, sometimes I do not feel well; sometimes I do not feel ... I say to myself that I do not want ... I do not want to get out of the bedroom, I do not want to comb my hair, I do not want to do anything, *nada, nada, nada*. Sometimes I feel a little better, I am in better spirits, and when I am in better spirits I do everything around the house very quick [inaudible].

Interviewer: and have you gone to psychotherapy or to a psychologist?

Maria: No, the only thing I have is the medicine for the depression and for sleeping, and there is also a group that a few of us attend, that is a therapy group. But I would like to have for me only [individual therapy].

Interviewer: Oh, ok, you do not have individual therapy.

(...)

And how does the group work for you?

Maria: Well, I like it.

Interviewer: And how is it that they did not give you individual [therapy], do you know?

Maria: Because sometimes they have, how do you say it? That like you have to wait ...

Interviewer: Like waiting lists or something?

Maria: That you have to wait a long time, yes. (María, age 61)

In spite of showing very high symptoms of depression and having a diagnosis of cancer, María does not receive individual mental health therapy; instead, her treatment consists of antidepressants and attending group therapy. Like other respondents who are not fluent in English, the inadequate access to individual talk therapy seems to be connected to language barriers and a shortage of Spanish speaking therapists relative to the number of potential clients in the area.

Antidepressants Work

A few interviewees reported that they have struggled with mental illness throughout their lives. The depression is described as being more chronic and complicated with other mental health diagnoses. These respondents also indicated never having sought help for their mental problems while living in Puerto Rico, and that they had waited too long to look for help once their condition had reached an advanced stage. In those cases, the subjects felt that drugs were beneficial to them — that they could not manage their condition without them.

Exemplary Case 6

Carmina, age 61, came to the United States with her parents and her ten younger siblings when she was still an adolescent. She remembers that it was close to Christmas time and it was very cold and snowy. Carmina was sent to Catholic school, but she had a hard time adjusting as she could not understand a word the teachers were saying, and often got into trouble because she did not know how to recite the mandatory prayers in English (acculturation = 15, 6th grade education). Carmina was not happy to be in Boston, she wanted to go back to Puerto Rico where the weather was warm and she enjoyed going to school, but she knew her parents would not let her go back, and she always did as she was told and kept her feelings to herself. After her unsuccessful school experience, she stayed home to help her mother raise her 10 siblings. Carmina reports that since childhood she suffered from *nervios* [nerves] but did not go to a psychiatrist until later when her condition was very advanced. In the United States, Carmina developed phobias that afflict her to this day; because of this she cannot venture outside her immediate neighborhood block and is afraid to be outside after dark. In 1968, Carmina had a terrible car accident in which she was thrown out of a car from a back seat window. As a result, she was in a coma for six months and had two operations in her head. She also hurt a leg and an arm and to this day she experiences loss of memory and pain from her old injuries. Carmina was married and had two children and reports that she started experiencing depression after she married and that her ex-husband gave her *malos ratos* [hard times]. She did not like being married and she wishes she had become a nun, an *hermanita de la caridad*, like her cousin. But because she did not have a school diploma she was told that she could not do so. She also wishes she could have continued her education so to have better jobs, instead of doing laundry, babysitting, and working in factories. She now lives in public housing on a very low income and cannot afford to buy many necessities such as clothes. She reports that she has received psychiatric treatment for years and she has stayed, twice, for short periods of time in a psychiatric hospital. In the past two years, Carmina has experienced several losses in her immediate family, the deaths of her mother and a sister that lived in the same building, as well as one other sister. As a consequence she went through a deep depression and reports that she tried to commit suicide through starvation, but all she managed to accomplish was losing a lot of weight. During the interview, Carmina reported that she still feels depressed and has suicidal ideas (CES-D = 28, PSS = 36).

> Interviewer: ... but with the psychiatrists that you have gone to and the doctors, do you feel they have helped you? What has your relationship with your psychiatrists been like?
>
> Carmina: Yes, they have helped me. Talking to them, making me understand ... Because, sometimes one does not understand ... They have helped me understand how is this, how is that ... how is life, that combined with the medication.
>
> Interviewer: So the medication helps you?
>
> Carmina: Yes. If it was not for that ... *MUCHACHA!* [girl!] [without the medication] I would have been ... I do not say I would be buried, but I would have been in a madhouse.

According to Carmina, the medications in combination with the talk therapy she received at the psychiatrist's office have helped her enormously. It is worth noting that Carmina did not report experiencing problems obtaining treatment. This could be explained by the severity of her mental health problems and the fact that she has a long history of mental illness. Indeed, she wished she had sought help earlier since, as mentioned, as she has been struggling with *nervios* since she was a child and still living in Puerto Rico.

Exemplary Case 7

When Aurora, age 69, was a young woman she lived in Puerto Rico with her four small children from two different marriages. She reports that the fathers of her children were *sinverguenzas* [a waste of time] and never helped her, so she had to fend for her family by herself. Aurora worked cleaning houses, in dining services, and later she was given a parcel of land and a house through a government program; in exchange, she had to work the land to make a living. Unfortunately, Aurora developed heart disease and problems with her *nervios* [nerves] – though she never went to a psychiatrist in Puerto Rico. Because of her health problems, she was unable to continue the strenuous kind of work she had been doing anymore. So one day, about forty years ago, Aurora decided to migrate to the US *pa echar palante* [to move ahead]. She worked in a factory assembling light bulbs (6th grade education or less, acculturation score = 10), but she continued having *nervios*, and one day in 1978 she felt very sick and was diagnosed with ventricular cardiac arrhythmia. After that, she stopped working and started collecting social security. Later, she gave her house to a son and was able to qualify for disability; thus, now she makes a little more than six hundred dollars a month and pays two hundred and eight dollars for the studio apartment in a public housing for seniors and disabled people where she has been living for the past six years. Aurora has experienced several losses in the recent past. One of her sons was found dead of a drug overdose in New York. Her mother, whom she had brought to the United States, died of cancer, and a sister also died of a heart attack. One brother was killed while being robbed for his social security money, and another brother killed his own toddler son. Even though she is herself very sick, Aurora still checks on a sister who has for years been interned in a mental institution nearby. Luckily, Aurora has the support of her ex-partner who comes by everyday to see her, and her living children with whom she says she has good relations. Aurora reports that she feels stressed out because, given her mobility problems, she needs a larger apartment with a bedroom. She suffers from several chronic health conditions including heart disease, digestive problems, an anxiety disorder and depression (CES-D = 16, PSS = 19).

Aurora: ... they gave me Zoloft 50 mg

Interviewer: Oh, Zoloft

Aurora: First they gave me half ...

Interviewer: Yes, to see how you tolerate it ...

Aurora: They say they gave me one of twenty-five, they gave me one of fifty and they have gone ... they have changed ... like four times ... and they have not changed the pills thank the Lord!

Interviewer: So you take Zoloft 50 mg.

Aurora: Aha, and I say, lucky me!

Interviewer: It makes you feel better?

Aurora: The Zoloft that ... that makes me feel more calmed down. You know, because here [apartment building for seniors] you are not your own boss, because you know that this belongs to the government, but here I say I have my *chavos* [money] and they cannot kick me out of here, they cannot scream at me, or anything like that. You know that .... (Aurora, age 69)

Aurora is content with the pharmacological treatment she receives. The current dosage is effective and was gradually increased to a working level; in fact, she did not experience any ill effects with the medication. However, it is also interesting to note that Aurora associates the rising of symptoms of anxiety/depression to her living conditions. Because she rents a studio in public housing for seniors and people with disabilities, she is afraid of being asked to leave if her nerves cause her to overreact (e.g., screaming) to potentially stressful situations. Thus, the medication helps her control her emotions while living in a stressful residential environment where she feels relatively powerless.

DISCUSSION

For decades, epidemiological studies have shown disproportionally high rates of depression and psychological distress among Puerto Ricans. Yet, very little is known about their experiences with treatment for depression and other mental disorders. Indeed, the process by which people come to realize of mental illness and how they seek mental health care are important research items that have not been sufficiently investigated, particularly among underserved minority groups (Bazargan et al., 2005b). Given the history of outpatient mental health services in the United States, especially as it relates to urban minority and immigrant populations we hypothesized that Puerto Rican elders in Boston would face problems obtaining quality depression treatment. Through the in-depth ethnographic interviews, we found that older Puerto Ricans feel that treatment for depression in the US context is too focused on pharmacological treatment that is not always adequate for their particular case.

In general, subjects identify problems that have been found to be correlates of depression in quantitative research. They believe that their depression is triggered or affected by social stressors that are not properly addressed, such as housing problems, financial problems, lack of jobs and activities and social isolation. Indeed, many subjects report that their depression is caused by difficult social circumstances and life events that are related to poverty, gender status, and ethnic minority status. The subjects also indicated that health problems and disability are major sources of stress; moreover, the fact that they already take multiple prescription drugs for other health conditions also contributes to their resistance to accept pharmacological treatment for depression. They believe that while psychotherapy helps people cope with life's difficulties, antidepressant medication is useful only in extremely severe cases of depression. Furthermore, antidepressant drugs are believed to be a kind of "dope," highly addictive, and with secondary effects that can damage other organs in the body and make their depression and general health even worse. The interaction between reported inadequate treatment options, cultural beliefs, low acculturation, language limitations, and complicated health profiles may also contribute to lack of trust in medications or lack of adherence to a prescribed regimen. For this reason, many avoid seeking help for their depression and, if they do, they resist taking antidepressants. As general guidelines indicate, depression treatment among the older population often requires addressing a range of needs that go beyond the strictly medical problems, such as living conditions and social isolation, that require the coordinated intervention of several agencies (NICE, 2004).

Previous studies have found that Hispanics prefer psychological treatment Over medication (Barzagan et al., 2005; Cooper et al., 2003), but to our knowledge, no study to date had addressed the reasons for avoiding pharmacological treatment and treatment in general. Given the lower availability of Latino and Spanish speaking mental health professionals to provide direct treatment, and the current national trend of treating depression at the primary care site by physicians, it is not surprising to find that older Puerto Ricans feel that the treatment options available to them are far from optimal. This – coupled with limited English ability, low acculturation, financial difficulties, and the belief that antidepressants are a kind of "dope" – may prevent many from adhering to treatment. One plausible interpretation for the persisting social norm of viewing use of antidepressants as carrying the same social connotations as if using illegal drugs ("dope") in this group may be that they have internalized majority stereotypes about Puerto Ricans and the poor as prone to be drug users. Thus, rejecting treatment through antidepressants may be an attempt to disassociate themselves from that negative image. This suggests that the use of antidepressants in US society has become more normalized; but there remain cultural niches where perceptions of the use of depression medications are seen through a different lens.

An emphasis on screening for depression and expansion of treatment must be accompanied by a parallel emphasis on reaching underserved minority populations (Bazargan et al., 2005a, 2005b). These would include taking measures to increase the representation of Latino mental health providers, especially in psychological and counseling services, but also in pharmaceutical services so that − when needed − Latino clients can obtain adequate education on the use of prescription drugs for depression. In the final analysis, one of the main lessons gained from this ethnographic exploration is the need to avoid simplistic interpretations of the expressed rejection of pharmacological treatment as just a "cultural" response. Puerto Ricans have been historically, and continue to be, a population that is underserved in the mental health arena, while they are also afflicted by multiple social and health problems. It is imperative to understand their reasons for avoiding drug therapies in order to continue make a dent on the treatment disparities for depression and other mental health ailments facing them by increasing the representation of Latino and/or culturally competent providers in the field of mental health.

FUNDING

This study was supported by the National Institute of Health grants R01 AG023394, and P50 HL105185 and by the Farnsworth Trust Fellowship in Aging Policy Research program (2006−2007).

REFERENCES

Aeran, P. A., Alvidrez, B. J., Robinson, G. S., & Scotia Hicks, B. S. (2002). Would older medi-cal patients use psychological services? *The Gerontologist*, *43*, 392−398.

Alegría, M., Canino, G., Rios, R., Vera, M., Calderon, J., Rusch, D., & Ortega, A. N. (2002). Inequalities in use of mental health services among Latinos, African Americans, and non-Latino whites. *Psychiatric Services*, *53*(12), 1547−1555.

Alegría, M., Perez, D. J., & Williams, S. (2003). The role of public policies in reducing mental health status disparities for people of color. *Health Affairs (Millwood)*, *22*, 51−64.

Angel, R., & Guarnaccia, P. J. (1989). Mind, body and culture: Somatization among Hispanics. *Social Science and Medicine*, *28*, 1229−1238.

Baer, R. D., Arteaga, E., Dyer, K., Eden, A., Gross, R., Helmy, H., ... Reeser, D. (2013). Concepts of race and ethnicity among health researchers: Patterns and implications. *Ethnicity & Health*, *18*(2), 211−225.

Baer, W. (1992). *The Puerto Rican economy and United States economic fluctuations.* Rio Piedras, Puerto Rico: Social Science Research Center, RVMBOS.

Balkrishnan, R. (2007, June 20). Challenges of appropriate prescribing, marketing and use of prescription medicines. *Diversity and aging in the 21st century conference,* Los Angeles, CA: AARP.

Bazargan, M., Calderon, J. L., Heslin, K. C., Mentes, C., Shaheen, M. A., Ahdout, J., & Baker, R. S. (2005a). A profile of chronic mental and physical conditions among African-American and Latino children in urban public housing. *Ethnicity & Disease,* *15,* S5–3–9.

Bazargan, M., Norris, K., Bazargan-Hejazi, S., Akhanjee, L., Calderon, J. L., Safvati, S. D., & Baker, R. S. (2005b). Alternative healthcare use in the under-served population. *Ethnicity & Disease, 15,* 531–539.

Biegel, D. E., Farkas, K. J., & Song., L.-y. (1997). Barriers to the use of mental health services by African-American and Hispanic elderly persons. *Journal of Gerontological Social Work, 29,* 23–44.

Borjas, G. J., & Bratsberg, B. (1996). Who leaves? The outmigration of the foreign born. *The Review of Economics and Statistics, 78,* 165–176.

Brody, A. L., Saxena, S., Silverman, D. H. S., & Aborzian, L. A. (1997). Brain metabolic changes in major depressive disorder from pre- to post-treatment with Paroxetine. *Psychiatry Research: Neuroimaging, 91,* 127–139.

Brody, H., & Hunt, L. M. (2006). BiDil: Assessing a race based pharmaceutical. *Annals of Family Medicine, 4*(6), 556–560.

Brown, C., & Schulberg, H. C. (1998). Diagnosis and treatment of depression in primary medical care practice: The application of research findings to clinical practice. *Journal of Clinical Psychology, 54,* 303–314.

Cohen, S., Kamarck, T., & Mermelstein, R. (1983). A global measure of perceived stress. *Journal of Health and Social Behavior, 24,* 386–396.

Cooper, L. A., Gonzales, J. J., Gallo, J. J., Rost, K. M., Meredith, L. S., Rubenstein, L. V., ... Ford, D. E. (2003). The acceptability of treatment for depression among African-American, Hispanic, and white primary care patients. *Medical Care, 41,* 479–489.

Dickey, B., Binner, P. R., Leff, S., Uyeda, M. K., Schlesinger, M. J., & Gudeman, J. E. (1989). Containing mental health treatment costs through program design: A Massachusetts study. *The American Journal of Public Health, 79,* 863–867.

DHHS. (1999). *Mental health: Culture, race and ethnicity.* A supplement to mental health: Report of the surgeon general. Bethesda, MD: National Institute of Mental Health.

Dowell, D. A., & Ciarlo, J. A. (1989). An evaluative overview of the community mental health centers program. In Rochefort (Ed.), *Handbook on mental health policy in the United States* (pp. 195–236). Westport, CT: Greenwood.

Dwight-Johnson, M., Sherbourne, C. D., Liao, D., & Wells, K. B. (2000). Treatment preferences among depressed primary care patients. *The Journal of General Internal Medicine, 15,* 527–534.

Falcón, L. M., & Tucker, K. (2000). Prevalence and correlates of depressive symptoms among Hispanic elders in Massachusetts. *Journal of Gerontology, 55*(B), S108–S116.

Fick, D. M., Cooper, J. W., Wade, W. E., Waller, J. L., MacLean, R., & Beers, M. H. (2003). Updating the beers criteria for potentially inappropriate use in older adults. *Archives of Internal Medicine, 163,* 2716–2724.

Gherovici, P. (2003). *The Puerto Rican syndrome.* New York, NY: Other Press.

Haberman, P. W. (1976). Psychiatric symptoms among Puerto Ricans in Puerto Rico and New York city. *Ethnicity, 3*, 133–144.

Hansen, M. C., & Cabassa, L. J. (2012). Pathways to depression care: Help-seeking experiences of low-income Latinos with diabetes and depression. *Journal of Immigrant and Minority Health, 14*, 1097–1106.

Karp, D. (1996). *Speaking of sadness: Depression, disconnection and the meanings of illness.* New York, NY: Oxford University Press.

Kemp, B. J., Staples, F., & Lopez-Aqueres, W. (1987). Epidemiology of depression and dysphoria in an elderly Hispanic population. Prevalence and correlates. *Journal of the American Geriatrics Society, 35*, 920–926.

Keyes, K. K., Martins, S. S., Hatzenbuehler, M. M., Blanco, C. C., Bates, L. L., & Hasin, D. (2012). Mental health service utilization for psychiatric disorders among Latinos living in the United States: The role of ethnic subgroup, ethnic identity, and language/social preferences. *Social Psychiatry & Psychiatric Epidemiology, 47*(3), 383–394.

Krause, N., & Carr, L. G. (1978). The effects of response bias in the survey assessment of the mental health of Puerto Rican migrants. *Social Psychiatry, 13*, 167–173.

Kuzawa, C., & Sweet, E. (2009). Epigenetics and the embodiment of race: Developmental origins of U.S. racial disparities in cardiovascular health. *American Journal of Human Biology, 21*(1), 2–15.

Malzberg, B. (1956). Mental disease among Puerto Ricans in New York City, 1949–1951. *The Journal of Nervous and Mental Disease, 123*, 262–269.

Maton, K. I., Kohout, J. L., Wicherski, M., Leary, G. E., & Vinokurov, A. (2006). Minority students of color and the psychology graduate pipeline: Disquieting and encouraging trends, 1989–2003. *American Psychologist, 61*(2), 117–131.

Miranda, J., & Cooper, L. A. (2004). Disparities in care for depression among primary care patients. *Journal of General Internal Medicine, 19*, 120–126.

Miranda, J., Schoenbaum, M., Sherbourne, C., Duan, N., & Wells, K. (2004). Effects of primary care depression treatment on minority patients' clinical status and employment. *Archives of General Psychiatry, 61*, 827–834.

NICE. (2004). *Depression: Management of depression in primary and secondary care.* National Clinical Guideline No. 23. London, UK.

O'Donnell, R. (1989). Functional disability among the Puerto Rican elderly. *Journal of Aging and Health, 1*(2), 244–264.

Olfson, M., Marcus, S. C., Druss, B., Elinson, L., Tanielian, T., & Pincus, H. A. (2002). National trends in the outpatient treatment of depression. *Journal of American Medical Association, 287*, 203–209.

Ramos, B. M. (2005). Acculturation and depression among Puerto Ricans in the mainland. *Social Work Research, 29*, 95–105.

Robinson, J., Gruman, C., Gaztambide, S., & Blank, K. (2002). Screening for depression in middle-aged and older Puerto Rican primary care patients. *Journals of Gerontology. Series A, 57*, M308–M314.

Rochefort, D. A. (1989). *Handbook on mental health policy in the United States.* Westport, CT: Greenwood.

Rodríguez-Galán, M. B., & Falcón, L. M. (2009). Perceived problems with access to medical care and depression among older Puerto Ricans, Dominicans, other Hispanics and a comparison group of non-Hispanic whites. *Journal of Aging and Health, 21*(3), 501–518.

Schulberg, H. C., Pilkonis, P. A., & Houck, P. (1998). The severity of major depression and choice of treatment in primary care practice. *Journal of Consulting and Clinical Psychology, 66,* 932–938.

Tucker, K. L., Mattei, J., Noel, S. E., Collado, B. M., Mendez, J., Nelson, J., ... Falcon, L. M. (2010). The Boston Puerto Rican health study, a longitudinal cohort study on health disparities in Puerto Rican adults: Challenges and opportunities. *BMC Public Health, 10,* 107.

Vander Stoep, A., & Link, B. (1998). Social class, ethnicity and mental illness: The importance of being more than earnest. *American Journal of Public Health, 88,* 1396–1402.

Vera, M., Alegría, M., Freeman, D., Robles, R. R., Rios, R., & Rios, C. F. (1991). Depressive symptoms among Puerto Ricans: Island poor compared with residents of the New York city area. *American Journal of Epidemiology, 134,* 502–510.

Virnig, B., Huang, Z., Lurie, N., Musgrave, D., McBean, A. M., & Dowd, B. (2004). Does medicare managed care provide equal treatment for mental illness across races? *Archives of General Psychiatry, 61,* 201–205.

Young, A. S., Klap, R., Sherbourne, C. D., & Wells, K. B. (2001). The quality of care for depressive and anxiety disorders in the United States. *Archives of General Psychiatry, 58,* 55–61.